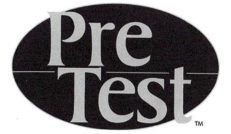

Anatomy, Histology, and Cell Biology

PreTest™ Self-Assessment and Review

Notice

Medicine is an ever-changing science. As new research and clinical experience broaden our knowledge, changes in treatment and drug therapy are required. The editors and the publisher of this work have checked with sources believed to be reliable in their efforts to provide information that is complete and generally in accord with the standards accepted at the time of publication. However, in view of the possibility of human error or changes in medical sciences, neither the editors nor the publisher nor any other party who has been involved in the preparation or publication of this work warrants that the information contained herein is in every respect accurate or complete, and they are not responsible for any errors or omissions or for the results obtained from use of such information. Readers are encouraged to confirm the information contained herein with other sources. For example and in particular, readers are advised to check the product information sheet included in the package of each drug they plan to administer to be certain that the information contained in this book is accurate and that changes have not been made in the recommended dose or in the contraindications for administration. This recommendation is of particular importance in connection with new or infrequently used drugs.

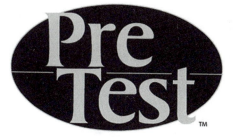

Anatomy, Histology, and Cell Biology

PreTest™ Self-Assessment and Review

Third Edition

Robert M. Klein, PhD
Professor and Associate Dean
Professional Development and Faculty Affairs
Department of Anatomy and Cell Biology
University of Kansas, School of Medicine
Kansas City, Kansas

George C. Enders, PhD
Associate Professor and Director
of Medical Education
Department of Anatomy and Cell Biology
University of Kansas, School of Medicine
Kansas City, Kansas

New York   Chicago   San Fr   London   Madrid   Mexico City
Milan   New Delhi   Singapore   Sydney   Toronto

The McGraw·Hill Companies

Anatomy, Histology, and Cell Biology: PreTest™ Self-Assessment and Review, Third Edition

1 2 3 4 5 6 7 8 9 0   DOC/DOC   0 9 8 7

ISBN-13: 978-0-07-147185-5
ISBN-10:   0-07-147185-5

This book was set in Berkeley by International Typesetting and Composition.
The editors were Catherine A. Johnson and Regina Y. Brown.
The production supervisor was Sherri Souffrance.
Project management was provided by International Typesetting and Composition.
The cover designer was Li Chan Chang/Pinpoint.
RR Donnelley was printer and binder.

This book is printed on acid-free paper.

Library of Congress Cataloging-in-Publication Data

Anatomy, histology and cell biology : PreTest self-assessment and review / [edited by] Robert M. Klein George C. Enders.—3rd ed.
    p. ; cm.
    i 9des bibliographical references and index.
    ISBҎ: 978-0-07-147185-5 (pbk. : alk. paper)
    1. Huᵥ   0-07-147185-5 (pbk. : alk. paper)
Examinatioᵥtomy—Examinations, questions, etc.   2. Embryology, Human—
4. Cytology⁻ᵗions, etc.   3. Histology—Examinations, questions, etc.
II. Enders, Geᵘᵗions, questions, etc.   I. Klein, Robert M. (Robert Melvin), 1949-
    [DNLM: 1. Añᵏ
Questions.   3. Hᵢᵥ
QM32.A646   20ᵗamination Questions.   2. Cytology—Examination
611.0076—dc22   ᵐmination Questions.   QS 18.2 A53603   2007]

                                                            2007000521

To my wife, Beth, and our children Melanie, Jeffrey, and David, for their support and patience during the writing and revision of this text, and to my parents, Nettie and David, for their emphasis on education and the pursuit of knowledge.

—RMK

To Sally Ling, M.D., an incredibly hard working and considerate person whom I am lucky enough to call my wife. She has given us three great kids, Carolyn, Tyler, and Robert who keep me on my toes, and to my mother and my father who always encouraged "the boys" to do our best.

—GCE

Student Reviewers

Jonathan Carnell
University of Kansas, School of Medicine
Class of 2009

Michael Curley
University of Wisconsin
School of Medicine and Public Health
Class of 2007

Nathan Heckerson
University of Kansas, School of Medicine
Class of 2009

Alicia K. Morgans
University of Pennsylvania, School of Medicine
Class of 2006

Andrew Schlachter
University of Kansas, School of Medicine
Class of 2009

Contents

High-Yield Facts

Embryology: Early and General

Cell Biology: Membranes

Cell Biology: Cytoplasm

Cell Biology: Intracellular Trafficking

Cell Biology: Nucleus

Integumentary System

Gastrointestinal Tract and Glands

Endocrine Glands

Reproductive Systems

Urinary System

Eye and Ear

Head and Neck

Thorax

Abdomen

Pelvis

Extremities and Spine

Preface

In this 3rd edition of *Anatomy, Histology, and Cell Biology: PreTest Self-Assessment and Review,* a significant number of changes and improvements have been made. This PreTest reviews all of the anatomical disciplines encompassing early embryology, cell biology, histology of the tissues and organs, as well as regional human anatomy of the head and neck, thorax, abdomen, pelvis, extremities, and spine. This edition represents a comprehensive effort to integrate the anatomical disciplines with clinical scenarios and cases. The authors' development of numerous clinical vignettes, integrating basic science disciplines with clinical medicine, will benefit students enrolled in medical schools with integrated curricula, as well as those students in discipline-based programs of study. The sections on cell biology and microscopic anatomy have been updated to include important new knowledge in Cell and Tissue Biology. There is also a greater focus on clinically-related questions, problems, and scenarios. New and improved light micrographs have been added and matching questions have been eliminated in favor of multiple-choice questions in keeping with recent changes in USMLE format. This 3rd edition is designed to help students prepare for USMLE Step 1, Subject Exams in Human Anatomy and Histology, and even USMLE Step 2 in which the NBME plans to add more Step 1 questions.

New for this 3rd edition is the addition of radiographs and MRIs. These radiological methods have become an important part of medical practice. It is imperative that students be able to recognize structures and relationships as part of their radiological anatomy knowledge base.

An updated High-Yield facts section is provided to facilitate rapid review of specific areas of Anatomy that are critical to mastering the difficult concepts of each subdiscipline: embryology, cell biology, histology of tissues and organs, regional human (gross) anatomy, pathology, and a brief review of neuroanatomical tracts.

Introduction

Each *PreTest Self-Assessment and Review* allows medical students to comprehensively and conveniently assess and review their knowledge of a particular medical school discipline, in this instance anatomy and cell biology. The 500 questions parallel the format and degree of difficulty of the questions found on the United States Medical Licensing Examination (USMLE) Step 1. Although the main emphasis of this PreTest is preparation for Step 1, the book will be very beneficial for medical students during their preclinical courses whether they are enrolled in a medical school with a problem-based, traditional, or hybrid curriculum. This PreTest focuses on an interdisciplinary approach incorporating numerous clinical scenarios so it will also be extremely valuable for students preparing for USMLE Step 2 who need to review their anatomical knowledge. Practicing physicians who want to hone their basic science skills and supplement their knowledge base before USMLE Step 3 or recertification will also find this book to be a good beginning in their review process.

This book is a comprehensive review of early embryology, cell biology, histology (tissue and organ biology), and human (gross) anatomy with some neuroanatomical topics covered through cases that integrate neuroanatomical tract information with regional anatomy of the head and neck. In keeping with the latest curricular changes in medical schools, as much as possible, questions integrate macroscopic and microscopic anatomy with cell biology, embryology, and neuroscience as well as physiology, biochemistry, and pathology. This PreTest begins with early embryology, including gametogenesis, fertilization, implantation, the formation of the bilaminar and trilaminar embryo, and overviews of the embryonic and fetal periods. This first section is followed by a review of basic cell biology, with separate chapters on membranes, cytoplasm, intracellular trafficking, and the nucleus. There are questions included to review the basics of mitosis and meiosis as well as regulation of cell cycle events. Tissue biology is the third section of the book, and it encompasses the tissues of the body: epithelium, connective tissue, specialized connective tissues (cartilage and bone), muscle, and nerve. Organ biology includes separate chapters on respiratory, integumentary (skin), digestive (tract and associated glands), endocrine, urinary, and male and female reproductive systems, as well as the eye and the ear. The topics in tissue and organ histology and cell biology include light and electron microscopic micrographs of appropriate structures that students should be able to identify. The last section of the book contains questions reviewing the basic concepts of regional anatomy of the head and neck, thorax, abdomen, pelvis, and extremities. For each section, appropriate x-rays, including MRIs, are included to assist the student in reviewing pertinent radiological aspects of the anatomy. Where possible, information is integrated with development and histology of the organ system.

Each multiple-choice question in this book contains four or more possible answer options. In each case, select the ONE BEST ANSWER to the question.

Each question is accompanied by an answer, a detailed explanation, and a specific page reference to an appropriate textbook. A bibliography listing sources can be found following the last chapter of this PreTest.

Acknowledgments

The authors express their gratitude to their colleagues who have greatly assisted them by providing light and electron micrographs as well as constructive criticism of the text, line drawings, and micrographs. They also acknowledge Eileen Roach for her painstaking care in the preparation of photomicrographs. Thanks to Drs. Amy Klion, Ann Dvorak, Anne W. Walling, Christopher Maxwell, Dale R. Abrahamson, Daniel Friend, David A. Sirois, David F. Albertini, Don W. Fawcett, Erik Dabelsteen, George Varghese, Giuseppina Raviola, H. Clarke Anderson, J.E. Heuser, John K. Young, Julia Neperud, K. Hama, Kristin M. Leiferman, Kuen-Shan Hung, Louis Wetzel, Michael J. Werle, Nancy E.J. Berman, Per-Lennart Westesson, Robert P. Bolender, Ronal R. MacGregor, Stanley L. Erlandsen, WenFang Wang, Wolfram Sterry, and Xiaoming Zhang for their contribution of micrographs and ideas for question development. Also, thanks to the Jeffrey Modell Foundation and The Primary Immunodeficiency Resource Center for use of the Martin Causubon case. The authors remain indebted to their students and colleagues at the University of Kansas Medical Center, past and present, who have challenged them to continuously improve their skills as educators.

—RMK
—GCE

High-Yield Facts

Embryology

Embryological development is divided into three periods:

The **Prenatal Period** consists of **gamete formation** and maturation, ending in fertilization.

The **Embryonic Period** begins with fertilization and extends through the **first 8 weeks** of development. It includes implantation, germ layer formation, and organogenesis. This is the critical period for susceptibility to **teratogens.**

The **Fetal Period** extends from the **third month** through birth.

THE PRENATAL PERIOD

The **development of gametes** begins with the duplication of chromosomal DNA followed by two cycles of nuclear and cell division **(meiosis).**

Genetic variability is assured by **crossing over** of DNA, **random assortment** of chromosomes, and **recombination** during the first meiotic division. Errors can result in duplication or deletion of all or part of a specific chromosome.

Spermatogenesis

The process of spermatogenesis is **continuous** after puberty and each cycle lasts about 2 months.

Spermatogonia in the walls of the seminiferous tubules of the testes undergo mitotic divisions to replenish their population and form a group of spermatogonia that will differentiate to form spermatocytes.

Primary spermatocytes are spermatogenic cells that have duplicated their DNA (4N) and enter meiosis.

Secondary spermatocytes result from the first meiotic division (2N).

Spermatids are formed by the second meiotic division (1N).

Spermiogenesis

During this phase, spermatids mature into sperm by losing extraneous cytoplasm and developing a head region consisting of an **acrosome** (specialized secretory granule) surrounding the nuclear material and grow a tail.

Oogenesis

Oogenesis begins in the fetal period in females and is a discontinuous process involving mitosis, meiosis, and maturation.

Oogonia undergo mitotic division and duplicate their DNA to form **primary oocytes,** but stop in the prophase of the first meiotic division until puberty.

The second meiotic division is not concluded until fertilization occurs.

Maturational events include retention of protein synthetic machinery in the surviving oocyte, formation of **cortical granules** that participate in events at fertilization, and development of a protective glycoprotein coat, the **zona pellucida.**

Fertilization

Fertilization occurs when sperm and oocyte cell membranes fuse. Following coitus, exposure of sperm to the environment of the female reproductive tract causes **capacitation,** removal of surface glycoproteins and cholesterol from the sperm membrane, enabling fertilization to occur.

Fusing of the first sperm initiates the **zona reaction.** Release of **cortical granules** from the acrosome causes biochemical changes in the zona pellucida and oocyte membrane that prevent polyspermy.

EMBRYONIC DEVELOPMENT

The embryo forms one **germ layer** during each of the first 3 weeks.

During the second week, the **blastocyst** differentiates into two germ layers, the **epiblast** and the **hypoblast.** This establishes the dorsal (epiblast)–ventral (hypoblast) body axis.

During the third week, the process of **gastrulation** occurs by which epiblast cells migrate toward the **primitive streak** and ingress to form the **endoderm** and **mesoderm** germ layers below the remaining epiblast cells (**ectoderm**).

Lateral body folding at the end of the third week causes the germ layers to form three concentric tubes with the innermost layer being the endoderm, the mesoderm in the middle, and the ectoderm on the surface.

GERM LAYER DERIVATIVES

Mesoderm Derivatives

The mesoderm is divided into four regions (from medial to lateral): axial, paraxial, intermediate, and lateral plate.

Axial mesoderm is located in the midline and forms the notochord.
Paraxial mesoderm forms **somites.** Somites are divided into **sclerotomes** (bone formation), **myotomes** (muscle precursors), and **dermatomes** (precursor of dermis).
Intermediate mesoderm gives rise to components of the genitourinary system.
Lateral plate mesoderm forms bones and connective tissue of the limbs and limb girdles (**somatic layer,** also known as **somatopleure**) and the smooth muscle lining viscera and the serosae of body cavities (**splanchnic layer,** also known as **splanchnopleure**).

Intermediate mesoderm is *not found* in the head region, and the lateral plate mesoderm is *not divided* into layers there.

GERM LAYER DERIVATIVES			
Ectodermal Derivatives	Epithelium of skin (superficial epidermis layer)		
	All nervous tissue: formed by neuroectoderm: Brain and spinal cord (neural tube) Peripheral nerves and other neural crest derivatives		
Endodermal Derivatives	Epithelial linings of:	The gastrointestinal tract	
		Organs that form as buds from the endodermal tube: Pharyngeal gland derivatives* Respiratory system Digestive organs (liver, pancreas) Terminal part of urogenital systems	
	Hypoblast Endoderm: Gametes migrate to gonads		
Mesodermal Derivatives	All connective tissue†	General connective tissue	
		Cartilage and bone	
		Blood cells (red and white)	
	All muscle types:	Cardiac, skeletal, smooth	
	Epithelial linings of:	Body cavities	
		Some organs: Cardiovascular system Reproductive and urinary systems (most parts)	

*Pharyngeal derivatives: palatine tonsils, thymus, thyroid, parathyroids.
†Some connective tissue in the head are derived from neural crest.

Ectoderm Derivatives

Formation of the primitive central nervous system is induced in the ectoderm layer by cells forming the **notochord** in the underlying mesoderm. The neural plate ectoderm (**neuroectoderm**) forms two lateral folds that meet and fuse in the midline to form the neural tube (**neurulation**). Cells from the tips of the folds (**neural crest**) migrate throughout the body to form many derivatives including the peripheral nervous system.

FORMATION OF THE HEAD REGION

Neural crest contributes significantly to formation of connective tissue elements in the head.

The bony skeleton of the head is comprised of the **viscerocranium** and the **neurocranium.**

The neurocranium (cranial vault) is composed of a base formed by **endochondral ossification** (chondrocranium) and sides and roof bones formed by **intramembranous ossification.**

The chondrocranium is derived from both **somitic mesoderm** (occipital) and neural crest.

The viscerocranium (face) is derived from the first two **pharyngeal (branchial) arches** (neural crest in origin).

LIMB FORMATION

The limbs form as ventrolateral buds under the mutual induction of ectoderm [apical ectodermal ridge (AER)] and underlying mesoderm beginning in the fifth week. *The AER influences proximal-distal development.*

Somatic lateral plate mesoderm (somatopleure) forms the bony and connective tissue elements of the limbs and limb girdles while skeletal muscle of the appendages is derived from **somites.**

Cranio-caudal polarity is determined by specialized mesoderm cells [zone of polarizing activity (ZPA)] that release inducing signals such as **retinoic acid.**

Homeobox genes are the targets of induction signals. They are named after their **homeodomain** called the homeobox which is a DNA-binding motif. Homeobox genes encode trancription factors that regulate processes such as segmentation and axis formation.

Rotation of the limb buds establishes the position of the joints, the location of muscle groups, and the pattern of sensory innervation (**dermatome map**).

MATURATION OF THE CENTRAL NERVOUS SYSTEM

Both neurons and glia develop from the original neurectoderm forming the neural tube.

Microglia *are the exception*: they develop from the monocyte-macrophage lineage of mesodermal (bone marrow) origin and migrate into the CNS.

Induction of regional differences in the developing CNS is regulated by retinoic acid (vitamin A). Overexposure of the cranial region to **retinoic acid** can result in "caudalization," i.e., development more similar to the spinal cord.

During development, the spinal cord and presumptive brainstem develop three layers: (1) a **germinal layer** or **ventricular zone**, (2) an **intermediate layer** containing **neuroblasts** and comprising gray matter, and (3) a **marginal zone** containing myelinated fibers (white matter). Other layers are added in the cerebrum and cerebellum by cell migration along glial scaffolds.

The notochord induces the establishment of **dorsal-ventral polarity** in the neural tube. Ventral portions of the tube will become the **basal plate** and give rise to motor neurons, whereas the dorsal portions become the **alar plates**, derivatives of which subserve sensory functions.

Meninges are formed by mesoderm surrounding the neural tube with contributions to the arachnoid and pia from neural crest.

Defects in the CNS may result from several causes including high maternal blood glucose levels and vitamin A overexposure and often involve bony defects (e.g., spina bifida and anencephaly). Defects are most common in the regions of neuropore closure. Folic acid, also known as folate, is a B-vitamin that can be found in some enriched foods and vitamin supplements. Women who take folate before pregnancy have a decreased risk of neural tube defects (NTDs) including spina bifida and anencephaly. The U.S. Public Health Service recommends that all women who could possibly become pregnant get 400 μg (or 0.4 mg) of folic acid every day. This could prevent up to 70% of NTDs. Folic acid is found in some foods, such as enriched breads, pastas, rice, and cereals (some with 100% of the daily requirement).

Fetal alcohol syndrome (FAS) is the most common cause of mental retardation; FAS includes the triad of growth retardation, characteristic facial dysmorphology and neurodevelopmental abnormalities. Alcohol rapidly crosses the placenta and the fetal blood-brain barrier. Damage is dependent on gestational age, alcohol dosage, and pattern of maternal alcohol abuse. Altered neural crest cell migration, differentiation and programmed cell death (apoptosis) are hypothesized mechanisms for the congenital dysmorphologies associated with FAS.

PERIPHERAL NERVOUS SYSTEM

Sensory neurons of the spinal ganglia, as well as autonomic postganglionic neurons and their supporting cells, are derived from **neural crest.** Focal deficiencies in neural crest cell migration may result in lack of innervation to specific organs or parts of organs. In **Hirschsprung disease** (aganglionic megacolon), failure of neural crest cells to migrate to a portion of the colon results in a localized deficiency in parasympathetic intramural ganglia that may cause a loss of peristalsis and bowel obstruction.

DEVELOPMENT OF THE HEAD AND NECK

The cartilages and bones of the face (viscerocranium) develop from the **pharyngeal (branchial) arches.** Each arch receives its blood supply from a specific aortic arch and its innervation from a specific cranial nerve (special or branchial visceral efferent fibers). The **third aortic arch** provides most of the adult **blood supply to the head and neck.** The **skeletal muscles** of the head and neck primarily arise from the pharyngeal arches and have a unique innervation (special visceral efferent).

The face develops from a midline **frontonasal prominence** and bilateral **maxillary and mandibular prominences.** Failure of the prominences to fuse results in various facial clefts.

Teeth originate from both ectodermal (enamel) and neurectodermal (neural crest: dentin, pulp, cementum, and periodontal ligament) derivatives.

DERIVATIVES OF PHARYNGEAL POUCHES AND CLEFTS		
Pouch 1:		Epithelial lining of middle ear canals and tympanic membrane
Pouch 2:		Epithelial lining of palatine tonsils
Pouch 3:	Ventral portion:	Epithelial components of thymus gland
	Dorsal portion:	Epithelial cells of inferior parathyroid glands
Pouch 4:	Ventral portion:	Epithelial "C" [parafollicular (interfollicular) cells of the thyroid gland]
	Dorsal portion:	Epithelial cells of superior parathyroid glands
Clefts 1:		External auditory canal
Clefts 2 → 4:		No derivatives

Pituitary

The anterior portion of the pituitary is derived from oral ectoderm arising from the roof of the oral cavity (Rathke's pouch) anterior to the buccopharyngeal membrane and migrating through the sphenoid anlagen to unite with a downgrowth of neuroectoderm (posterior pituitary).

Eye

The eye is derived from three different germ layers:

Neuroectoderm: Vesicular outgrowths of the forebrain differentiate into retina and optic nerve.

Surface ectoderm: Contributes to the **lens, cornea,** and epithelial coverings of the lacrimal glands, eyelids, and **conjunctiva.**

Mesoderm: The **sclera** and **choroid** are derived from **lateral plate mesoderm.**

The **extraocular muscles** are derived from myoblasts of the **cranial somitomeres.**

Structures of the **outer and middle ear** are derived from the **first and second pharyngeal arches** and the **first pharyngeal cleft.**

Structures of the **inner ear** are derived from the **ectodermal otic placode,** *not neuroectoderm.*

Maternal rubella can cause defects in both eye (fourth to sixth weeks of gestation) and ear (seventh to eight weeks).

FORMATION OF THE CARDIOVASCULAR SYSTEM

All components of the cardiovascular system, including the epithelia, are derived from **splanchnic lateral plate mesoderm.**

The heart tubes forming on either side of the endodermal tube are brought together by **lateral body folding.**

Looping of the heart tube occurs while the tube is being divided into left and right portions by the interatrial and interventricular septa.

In the interatrial septum, the **septum primum** and **septum secundum** do not close off the **foramen ovale** until birth.

Failure of the **atrioventricular endocardial cushions** to fuse can result in septal and valve defects.

Neural crest cells contribute to septation of the truncus arteriosus and the formation of the aortic and pulmonary outflows, as well as the aortic arches.

The "**Tetralogy of Fallot**" is the most common defect of the conus arteriosus/truncus arteriosus and is due to unequal division of the conus due to anterior displacement of the conotruncal septum. The mnemomic **IHOP** is useful to remember the four cardiovascular alterations which comprise the Tetralogy: 1) interventricular septal defect, 2) hypotrophy of the right ventricle, 3) overriding aorta, and 4) pulmonary stenosis.

Vasculature

Vasculogenesis versus Angiogenesis

The endothelial lining of most blood vessels forms by coalescence of vascular endothelial progenitors (**angioblasts**) of mesodermal origin. The endothelial cells proliferate, migrate, differentiate, and organize into tubular structures with subsequent vacuolization to form a lumen. Subsequently, **periendothelial** cells form from local mesoderm and differentiate into muscle and connective tissue elements (i.e., **smooth muscle, fibroblasts**, and **pericytes**). That process is known as **vasculogenesis** and occurs in both embryonic and adult tissues. Vasculogenesis is the *de novo* formation of blood vessels and differs from angiogenesis, initiated in a pre-existing vessel. Both of those processes are regulated in part by **vascular endothelial growth factor (VEGF)**, which induces chemotactic (migratory) and proliferative responses in endothelial cells. Uterine angiogenesis occurs in adult women during each menstrual cycle. Angiogenesis also is a prominent characteristic of inflammation, pathology such as **diabetic retinopathy,** wound repair, placental development during embryogenesis, and tumor formation. Molecular triggers for angiogenesis include the **cytokines,** small, extracellular signal proteins or peptides that function as local mediators in cell-cell communication. For example, during inflammation or hypoxia, cytokines induce endothelial cell proliferation and differentiation and stimulate **matrix metalloproteinases** that digest type IV collagen in the basement membrane creating a new branch point in the vessel.

Tumor angiogenesis mimics the process observed during inflammation. Tumor angiogenesis has become a potential target in cancer treatment. Tumors produce **antiangiogenic factors** such as **endostatin** and **angiostatin,** which are derived from type XVIII collagen and plasminogen respectively. Pharmaceutical agents modeled after these anti-angiogenic peptides are being developed to inhibit tumor growth.

Development of the Vasculature

The paired doral aortae and the five aortic arches form an early symmetric arterial system. Regression of portions of these vessels later results in the asymmetrical adult arterial system.

The **vitelline arteries** connect the yolk sac to the abdominal dorsal aorta. They will form the arteries of the GI tract: **celiac, superior mesenteric**, and **inferior mesenteric**.

Blood islands are the first sites of **hematopoiesis** and seed other hematopoietic tissues.

The paired **umbilical arteries** develop from the caudal end of the dorsal aorta and invade the mesoderm of the placenta. They carry deoxygenated blood from the fetus to the placenta.

The **caval venous system** is derived mostly from the right anterior and posterior **cardinal veins**.

The **vitelline veins** form the veins of the digestive system, including the **portal vein**, and the terminal part of the inferior vena cava.

No components of the **umbilical veins** remain patent after closure of the ductus venosus.

DEVELOPMENT OF THE HEMATOPOIETIC SYSTEM

Onset of **hematopoiesis** begins with formation of blood islands in the wall of the **yolk sac** (derived from the hypoblast) during week 3.

Pluripotent stem cells from the blood islands seed the other hematopoietic sites. These are, in succession, the **liver** (week 5), **spleen** (week 5), and **bone marrow** (month 6).

All components of hematopoietic organs are derived from **mesoderm** except for the **epithelium of the thymus**, which is derived from **endoderm** of the **third pharyngeal pouch**.

DEVELOPMENT OF THE DIGESTIVE SYSTEM

The epithelium of the digestive tract and associated organs is formed by the **endodermal tube**, whereas connective tissue and smooth muscle are derived from **splanchnic lateral plate mesoderm**. The mesoderm induces regional specialization in the endoderm.

The midgut endoderm is the last to fold into a tube and remains connected to the yolk sac via the yolk stalk.

Formation of the mesodermal **urorectal septum** divides the cloaca into the **urogenital sinus** and **primitive rectum**.

Cell proliferation results in closure of the endodermal tube lumen during week 6. The lumen is reopened by **recanalization** in week 8.

Failure to recanalize can result in **stenosis**, preventing the passage of amniotic fluid swallowed by the fetus causing **polyhydramnios**.

Peristalsis begins in week 10 when neural crest cells invade the muscular layer to form the enteric nervous (autonomic) system. Failure of neural crest cell migration to the distal hindgut results in **aganglionic megacolon (Hirschsprung disease)**, which may cause fatal intestinal obstruction.

The adult pattern of GI organ distribution is achieved by **physiologic herniation** and then retraction of the midgut during the second month.

Failure of the midgut loop to return to the abdominal cavity may result in an **omphalocele** or **umbilical hernia.**

Associated digestive organs (liver, gallbladder, and pancreas) originate as outgrowths of the endodermal tube. Connective tissue components of the liver are derived from both splanchnic and somatic **(septum transversum)** lateral plate mesoderm. Lateral plate mesoderm also forms the peritoneum and mesenteries of the abdominal cavity.

FORMATION OF THE RESPIRATORY SYSTEM

The first part of the respiratory system is lined by ectoderm derived from the nasal **ectodermal placodes.**

In the fourth week, a **respiratory diverticulum** arises as an outgrowth of the ventral **endodermal tube.**

Endoderm will form the respiratory epithelium, whereas **splanchnic lateral plate mesoderm** will form connective tissue elements including cartilage, smooth muscle, and blood vessels.

Mesoderm directs the branching pattern of the developing airways.

The **diaphragm** forms from the **septum transversum,** the two **pleuroperitoneal membranes,** the **dorsal mesentery** of the **esophagus** (where the **crura** develop), and the muscular parts of the **dorsal and lateral body wall.**

Although most **alveoli** do not form until after birth, the lungs are capable of sufficient gas exchange after 6.5 months of gestation. **Respiratory distress syndrome (RDS)** develops in premature births because of immaturity of the Type II pneumocytes that produce **surfactant.** Surfactant is essential for expansion of the pulmonary alveoli; it lowers the **air-interface surface tension** and prevents the alveoli from collapsing at the end of expiration. Without surfactant, premature babies suffer from RDS with rapid breathing, chest wall retractions, grunting noise with each breath, and nasal flaring.

Abnormal septation of the trachea and esophagus can result in stenosis, atresia, or tracheoesophageal fistulas (TEFs).

DEVELOPMENT OF THE URINARY SYSTEM

Epithelial structures of the urinary system are derived from two sources: **intermediate mesoderm** and **urogenital sinus endoderm.**

Three pairs of kidneys develop in cranio-caudal sequence in the urogenital ridge of intermediate mesoderm: **pronephros, mesonephros,** and **metanephros.**

The caudal end of the mesonephric duct gives rise to the ureteric bud. The **ureteric bud** induces surrounding intermediate mesoderm to form the **metanephric cap,** which forms the excretory units of the kidney. The ureteric bud will form the collecting ducts.

During kidney development, **epithelial-mesenchymal interactions** occur reciprocally between the epithelium of the ureteric bud and the mesenchyme of the metanephric cap (blastema) to convert the **mesenchyme** of the metanephric cap into an **epithelium.** Those complex inductions are regulated by a cascade of growth factors that allow a **dialogue between the epithelium and mesenchyme** and the eventual formation of urine-producing (nephron) and collecting portions (i.e., collecting ducts, calyces, and pelves) of the developing kidney.

The epithelial lining (transitional epithelium) of the **ureters,** as well as their muscular and connective tissue components, are derived from **intermediate mesoderm.**

The transitional epithelium of the **bladder** and most of the **urethra** are derived from hindgut **endoderm of the urogenital sinus.** Connective tissue and muscle are derived from splanchnic lateral plate mesoderm.

DEVELOPMENT OF THE REPRODUCTIVE SYSTEMS

Intermediate mesoderm forms the epithelia, connective tissues, and smooth muscle of the indifferent **sex cords** and their ducts.

The **endoderm of the urogenital sinus** gives rise to the epithelia of distal organs of the reproductive system and the external genitalia. As in the urinary system, connective tissue and smooth muscle of these terminal elements are provided by splanchnic lateral plate mesoderm.

Germ cells migrate from their origins in yolk sac endoderm into the indifferent sex cords of the **urogenital ridge** by week 6. Further differentiation of both the immature sex cords and the germ cells occurs.

The **Sry gene** on the **Y chromosome** directs the differentiation of the medullary sex cords into **testes.** If this gene *is not* present, the cortical sex cords will develop as ovaries.

Sertoli cells produce **Müllerian inhibiting substance** which causes the apoptosis of **paramesonephric (Müllerian) duct** structures in the male fetus. **Leydig cells** produce **testosterone** and other sex hormones that regulate further male differentiation.

In the absence of testosterone, **follicular cells** and **oogonia** develop. Two pairs of genital ducts develop in both sexes. **Mesonephric (Wolffian) ducts** develop first as part of the urinary system.

Paramesonephric (Müllerian) ducts develop next and are open to the pelvic cavity at their cranial ends, and connect to each other and then to the urogenital sinus via a sinovaginal bulb at their caudal ends. The mesonephric system will persist in the male and the paramesonephric system in the female. In males, the mesonephric system gives rise to the efferent ductules, epididymis, ductus deferens, seminal vesicles and ejaculatory ducts. In females the paramesonephric system gives rise to the oviduct, uterus and upper part of the vagina.

In **males**, the **urogenital sinus endoderm** gives rise to the epithelia of the **urethra** and associated **prostate** and **bulbourethral glands.**

In the **female**, the endoderm of the **urogenital sinus** is the origin of the epithelium of the **lower vagina**, the upper portion being formed by the **paramesonephric ducts.**

Male differentiation of external genitalia requires androgens. Female differentiation is the intrinsic pathway and occurs in **the absence of androgens and/or functioning androgen receptors.**

DEVELOPMENT OF THE PLACENTA AND FETAL MEMBRANES

The fetal portion of the placenta forms from the **trophoblast.**

Syncytiotrophoblast cells are in direct contact with maternal tissue, whereas the embryo proper is separated from the **cytotrophoblast** by **extraembryonic mesoderm** (together, the **chorion**).

Primary villus: syncytiotrophoblast with a cytotrophoblast core.

Secondary villus: Cytotrophoblast core invaded by extraembryonic mesoderm.

Tertiary villus: Fetal blood vessels invade the mesoderm (week 3).

The presumptive **umbilical blood vessels** form in the wall of the **allantois,** an endodermal outpocket of the urogenital sinus.

The **amnionic membrane** develops from **epiblast** and is continuous with embryonic ectoderm. The lining of the **yolk sac** develops from **hypoblast** and is continuous with embryonic endoderm.

The yolk sac gives rise to the first **blood islands** that will form the **vitelline vessels.**

Passive immunity is transfered to the fetus by transport of **immunoglobulin G** (IgG) from the maternal to the fetal circulation. Excess amniotic fluid is swallowed by the fetus, absorbed by the fetal GI tract, transferred to the fetal circulation, and finally crosses the placental membranes to the maternal circulation.

Hormones secreted by the placenta include chorionic gonadotropin (HCG), estrogen, progesterone, and chorionic somatostatin (placental lactogen).

High-Yield Facts

Histology and Cell Biology

CELL MEMBRANES

Cell membranes consist of a **lipid bilayer** and associated proteins and carbohydrates. In the bilayer, the hydrophilic portions of the lipids are arranged on the external and cytosolic surfaces, and the **hydrophobic tails** are located in the interior. **Transmembrane proteins** are anchored to the core of the bilayer by their hydrophobic regions and can be removed only by detergents that disrupt the bilayer. **Peripheral membrane proteins** are attached to the surface of the membrane by weak electrostatic forces and are easy to remove by altering the pH or ionic strength of their environment.

CYTOPLASM AND ORGANELLES

Cytoplasm is a dynamic fluid environment bounded by the cell membrane. It contains various membrane-bound organelles, nonmembranous structures (such as lipid droplets, glycogen, and pigment granules), and structural or cytoskeletal proteins in either a soluble or insoluble form. The **endoplasmic reticulum (ER)** is a continuous tubular meshwork that may be either **smooth (SER) or rough (RER)** where studded with ribosomes. RER is involved in protein synthesis while the SER is involved in sterioid synthesis and detoxification. The discoid stacks (**CGN, *cis*, medial, *trans*, and TGN** as one moves from the RER-side to the secretory vesicle-side) of the **Golgi apparatus** are involved in packaging and routing proteins for export or delivery to other organelles, including lysosomes and peroxisomes. **Lysosomes** degrade intracellular and imported debris, and **peroxisomes** oxidize a variety of substrates, through beta-oxidation and are the sole source of **plasmalogens**. Targeting sequences include **KDEL**, which targets ER proteins from the Golgi to the ER, and **mannose 6-phosphate**, which targets proteins to the lysosome. **Mannose 6-phosphate receptors** are found in the Golgi and in lysosomes. In the absence of mannose 6-phosphate on lysosomal enzymes (**I-cell disease**) they follow the default pathway and are secreted from the cell. Lysosomal enzymes are specific for substrate; the absence of specific enzymes results in **lysosomal storage diseases** such as **Tay-Sach's**. Secretory granules leave the **TGN** to dock with the plasma membrane. In that process, **v-SNARE** on the vesicle docks with **t-SNARE** on the cell membrane and requires **Rab GTPase**-activity, linking to tethering proteins, and eventually to a receptor protein in the cell membrane. **Receptor-mediated endocytosis** is the process that permits selective uptake of molecules into the cell using **clathrin-coated pits and vesicles.** Molecules not recycled to the cell membrane enter **early endosomes** and subsequently **late endosomes** by way of **multivesicular bodies (MVBs).** The late endosome is more acidic than the early endosome and generally leads to degradation of the molecules in lysosomes. There are several major pathways for shuttling of receptors and ligands.

- The internalized ligand-receptor complex dissociates in the early endosome with recycling of receptors [e.g., low density-lipoprotein (LDL)-LDL-receptor complex].
- Receptor and ligand are recycled (e.g., iron-transferrin-transferrin receptor-complex).
- The internalized ligand-recepetor complex dissociates in the late endosome and is degraded in the lysosome (e.g., growth factors such as epidermal growth factor).
- Internalized ligand-receptor passes through the cell (transcytosis) and is released at another surface (e.g., IgA uptake by small intestinal enterocytes).

Only the **nucleus,** which is the repository of genetic information stored in deoxyribonucleic acid (DNA), and the **mitochondria,** which are the storage sites of energy for cellular function in the form of adenosine triphosphate **(ATP),** are enclosed in double membranes. Also included in the cytoplasm are three classes of proteins that form the **cytoskeletal infrastructure: actin bundles** that determine the shape of the cell; **intermediate filaments** that stabilize the cell membrane and cytoplasmic contents; and **microtubules (tubulin),** which use molecular motors (i.e., dynein and kinesin) to move organelles within the cell.

NUCLEUS

The nucleus consists of a **nuclear envelope** that is continuous with the ER, chromatin, matrix, and a **nucleolus** the site of ribosomal ribonucleic acid (rRNA) synthesis and initial ribosomal assembly. The nuclear envelope contains pores for bidirectional transport and is supported by intermediate filament proteins, the **lamins. Chromatin** consists of **euchromatin** (eu = true), which is an open form of DNA that is actively transcribed, and **heterochromatin** that is quiescent. There is a sequential packing of chromatin beginning with the DNA double helix, which is combined with **histones** to form the **nucleosomes**, the smallest unit of chromatin structure. This is the **"beads on a string"** structure with the histones forming the octamer arrangment of paired H2A, H2B, H3, and H4. **H1** is the **linker histone**. The nucleosomes are connected by strands of protein free DNA, so called **linker DNA**. Nucleases degrade the linker DNA, but nucleosome particles are protected against micrococcal nuclease activity because of the close interaction of DNA with histone proteins. The next orders of packing are the 30 nm chromatin fibril, the chromatin fiber with loops of chromatin fibrils, and chromatin fibers loosely or tightly packed in euchromatin and heterochromatin respectively.

During **cell division**, DNA is accurately replicated and divided equally between two daughter nuclei. Equal distribution of chromosomes is accomplished by the **microtubules of the mitotic spindle**. The separation of cytoplasm (**cytokinesis**) occurs through the action of an **actin contractile ring**. The cell cycle consists of interphase (**G$_1$, S, and G$_2$**), and the stages of mitosis (M): **prophase, prometaphase, metaphase, anaphase, and telophase.** The cell cycle is regulated at the G$_1$/S and G$_2$/M boundaries (checkpoints) by phosphorylation of complexes of a protein kinase [**cyclin-dependent kinase (Cdk)** protein] and a **cyclin (cytoplasmic oscillator).** For example, the G$_2$/M interface is regulated by **M-Cdk complex** (formerly called **Mitosis Promoting Factor, MPF**), which is responsible for the phosphorylation of **spindle proteins, histones, and lamins.** Phosphorylation of **lamins** results in their breakdown as well as the dissolution of the nuclear envelope. There are different cyclins and Cdks for each of the cell cycle checkpoints. Overarching the Cdks are the **Cdk inhibitors** that form an additional regulatory layer at each of the cell cycle checkpoints. Study of the cell cycle is critical to an understanding of the regulation of abnormal proliferation as occurs in cancer cells. Two **tumor suppressor genes** that have been well studied are **retinoblastoma gene (Rb)** and **p53.** Rb is active (suppressing growth) in the hypophosphorylated state and inactive in the hyperphosphorylated form. In its nonphosphorylated form Rb serves as a brake on the cell cycle at the G$_1$/S interface by binding to the **transcription factor, E2F.** Stimulation by growth factors results in phosphorylation and release of the brake; E2F is free to turn on transcription of cell cycle genes, allowing cells to traverse the G_1/S interface. **Mutations in Rb occur in tumors**; a mutation has the same effect as inactivating Rb leading to uncontrolled cell proliferation as E2F trancribes cell cycle genes. **p53 is a protective gene** or molecular policeman, which prevents the replication of damaged DNA and stimulates repair. p53 acts as a transcription factor and also works through the Cdk inhibitors to arrest the cell cycle at the G_1/S interface. **p53 mutations are found in many human tumors.**

INTRACELLULAR TRAFFICKING

The key event in exocytosis is translocation of newly synthesized protein into the cisternal space of the rough ER (**signal hypothesis**). Proteins and lipids reach the Golgi apparatus by vesicular transport. Using carbohydrate-sorting signals, proteins are sorted from the *trans*-face of the Golgi apparatus to secretory vesicles, the cell membrane, and **lysosomes**. Lysosomal enzymes are sorted by using a **mannose-6-phosphate** signal recognized by a receptor on the lysosomal membrane. Absence of mannose 6-phosphate results in **default to the secretory pathway and release of enzymes by exocytosis.** Nuclear and mitochondrial-sorting signals (positively charged amino acid sequences) are recognized by those organelles.

Endocytosis involves transport from the cell membrane to lysosomes using endosome intermediates. The process originates with a **clathrin-coated pit** that invaginates to form a **coated vesicle** that fuses with an **endosome**. This internalization can be **receptor-mediated** (e.g., uptake of cholesterol). Endosomes subsequently fuse with lysosomes. Internalized receptor/ligand complexes may be conserved, degraded, or recycled.

EPITHELIUM

Epithelial cells line the free external and internal surfaces of the body. Epithelia have a paucity of intercellular substance and are interconnected by **junctional complexes.** Components of the junctional complex include the *zonula occludens* (tight junction), which prevents leakage between the adjoining cells and maintains apical/basolateral polarity; *zonula adherens*, which links the actin networks within adjacent cells; and *macula adherens* (desmosome), which links the intermediate filament networks of adjacent cells. Epithelial cells also form a firm attachment to the **basal lamina,** which they secrete. **Gap junctions** or **nexi** permit passage of small molecules directly between cells. Apical specializations are prominent in epithelia and include **microvilli** that increase surface area; **stereocilia**, which are non-motile modified microvilli; and **cilia and flagella**, which are motile structures. Cilia and flagella have the classic "**9 + 2**" microtubular arrangement emanating from **basal bodies**. The basal surface may be modified with infoldings that house numerous mitochondria as found in proximal and distal tubule cells of the kidney and striated duct cells of the salivary glands. Those cells are involved in extensive ion transport.

CONNECTIVE TISSUE

Connective tissue consists of cells and a matrix (fibers and ground substance). The cells include **fibroblasts** (the source of collagen and other fibers), **plasma cells** (the source of antibodies), **macrophages** (the cells responsible for phagocytosis), **mast cells** (the source of heparin and histamine), and a variety of transient blood cells: **lymphocytes (B and T)**, **eosinophils, basophils**, and **neutrophils (PMNs)**. B cells are involved in humoral immunity and T cells in **cell-mediated immunity** as well as **humoral immunity** (helper T cells). Neutrophils phagocytose bacteria; the dead neutrophils are a major component of pus. Basophils, like mast cells, release histamine although they originate from a different bone marrow stem cell. Eosinophils are involved in response to parasitic infection. Eosinophilic granules contain a crystalline core of major basic protein, which is toxic for parasites and histaminase, which breaks down histamine and limits the allergic response. **Type I collagen** and elastin make up the predominant fibers found in connective tissue. Ground substance includes proteoglycans and glycoproteins that organize and stabilize the fibrillar network. **Type II collagen** is associated with hyaline cartilage; **type III collagen** forms the collagenous component of reticular connective tissue found in highly cellular organs, such as the liver and lymphoid organs. **Type IV collagen** forms a **sheet-like meshwork** or **insoluble scaffolding** of the basal lamina. Other types of collagen exist and include the **fibril-associated collagens** with interrupted triple helices (**FACIT**). Collagen fibrils are connected to other extracellular matrix molecules by the FACIT collagens.

SPECIALIZED CONNECTIVE TISSUES: BONE AND CARTILAGE

Bone contains three major cell types: **osteoblasts** that secrete **type I collagen** and noncollagenous proteins; **osteocytes**, which maintain mature bone; and **osteoclasts,** which resorb bone by acidification. Osteoclastic activity uses **protons** (H^+) derived from carbonic acid formed by the enzyme **carbonic anyhydrase.** Carbonic anhydrases are zinc-containing enzymes that catalyse the reversible reaction between carbon dioxide hydration and bicarbonate dehydration:

$$H_2O + CO_2 \leftrightarrow H^+ + HCO_3^-$$

In the region of the **ruffled border, protons and lysosomal enzymes,** such as acid phosphatase, are released into a sealed zone (Howship's lacuna). Breakdown of bone occurs due to the **acidification of this extracellular compartment** that is analogous to an intracellular secondary lysosome. Bone deposition is regulated primarily by **parathyroid hormone (PTH),** which is secreted in response to low serum calcium levels. PTH increases serum calcium as summarized below. The increased serum calcium inhibits PTH secretion by negative feedback. PTH stimulates:

- **osteoclasts** to resorb bone (through PTH receptors on osteoblasts),
- renal synthesis of **1,25-dihydroxycholecalciferol,** which in turn increases intestinal absorption of Ca^{++}.
- **intestinal absorption of Ca^{++}.**

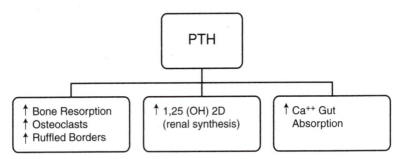

PTH regulates osteoclasts by an indirect mechanism through **PTH receptors** on osteoblasts. There are *no* PTH receptors on osteoclasts. PTH stimulation of osteoblasts releases **macrophage colony-stimulating factor (M-CSF)** and **RANK-L.** M-CSF stimulates differentiation of **monocytes into osteoclasts.** RANK-L is found in both membrane and soluble forms and binds to **RANK (receptor for activation of nuclear factor kappa B)** on osteoclasts and osteoclast precursors stimulating osteoclastic activation/ruffled border formation. **Osteoprotegerin (OPG) is a decoy receptor for**

RANK-L, binds RANK-L, and leads to inhibition of osteoclastic activity. Those molecules create the link between osteoblasts and osteoclasts known as the **ARF (activation-resorption-formation)** cycle in which activation of osteoclasts is inextricably linked to osteoblasts. This has been one of the problems in treating **osteoporosis** in which osteoclastic activity dominates osteoblastic activity. Growth factors such as transforming growth factor-beta (TGF-β) and insulin-like growth factors also play a role in differentiation of osteoblasts and osteoclasts. TGF-β is found in an inactive form in the bone matrix and is activated by acid produced by osteoclasts. TGF-β then inhibits osteoclast differentiation and stimulates osteoblastic activity.

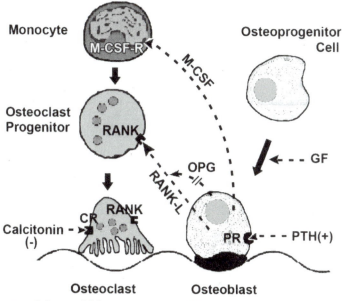

GF = growth factors, OPG = osteoprotegerin, PR = parathyroid hormone receptor, PTH = parathyroid hormone, RANK = receptor for activation of nuclear factor kappa B, RANK-L = ligand for RANK, M-CSF = macrophage colony-stimulating factor, M-CSF-R = MCSF receptor.

Calcitonin opposes the actions of PTH, but plays a lesser role overall.

Bone is highly vascular and mineralized with **hydroxyapatite**. In contrast, the three types of cartilage are avascular and contain chondrocytes that synthesize fibers and ground substance. **Hyaline cartilage** covers articular surfaces and forms the cartilage model in long bone development. **Elastic cartilage** is found in the pinna of the ear and in the epiglotlis, while **fibrocartilage** is an intermediate form found in the intervertebral disc, pubic symphysis, and connecting tendon and bone. Hyaline cartilage contains matrix comprised of type II collagen electrostatically bound to proteoglycans. Elastic cartilage contains type II collagen and elastic fibers, and fibrocartilage, like bone, contains type I collagen.

MUSCLE AND CELL MOTILITY

Skeletal and cardiac (striated) muscle contract by sliding **myosin** and **actin** filaments past each other in a process facilitated by ATP. Myosin contains a motor that interacts with the actin filament and allows myosin to ratchet along the actin. The filaments are arranged in a banded pattern in individual sarcomeres, which act in series. Specialized invaginations of the plasma membrane **(T tubules)** spread the surface depolarization to the interior of the cell to release calcium from the **sarcoplasmic reticulum,** initiating contraction. **Troponin** and **tropomyosin** are specialized proteins that permit contraction of skeletal and cardiac muscle to be regulated by calcium. Skeletal muscle is a syncytium, while cardiac muscle consists of individual cells connected by intercalated disks. The organization of striated muscle is shown below:

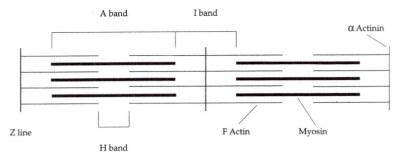

Sarcomere

Extrafusal muscle fibers generate the force of contraction while intrafusal fibers (both IA and II-type fibers (receptors) serve as sensory detectors signaling muscle location (proprioception) and the rate of contraction.

Smooth muscle contraction closely resembles the cell motility exhibited in other cell types. It also occurs through the action of actin and myosin, which are arranged in a lattice-like pattern. Troponin is *not* present in smooth muscle.

NERVOUS SYSTEM

Myelin, which insulates neuronal projections and permits rapid (saltatory) conduction, is produced by **oligodendroglia (oligodendrocytes)** in the central nervous system (CNS) and by **Schwann cells** in the **peripheral nervous system (PNS)**. **Microglia** are brain macrophages. **Astrocytes** have a complicated role in physical and metabolic support of neurons. Astrocytes **induce and maintain the blood-brain-barrier**, but they *do not* constitute the **barrier function** of the blood-brain barrier which is established by **endothelial tight junctions (zonula occludens)**. Neurons conduct electrochemical impulses and move neurotransmitters to their synaptic termini by **axoplasmic transport**. Transneuronal transmission is accomplished by calcium-regulated release of **synaptic vesicles**. Neurons also synapse with muscle cells. A typical contact between a myelinated neuron and skeletal muscle **(neuromuscular junction)** is shown below.

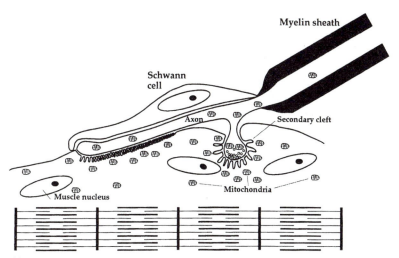

Neuromuscular junction. Axonal terminals (telodendria) rest in shallow depressions (primary clefts) on the surface of the striated muscle fiber. Secondary clefts increase the surface area for interaction with a neurotransmitter (acetylcholine). Muscle cell nuclei and mitochondria are abundant near the junction.

In the **cerebral** and **cerebellar** cortices, **gray matter** (cell bodies and immediately adjacent processes) is located peripherally and white matter centrally; this pattern is reversed in the **spinal cord.** Cerebellar cortex consists of **molecular, Purkinje,** and **granular** layers [**mnemonic: miles per gallon (MPG)**] with extensive arborization of the neuronal processes. The **cerebral cortex** consists of a homogenous layer I with multiple deeper layers of large **pyramidal** and other types of **neurons.** The number of layers varies, depending on the cortical region. Neuronal cell bodies **(perikarya)** are also localized in **ganglia** in the peripheral nervous system and **autonomic nervous system (ANS).**

CARDIOVASCULAR SYSTEM, BLOOD, AND BONE MARROW

Blood vessels are comprised of three layers or tunics: intima, media, and adventitia. In large arteries close to the heart, the *tunica media* contains high amounts of elastin to buffer the heart's pulsatile output. Smaller muscular arteries distribute blood to organs and capillary beds; their contractions are mediated by both the **sympathetic nervous system (SNS)** and by humoral factors. **Endothelial cells** lining the vascular lumen secrete **vasoactive substances** that regulate relaxation and contraction of the underlying smooth muscle. For example, **endothelin 1** is a **potent vasoconstrictor; nitric oxide** is **synthesized** from **L-arginine** and induces relaxation of the smooth muscle through a **cGMP**-dependent mechanism. **Prostacyclin,** also synthesized by endothelial cells, is a smooth muscle relaxant that functions through a **cAMP**-dependent mechanism. Prostacyclin **inhibits platelet adhesion** and **prevents intravascular clot formation.** Endothelial cells produce molecules that regulate fibrinolysis and thrombogenesis. Endothelial cell-derived factors are stored in intracellular granules and released into the blood stream upon stimulation. There are two contrasting factors, **fibrinolytic tissue-type plasminogen activator (tPA)** and **von Willebrand factor (vWF).** In contrast to tPA, vWF induces **coagulation and thrombus formation.** Endothelial cells also produce **tissue factor,** the only nonplasma protein in the clotting cascade, which initiates the common blood clotting pathway. **E-selectin** expression on endothelial cells modulates **extravasation** of **monocytes** and **neutrophils. Chemokines (chemoattractant cytokines)** induce expression of E-selectins on the endothelium under normal conditions and following inflammation. **Smooth muscle cells** undergo **hyperplasia** and **hypertrophy** in hypertension. The heart contains specialized cardiomyocytes that function as impulse-generating and conducting cells regulated by the ANS. The **heart** also functions as an **endocrine organ**, releasing **atrial natriuretic factor** [peptides (ANP or ANF)] in response to **increased plasma volume**. ANPs reduce plasma volume by (1) increasing urinary sodium (**natriuretic**) and water excretion (**diuretic**), (2) inhibiting **aldosterone** synthesis and **angiotensin II** production, and (3) inhibiting **vasopressin** release from the neurohypophysis.

Blood cells include **erythrocytes**, which are specialized for oxygen transport; **lymphocytes** that function in cellular and humoral immune responses; **neutrophils**, which are early responders to acute inflammation; **monocytes** that are the precursors of tissue macrophages; **eosinophils**, which respond to parasitic infection and release histaminases to counteract basophils and mast cells; and **basophils**, which contain histamine and heparin and assist mast cell function.

Bone marrow is the site of blood cell development in adults. The erythrocyte lineage includes the following stages: proerythroblasts → basophilic erythroblasts → polychromatophilic erythroblasts → orthochromatophilic erythrocytes. The white cell series includes myeloblasts → promyelocytes → myelocytes → metamyelocytes → mature granular leukocytes.

LYMPHOID SYSTEM AND CELLULAR IMMUNOLOGY

Functional cells include **B lymphocytes** (humoral immunity), **T lymphocytes** (cellular immunity), **macrophages** (phagocytic and one of several types of antigen-presenting cells), and **mast cells**.

Immunity and T and B cells

There are two types of immunity:

- **Innate immunity** is the first-line of defense and comprises basic mechanisms of host defense including **barriers** (e.g., skin, **zonula occludens/tight junctions**) and **phagocytic cells** such as **macrophages** and **neutrophils**. Innate immunity is *not* specific for particular pathogens or individuals of the species.
- **Adaptive immunity** is a response **to antigenic challenge** and possesses four essential characteristics which are *not* part of innate immunity:
  - **Specificity of response to antigen**
  - **Memory**
  - **Diversity**
  - **Recognition of self versus nonself**

Lymphocytes display the four attributes listed above. There are two types of lymphocytes: B cells and T cells. B cells are involved in humoral immunity. On first exposure to an antigen it recognizes on its surface, a naïve B cell proliferates to produce a memory B cell and a plasma cell that is the effector, synthesizing antibodies for release. T cells are unable to recognize antigen on their own. T cells require antigen-presenting cells (**macrophages, dendritic cells,** and **B cells**) to process antigen and bind it to membrane proteins known as **major histocompatibility molecules (MHC).** **Class I MHC** is found on virtually all cells of the body, while **Class II MHC** is specific for **antigen-presenting cells (APCs).** On first encounter with a specific antigen-MHC II complex, the T cell proliferates resulting in a memory T cell and an effector T cell. There are several sub-types of T cells:

- **T$_H$ cells,** which express the specific glycoprotein, CD4, are called CD4$^+$
- **T$_C$ cells,** which express the specific glycoprotein, CD8, are called CD8$^+$
- **T$_{reg}$ cells,** (suppressor T cells) are critical for maintenance of **immunological tolerance.**

The T$_H$ cell secretes cytokines (small protein or peptide intercellular communication molecules) that activate T$_C$ cells, B cells, and macrophages. Release of cytokines by **T$_H$ cells** induces **T$_C$ cells** to proliferate and differentiate into effector cells. In that case the effectors are **cytotoxic T lymphocytes (CTLs)** that recognize Class I MHC-antigen complex on the surface of altered self cells (e.g., cells of a foreign tissue graft or self cells infected with virus). CTLs recognize altered self-cells and form a conjugate with them; the target cell is killed by release of **perforins** (pore-forming proteins) and serine proteases **(granzymes)** leading to **apoptosis** of the target.

T$_H$ cells are regulated by APCs that internalize antigen and then process it through the secretory pathway to a membrane-bound MHC II-antigen complex. The T$_H$ cell is activated by a co-stimulatory signal from the APC. Cytokines from T$_H$ cells are required for B cells to proliferate and differentiate into a memory B cell and an antibody-producing plasma cell. Two of the key cytokines involved in the interaction of those cells are IL-1 produced by activated macrophages and IL-2 that regulates T cell, but also B cell proliferation. Another critical cytokine is **interferon-gamma (IFN-γ)** that activates macrophages and is secreted by activated T$_H$ cells. There are two profiles of cytokines produced by T$_H$ cells:

- T_H1 response is primarily directed toward macrophages and T cells and the support of the inflammatory response.
- T_H2 response is primarily directed toward B cells and therefore antibody responses.

T_{reg} cells are CD4$^+$, express CD25 and produce IL-10 and TGF-beta, lymphokines that are both strong immunosuppressants inhibiting T_H1 and T_H2 cells.

NK cells are not T cells, but kill cellular targets such as tumor cells in a nonspecific manner.

Organs

Lymphoid organs may be either primary (bone marrow and thymus) or secondary (lymph nodes and dispersed lymphatic nodules, spleen, and tonsils). The B lymphocytes are educated in the bone marrow [differentiation of antigen-binding receptors (antibodies)] and are seeded to specific B cell regions of the secondary lymphoid organs, while T lymphocytes are educated in the thymus [differentiation of T cell receptors (TcR)] and are seeded to T cell-dependent regions of the secondary lymphoid organs.

The thymus is recognized by lobulation, separate cortex and medulla in each lobule, the absence of germinal centers, and the presence of Hassall's corpuscles. The lymph nodes, which filter lymph and blood, are characterized by a central medulla consisting of cords with many plasma cells and a cortex containing primary and secondary follicles. The spleen, which filters blood, is characterized by red and white pulp. The tonsils are characterized by crypts with an epithelial lining on one side. That lining is stratified squamous epithelium in palatine tonsils and pseudostratified epithelium on pharyngeal tonsils.

RESPIRATORY SYSTEM

The respiratory epithelium consists of conducting pathways (nasal cavities, naso- and oropharynx, larynx, trachea, bronchi, and bronchioles) and respiratory portions (respiratory bronchioles and alveoli). The nasal epithelium includes a region of specialized olfactory receptors. Ciliated cells appear in all portions of the respiratory system except the respiratory epithelium and move mucus and particulates toward the oropharynx (mucociliary escalator). Gas exchange in the lungs takes place across a minimal barrier consisting of the capillary endothelium, a joint basal lamina, and an exceedingly thin alveolar epithelium consisting primarily of type I pneumocytes. **Type II pneumocytes** are responsible for the secretion of surfactant, a primarily lipid substance that facilitates respiration by reducing alveolar surface tension. The type II pneumocyte is recognizable at the EM level by the presence **lamellar bodies** that contain surfactant comprised primarily of **lecithin (Dipalmitoylphosphatidylcholine, DPPC)** as well as some cholesterol and sphingomyelin. Although surfactant is produced beginning at about the 28th week, premature babies born before 30 weeks are likely to suffer from **respiratory distress syndrome (RDS)** because of the absence of surfactant. There are a variety of treatments for RDS including the administration of artificial surfactant and ventilation for the premature infant. In **cystic fibrosis, mutations in the cystic fibrosis transmembrane conductance regulator (CFTR) result in defective Cl⁻ transport and increased Na⁺ absorption.** HCO_3^- transport through the CFTR is also defective. The result is thick, more viscous (less watery) mucus in the airways that promotes bacterial infections and reduces the effectiveness of the mucociliary escalator.

INTEGUMENTARY SYSTEM

The epidermis of thick skin consists of five layers of cells **(keratinocytes)**: *stratum basale* (proliferative layer), *stratum spinosum* (characterized by tonofibrils and associated desmosomes), *stratum granulosum* (characterized by keratohyalin granules), *stratum lucidum* (a translucent layer *not* obvious in thin skin), and *stratum corneum* (characterized by dead and dying cells with compacted keratin). Specialized structures of the skin include hair follicles (found only in thin skin), nails, and sweat glands and ducts. Nonkeratinocyte epidermal cells include **melanocytes** (derived from **neural crest**), **Langerhans cells** (antigen-presenting cells derived from monocytes), and **Merkel cells** (sensory mechanoreceptors). Various sensory receptors and extensive capillary networks are found in the underlying dermis. There are skin diseases with a cell biological etiology. Psoriasis is a disease characterized by dermal and epidermal infiltration of inflammatory cells. Those cells release cytokines, which cause hyperplasia of the epidermis. Proliferation occurs throughout the epidermis and *is no* longer restricted to the basal layer and there is a thickening of the stratum corneum with nucleated keratinocytes present. **Pemphigus** is an autoimmune disease in which **autoantibodies** are produced to the **desmogleins**, members of the cadherin family. The desmosomes break apart resulting in blistering of the skin. The basal layer remains intact and attached to the basal lamina because the hemidesmosomes *do not* contain cadherins. In contrast, **bullous pemphigoid** is a disease in which the antigen recognized by the autoantibodies is the **BP (bullous pemphigoid) antigen** involved in the linkage of the basal layer to the basal lamina. Bullous pemphigoid is also a blistering disease, but the blistering occurs at the epidermal-dermal junction.

GASTROINTESTINAL TRACT AND GLANDS

The epithelium of the gastrointestinal (GI) tract is simple and columnar throughout, except for the stratified squamous epithelia in regions of maximal friction (esophagus and anus). The **stomach** is a grinding organ with glands in the fundus and body that produce mucus (surface and neck cells), pepsinogen (chief cells), and acid and intrinsic factor (parietal cells). Intrinsic factor binds to vitamin B_{12} and is required for uptake of that vitamin from the intestine. The parietal cell functions in a similar fashion to the osteoclast in using carbonic anhydrase to produce protons that are pumped into the **intracellular canaliculi,** which are lined by **microvilli** in the **active parietal cell.** In the **inactive parietal cell, the proton pumps are sequestered in tubulovesicles in the cytosol.**

The **small intestine** is an absorptive organ with folds at several levels (**plicae, villi,** and **microvilli**) that increase surface area for more efficient absorption. The microvilli also contain specific enzymes for the breakdown of **sugars (disaccharidases), lipids (lipases),** and **peptides (peptidases).** The major digestive processes in the small intestine occur through the action of the **pancreatic juice,** which contains **trypsinogen, chymotrypsinogen, procarboxypeptidases, amylase, lipase,** and other enzymes. **Trypsinogen** is activated by **enterokinase** found on the microvilli. Lipids are broken down to **triglycerides** in the small intestinal lumen which are subsequently degraded to **glycerol, fatty acids,** and **monoglycerides** that are transported into the enterocyte. Once in the cytosol of the enterocyte, the **SER** resynthesizes the **triglycerides,** which are coupled with protein to form **chylomicra.** The chylomicra are exocytosed into the **lacteals** and travel to the cisterna chyli and through the thoracic duct to the venous system. They return to the liver through the arterial system (hepatic artery). In the liver the lipid processing is similar, but reversed to form **very low density lipoprotein (VLDL)** from chylomicra. Other digested materials travel through the **hepatic portal vein** to the liver where hepatocytes process the digested nutrients. Cell types in the small intestine include **enterocytes (absorption), Paneth cells (production of lysozyme, defensins, and cryptidins),** goblet cells (mucus), and enteroendocrine cells (secretion of peptide hormones). All of those cells originate from a single **stem cell in the crypt.** New cells are born in the crypt, move up the villus, die by **apoptosis,** and are sloughed off at the tip. The primary function of the **colon,** which appears histologically as **crypts with prominent goblet cells** and *no* villi, is water resorption.

The major salivary glands **(parotid, submandibular,** and **sublingual)** are exocrine glands that secrete **amylase** and mucus, primarily **regulated by the autonomic nervous system.** In contrast, the **pancreas** has both **exocrine (acinar cells)** and **endocrine (islet cells)** components that synthesize pancreatic juice and blood sugar–regulating hormones, respectively. The exocrine pancreas is primarily regulated by the hormones cholecystokinin (CCK) and secretin, which primarily regulate acinar and ductal secretion, respectively.

The **liver** is also a dual-function gland whose exocrine product is **bile,** synthesized by hepatocytes, and transported by a duct system to the gallbladder for storage and concentration. Bile **emulsifies lipids** for more efficient enzymatic access. The endocrine products include **glucose** and **major blood proteins (albumin, fibrinogen, coagulation proteins).** The liver subserves numerous other functions including synthesis of cholesterol and **detoxification of lipid-soluble drugs,** such as **phenobarbital** by the **SER** (using the **P450 enzyme system). Alcohol detoxification** is one of the major processes carried out in the hepatocyte. Alcohol detoxification involves alcohol dehydrogenase **(ADH), MEOS** (microsomal ethanol oxidation system, P450 enzymes in the SER), and catalase in peroxisomes. The primary metabolic pathway is ADH. At higher alcohol levels the MEOS and even catalase systems are activated. The **bile canaliculus** is defined as **apical,** the **junctional complexes** as **lateral,** and the blood surface with the **space of Disse** and **hepatic sinusoids** is considered **basal.** The sinusoids are lined by **hepatic stellate cells,** endothelial cells, and **Kupffer cells.** The **hepatic stellate cells** are affected following chronic alcohol toxicity and are converted into **myofibroblasts** during the onset of **cirrhosis.** Those cells synthesize large quantities of collagen and are responsible for the fibrotic changes observed in cirrhosis. The **Kupffer cells** are the **antigen-presenting cells** of the liver and are derived from monocytes. Hepatocytes are arranged in interlocking cords and plates so there are several ways of analyzing the histological organization of the liver. The **classic lobule** emphasizes the **endocrine** function of the liver; the **portal lobule** emphasizes the **exocrine** function of the liver, and the **liver acinus** focuses on actual **blood supply** and regeneration.

ENDOCRINE GLANDS

The **pituitary (hypophysis)** is formed from two embryonic sources. The **adenohypophysis** is derived from the **oral ectoderm** of Rathke's pouch and is regulated through a **hypophyseal portal system** carrying factors that stimulate or inhibit secretion. The **anterior pituitary** contains **acidophils,** which produce **prolactin** and **growth hormone (GH),** and **basophils** that produce **luteinizing hormone (LH), follicle-stimulating hormone (FSH), thyroid-stimulating hormone (TSH), adrenocorticotropic hormone (ACTH),** and **melanocyte-stimulating hormone (MSH).** The **neurohypophysis** is derived from the floor of the diencephalon and consists of astrocyte-like glial cells **(pituicytes)** and expanded terminals of nerve fibers originating in the hypothalamus. The neurohypophysis contains the hormones **vasopressin** and **oxytocin,** which are synthesized primarily in the **supraoptic** and **paraventricular** nuclei respectively.

The **adrenal gland** consists of two parts. The **adrenal cortex,** derived from **intermediate mesoderm,** and covered by a connective tissue capsule, consists of three zones: the *zona glomerulosa* produces **aldosterone** (a mineralocorticoid) and is regulated primarily by **angiotensin II;** the *zona fasciculata* and *zona reticularis* produce glucocorticoids (e.g., cortisol) and weak androgens and are regulated primarily by **ACTH.** The **adrenal medulla,** derived from the **neural crest,** synthesizes **epinephrine** and **norepinephrine** (see figure on the following page). Most of the blood that reaches the adrenal medulla has passed through the adrenal cortex and contains glucocorticoids that regulate the norepinephrine/epinephrine balance in the adrenal medulla through regulation of phenylethanolamine-N-methyl-transferase. The **fetal adrenal cortex** functions to produce **dehydroepiadrosterone,** an androgen that is transported to the placenta where it serves as a precursor of estrogen.

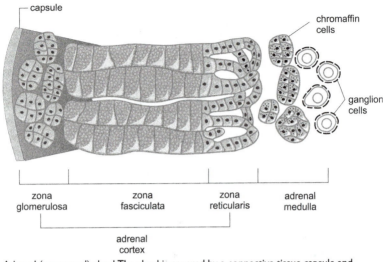

Adrenal (suprarenal) gland. The gland is covered by a connective tissue capsule and divided into a cortex containing steroid-producing cells with prominent lipid droplets and a medulla containing chromaffin cells that secrete catecholamines and neuropeptides.

There are a number of adrenal hormonal disorders. **Congenital viriliz-ing adrenal hyperplasia** results from the deficiency of an enzyme required for cortisol production. The result is elevated ACTH and secretion of dehy-droepiandrosterone from the fetal cortex causing masculinization (virilizing) of the female genitalia. The fetal adrenal cortex is a key component of the fetal-placental unit. **Hypercortisolism** or **Cushing's syndrome** is five times more common in women than men. Cushing's syndrome may be caused by a tumor in the corticotrophs of the anterior pituitary (Cushing's disease), an adrenal adenoma, or administration of exogenous glucocorticoids. **Addi-son's disease** is **primary chronic adrenal insufficiency** and is most often caused by **autoimmune mechanisms** leading to atrophy of the adrenal cor-tex. Elevated ACTH levels lead to hyperpigmentation especially in exposed areas of the skin or at pressure points such as the elbows and knuckles.

The **thyroid gland** is characterized by an extracellular hormone pre-cursor (iodinated thyroglobulin) stored in its follicles. The follicular cells endocytose the storage product to form the thyroid hormones [triiodothy-ronine (T_3) and thyroxine (T_4)]. Scattered between the follicular cells are

"C" cells (parafollicular cells), which secrete **calcitonin,** a hormone that reduces blood calcium levels. Diseases of the thyroid include **Hashimoto's thyroiditis,** an autoimmune disease, in which autoantibodies to thyroglobulin and thyroid peroxidase (antimicrosomal antibodies) are produced. Binding of antibodies to those molecules interferes with their uptake and function respectively. Infiltrating T cells and autoantibodies destroy the **thyroid follicular cells** resulting in **hypothyroidism.** In Hashimoto's thyroiditis autoantibodies are also produced to the **thyroid-stimulating hormone (TSH) receptor.** In that case, the autoantibody recognizes an epitope which results in **blocking the activity of TSH.** In contrast, in **Graves' disease** autoantibodies are produced to the **TSH receptor,** but they are **long-acting thyroid stimulating (LATS) antibodies.** The result is unregulated activation of the receptor and overproduction of thyroid hormones **(hyperthyroidism).**

The **parathyroid gland** consists primarily of chief cells that secrete **parathyroid hormone (PTH)** that increases blood calcium levels by stimulating ruffled border activity in osteoclasts and decreasing renal Ca^{++} excretion and increasing intestinal absorption.

The pineal gland contains pinealocytes that secrete melatonin and is innervated by postganglionic sympathetic fibers. Darkness stimulates the production of melatonin in the pineal.

The **pancreas** is both an exocrine and endocrine gland. Endocrine cells of the pancreatic islets secrete primarily **insulin** and **glucagon,** hormones that **regulate blood sugar by lowering and increasing gluocse respectively.** Blood entering the islets bypasses the peripherally located glucagon-secreting cells to reach the more centrally-located insulin-producing **beta cells.** Blood leaving the beta cells contains insulin that influences glucagon secretion from the **alpha cells.** Blood leaving the islets travels to the surrounding exocrine pancreas and influences secretion from the acini. In **type I diabetes mellitus** formerly known as insulin-dependent diabetes mellitus (IDDM) an autoimmune reaction results in **destruction of beta cells** and the absence of insulin. Type II diabetes, formerly known as non-insulin-dependent diabetes, is the most common form of diabetes mellitus. Type II diabetes can occur at any age and is reaching epidemic proportions in the United States. **Type II diabetes** begins with **insulin resistance,** a condition in which adipocytes, muscle cells, and hepatocytes *cannot* efficiently use insulin because of a decrease in insulin receptors or defective glucose transporter function. The beta cells are overworked and eventually lose their ability to secrete enough insulin in response to meals. Individuals who are overweight and inactive have an increased chance of developing type II diabetes. Scattered through several organ systems (e.g., digestive and respiratory systems) are **enteroendocrine cells,** which synthesize peptide hormones for local regulation.

URINARY SYSTEM

The **filtration apparatus** of the renal glomeruli consists of an expanded basement membrane and slit pore associated with **podocytes.** Epithelial cells of the **proximal tubule** are specialized for absorption and ion transport. They remove most of the **sodium** and **water** from urine, as well as virtually all of the amino acids, proteins, and glucose. The **brush border** of the proximal tubule cells contains proteases. The cells of the **distal tubule,** under the influence of **aldosterone, resorb sodium and acidify the urine.** Specialized cells of the distal tubule (the **macula densa**) monitor ion levels in the urine and stimulate the **juxtaglomerular (JG) cells** of the **afferent arteriole** to secrete **renin,** an enzyme that cleaves **angiotensinogen** to a precursor of **angiotensin II.** **Collecting ducts** contain light and dark (intercalated) cells; they are sensitive to **antidiuretic hormone (ADH)** and are the **final mechanism for concentrating urine.** Transitional epithelium (allowing for stretch) is found lining the calyces, renal pelvis, ureters, and urinary bladder.

MALE REPRODUCTIVE SYSTEM

The **testes** produce **sperm** and **testosterone** under the influence of **luteinizing hormone (LH)** and follicle-stimulating hormone **(FSH),** secreted by **gonadotrophs** of the **anterior pituitary.** The testicular epithelium contains **Sertoli cells** and precursors of sperm. **Spermatogenesis** involves the following lineage: **spermatogonia (germ cells)** → (**spermatocytogenesis**) → **primary spermatocytes** → **secondary spermatocytes** → (**completion of meiosis**) → **spermatids (spermiogenesis)** → **mature sperm.** **Sertoli cells** perform several functions: (1) **maintenance of the blood-testis barrier,** (2) **phagocytosis,** and (3) **secretion of androgen-binding protein** and **inhibin,** as well as **Müllerian inhibiting hormone** in the fetus.

The **epididymis,** like most of the male duct system, is lined by a pseudostratified epithelium characterized by modified microvilli (**stereocilia**).

The **seminal vesicles** produce **fructose** and other molecules that **activate spermatozoa.** The **prostate** is a **fibromuscular** organ that produces the **enzymes** responsible for the liquefaction of the **ejaculate.** Virtually all males over 70 show some form of **prostatic hypertrophy. Prostatic malignancies are the second most common form of cancer in males.**

FEMALE REPRODUCTIVE SYSTEM

The ovaries produce ova, **estrogen,** and **progesterone** under the influence of **LH** and **FSH.** **Oocyte (germ cell)** maturation involves several stages of **follicular development (granulosa cells plus the oocyte):** primordial follicle → primary follicle → secondary follicle → mature, or Graafian, follicle. In the **secondary follicle,** the **stroma differentiates into a theca.** The *theca interna* synthesizes **androgens,** which are converted into **estradiol** by **granulosa cells.** After **ovulation,** these **thecal cells** form the *theca lutein;* the **granulosa cells** become the *granulosa lutein,* which produces **progesterone** (see figure below). **Human chorionic gonadotropin (hCG)** in the placenta maintains the **corpus luteum of pregnancy.**

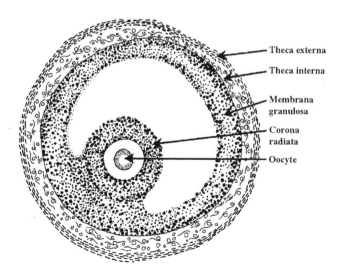

Theca externa
Theca interna
Membrana granulosa
Corona radiata
Oocyte

The **uterine endometrium** goes through a monthly cycle during which the **functionalis** is lost and replaced from the **basalis**. The **menstrual phase** occupies the first four days of the cycle (in the absence of hCG), followed by the **proliferative phase** under the influence of FSH (days 5 to 14) and then the **secretory phase** under the influence of LH (days 15 to 28). During this phase, endometrial cells accumulate glycogen preliminary to the synthesis and secretion of glycoproteins.

The **vaginal epithelium** is made up of stratified squamous cells and varies with maturity, phase of the menstrual cycle, pregnancy, and cancer (detected by vaginal Pap smear).

When fertilization and implantation occur, the placenta, consisting of the **chorion (fetal part)** and **decidua basalis (maternal part)**, is established for O_2/CO_2 exchange, as well as its endocrine role (e.g., conversion of androgens to estradiol, placental lactogen secretion). During parturition, oxytocin secreted by the neurohypophysis stimulates the contraction of uterine smooth muscle.

The **breast (mammary gland)** is a resting alveolar gland except during pregnancy, when the **lactiferous ducts** proliferate and **milk** production is initiated. Milk synthesis and ejection are under the influence of **prolactin** and **oxytocin**.

EYE

The photosensitive layer of the retina is derived from the inner layer of the **optic cup** and contains the **rod** and **cone** cells involved in visual signal transduction. **Rhodopsin** is a visual pigment found within lamellar disks of the outer segment of the rod cell. Rhodopsin consists of **retinal** and **opsin**; photons induce an isomeric change in retinal, leading to dissociation of the retinal/opsin complex. The resulting decrease in the intracellular second messenger, guanosine 3'5'-cyclic monophosphate (**cGMP**), directs closure of membrane sodium channels and leads to **hyperpolarization** of the photoreceptor cell. This signal is transmitted to interneurons within the retina and finally to ganglion cells. The fovea defines the center of the retina, and is the point of sharpest visual acuity. The **fovea** contains all cones and is directed toward whatever object you wish to see or read, for example, these PreTest words at this very moment.

The **lens** arises from **surface ectoderm** during development. Production of lens fibers (elongated, protein-filled cells) continues throughout life without replacement. Increased opacity of the lens (**cataract**) may be

caused by congenital factors, excess ultraviolet (UV) radiation, or high glucose levels.
The **choroid** and **sclera** are the supportive, protective coats of the eye.
The **aqueous humor,** produced by processes of the ciliary body, flows between the lens and iris to the anterior chamber of the eye toward the **iridocorneal angle,** where it is drained into the **canal of Schlemm.** Blockage of the canal of Schlemm or associated structures leads to **increased intraocular pressure** and **glaucoma.**

EAR

The ear functions in two separate but related signal transduction systems, **audition** and **equilibrium.** The **external ear,** largely formed from the **first two branchial arches,** funnels sound to the **tympanic membrane.** The **middle ear** is made up of the **malleus, incus, and stapes** formed from the **first two arch cartilages.** The **internal ear** consists of a **membranous** and a **bony labyrinth** filled with **endolymph** and **perilymph,** respectively. The **saccule (ventral)** and **utricle (dorsal),** parts of the membranous labyrinth, form from the **otic vesicle** (an ectodermal invagination). The **cochlea** contains three spaces, the *scala vestibuli, scala media* (**cochlear duct,** which extends from the **saccule**), and *scala tympani.* The **semicircular canals** (which extend from the **utricle**) contain the *cristae ampulares,* made up of **cupulae** with **hair cells** embedded in a gelatinous matrix that respond to **changes in direction** and **rate of angular acceleration.** The hair cells are located within the **organ of Corti** and respond to **different frequencies.** In the **saccule** and **utricle,** the **maculae,** along with **stereocilia, kinocilia,** and **otoconia** (crystals of protein and calcium carbonate), detect **changes in position** with reference to gravity.

High-Yield Facts

Neural Pathways

ASCENDING PATHWAYS

Cells in the spinal cord receive inputs from ipsilateral structures. Pathways to the thalamus cross to terminate on the contralateral side.

The major ascending pathways are the dorsal (posterior) columns and the anterolateral system.

Pain, Temperature, and Tactile
- Simple receptors, unmyelinated, or poorly myelinated fibers.
- Enter via dorsal root and may ascend or descend a few segments.
- Secondary fibers cross the midline in the ventral commissure and ascend in ventral and lateral funiculi (ventral and lateral spinothalamic tracts).
- Terminate in ventral posterior lateral nucleus of thalamus.
- Tertiary fibers project via the internal capsule to terminate in the postcentral gyrus.
- Injury to the spinothalamic tracts results in loss of pain and temperature sensation on the opposite side of the body.
- Syringomyelia interrupts pain and temperature fibers crossing in the ventral white commissure and thus results in bilateral sensory deficit.

Proprioception, Tactile Discrimination, and Stereognosis
- Primary fibers arising from more complicated receptors are generally well myelinated.
- Afferents enter the spinal cord via the dorsal root and ascend in the dorsal funiculus. The dorsal funiculus divides into a medial fasciculus gracilis (sacral, lumbar, and lower thoracic inputs) and a lateral fasciculus cuneatus (upper thoracic and cervical inputs). Both fasciculi terminate in corresponding nuclei in the medulla.
- Secondary fibers from the nucleus gracilis and nucleus cuneatus cross the midline and ascend in the medial lemniscus to terminate in the ventral posterior lateral nucleus of the thalamus.
- Tertiary fibers terminate in the postcentral gyrus.
- Muscle spindle information is sent to the cerebellum via two major pathways. The dorsal spinocerebellar tract originates from Clarke's

nucleus in the thoracic cord and enters the cerebellum via the inferior cerebellar peduncle. The ventral spinocerebellar tract originates from spinal cord gray matter and enters the cerebellum via the superior cerebellar peduncle.

- Interruption of primary fibers in the dorsal funiculus will cause loss of proprioception, and so forth, on the same side of the body as the lesion.
- Interruption of secondary fibers in the medial lemniscus will give rise to contralateral deficits.
- Tabes dorsalis and pernicious anemia attack the dorsal funiculi.

Trigeminal Pathways
- Primary trigeminal fibers enter at the level of the pons.
- Primary afferents of the descending root terminate in the spinal trigeminal nucleus.
- Secondary fibers ascend through the medulla and pons as the trigeminal lemniscus to terminate in the ventral posterior medial (VPM) nucleus of the thalamus.
- The ascending root primary tactile afferents terminate in the main sensory nucleus of CN V.
- Secondary fibers ascend in the trigeminal lemniscus to the VPM.
- The cell bodies of the primary proprioceptive afferents from the muscles of mastication are located in mesencephalic nucleus of V, and thus are "like" dorsal root ganglion cells embedded in the brain. They project to the motor nucleus of V for a monosynaptic jaw jerk reflex.
- Lesion of the descending root of V and the adjacent lateral spinothalamic tract on one side of the medulla will result in pain and temperature deficits on the contralateral side of the body and the ipsilateral side of the head.

Vestibular Pathways
- Primary afferents terminate in the vestibular nuclei and in the cerebellum on the same side.
- Secondary fibers ascend or descend in the medial longitudinal fasciculus or the ventral funiculus of the spinal cord.
- Unilateral lesions of the vestibular system result in movement of the head, body, and eyes (nystagmus) to the affected (ipsilateral) side. Symptoms include vertigo, nausea, and a tendency to fall to the affected side.

Visceral Afferents

- Primary general visceral afferents have cell bodies in the dorsal root ganglia and terminate in the dorsal horn. Ascending secondary neurons make abundant reflex connections with autonomic and somatic pathways and terminate in the reticular formation and intralaminar thalamic nuclei.
- Central processes of primary general visceral afferents associated with cranial nerves VII, IX, and X enter the solitary fasciculus and terminate in the nucleus of the solitary tract. Secondary fibers make reflex connections with visceral motor nuclei. Taste is represented in the thalamus in a region medial to the VPM nucleus.

DESCENDING (MOTOR) PATHWAYS

- In the brain, the cell bodies of general somatic efferent neurons are located in columns ventral to the cerebral aqueduct and fourth ventricle and ventrolateral to the central canal. Special visceral efferents (associated with branchial archderived muscle) are located lateral and ventral to the general somatic efferents. In the spinal cord, they originate in the ventral horn.
- These are lower motor neurons, or the "final common pathway." Total, or flaccid, paralysis results from destruction of peripheral nerves or motor nuclei. Destruction of upper motor neurons (from higher centers) results in spastic paralysis: initally hyporeflexia and later hyperreflexia.

Cerebellar Pathways

- The dentate nucleus receives fibers from the Purkinje neurons of the cerebellum and projects via the superior peduncle to the reticular formation (descending limb) and to the basal ganglia/thalamus-motor cortex (ascending limb).
- The cerebellum is involved with coordination of fine movements.
- Lesions to the cerebellum or superior peduncle result in ataxia, hypotonia, hyporeflexia, and/or intention tremor on the same side as the lesion.

CORTICOSPINAL (PYRAMIDAL) PATHWAYS

- Fibers arise from pyramidal neurons in layer 5 of the precentral gyrus and premotor areas and descend through the internal capsule and basis pedunculi, cross at the spinomedullary junction and form the lateral corticospinal tract in the lateral funiculus of the spinal cord. They terminate on lower motor neurons in the ventral horn or on interneurons.
- Most muscles are represented in the contralateral motor cortex. However, some (such as the muscles of the upper face and the muscles of mastication and muscles of the larynx) are represented bilaterally.

- With the noted bilateral exceptions, lesion of the pyramidal tract above the decussation results in spastic paralysis, loss of fine movements, and hyperreflexia on the contralateral side.
- Lesion of the corticospinal tract in the cord results in ipsilateral deficits.

The Extrapyramidal (Basal Ganglia) System

- The basal ganglia (caudate, putamen, globus pallidus) and associated nuclei (e.g., substantia nigra) do not project directly to medullary or spinal lower motor neurons, but to the motor cortex.
- The system controls coarse, stereotyped movements. Lesions result in altered muscle tone (usually rigidity), paucity of movement, and the appearance of rhythmic tremors and writhing or jerky movements.

Reticular Pathways

- Nuclei of the reticular system send ascending projections to the hypothalamus and thalamus as well as descending projections to the motor nuclei of cranial nerves, and the intermediate gray of the spinal cord.
- The reticular formation has reciprocal connections with most other areas of the CNS and produces both faciliatory and inhibitory effects on motor systems, receptors, and sensory conduction pathways.

High-Yield Facts

Anatomy

UPPER EXTREMITY

- **Axillary nerve injury** often results from shoulder joint dislocation or fractures at the surgical neck of the humerus. The injury causes deltoid muscle paralysis and skin anesthesia over the lateral deltoid region. Shoulder contour may be lost with time as the deltoid atrophies. Arm abduction is lost when the arm is abducted beyond the first 15 degrees.

- **Midhumeral fracture** may involve the deep brachial artery and the radial nerve as they wind about the posterior aspect of the humerus. Arterial injury produces ischemic contracture; nerve injury paralyzes the wrist extensors and extrinsic extensors of the hand ("wrist-drop").

- Except on the ulnar side (flexor carpi ulnaris and 4–5 flexor digitorum profundus), the **forearm flexor compartment** is innervated by the median nerve.

- **Scaphoid fracture** is the most common hand bone break because it transmits forces from the abducted hand directly to the radius. Because the blood supply enters distally, the **proximal portion** of the scaphoid is especially **prone to avascular necrosis.**

- **Lunate dislocation** is most common in falls on the out-stretched hand, compressing the median nerve within the carpal tunnel and producing carpal tunnel syndrome.

- **Extension** of the medial four digits at the **metacarpophalangeal joints** and **interphalangeal joints** is accomplished by the extensor digitorum in the forearm, innervated by the radial nerve. In addition, extension of the inter-phalangeal joints of the medial four digits is carried out by the lumbricals, which are innervated by both the median nerve (lumbricals 1–2 on the lateral side) and ulnar nerve (lumbricals 3–4 on the medial side). Lumbricals also flex the metacarpophalangeal joints of the medial four digits.

- **Proximal phalangeal flexion** at the metacarpophalangeal joint is by: (a) the interossei (ulnar nerve) and lumbricals muscles; (b) the flexor digitorum superficialis (median nerve) muscle; (c) the flexor digitorum profundus (medial and ulnar nerves) muscles. **Middle phalangeal flexion** at the proximal interphalangeal joint is by (b) and (c). **Distal phalangeal flexion** at the distal interphalangeal joint is by (c).

- **Digital abduction** is a function of the dorsal interossei ("DAB"—dorsal abduction); digital adduction is a function of palmar interossei ("PAD"—palmar adduct).
- The **ulnar artery** is the principal supply to the superficial palmar arch in the hand.
- **Lymphatic drainage** from the palmar hand and digits is toward the dorsal subcutaneous space of the hand, explaining the extreme swelling of this region that accompanies infections of the digits or volar surface.
- **Radial sensory function** is tested in the web space of the thumb; **ulnar sensory function** is tested along the fifth digit. The **digital branches** of the median and ulnar nerves lie along the sides of the fingers where they may be anesthetized (see figure below).

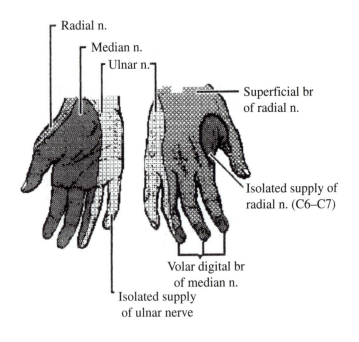

NERVE FUNCTION, TESTS, AND DYSFUNCTION

Nerve	Muscle Group	Reflex Test	Sign or Functional Deficit
Long thoracic	Serratus anterior		Wing scapula
Suprascapular	Supraspinatus, infraspinatus		Difficulty initiating arm abduction
Axillary	Deltoid		Inability to fully abduct arm
Radial	Extensors of forearm, wrist, proximal phalanges, and thumb	Triceps and wrist extension reflexes	Loss of arm extension; loss of forearm extension, supination, abduction; loss of wrist extension (**wrist-drop**); loss of proximal phalangeal extension and thumb extension
Musculocutaneous	Flexors of arm, forearm	Biceps reflex	Weak arm flexion, weak forearm flexion, weak forearm supination
Median	Wrist and hand flexors	Wrist flexion reflex	Paralysis of flexor, pronator, and thenar muscles; inability to fully flex the index and middle fingers (**sign of benediction**)
Ulnar	Wrist and hand flexors, phalangeal extensors		Inability to flex the 4th and 5th fingers- (**clawhand**); loss of thumb adduction

BACK

- **Fracture of the dens** of the axis with posterior dislocation may crush the spinal cord at the level of the first cervical vertebra with terminal paralysis of respiratory musculature.
- The **cruciform ligament** is the principal structure preventing subluxation at the atlantoaxial joint because the articular surfaces between the axis and atlas are nearly horizontal and there is no intervertebral disk.
- **Herniation** usually occurs in the L4/L5 or L5/S1 **intervertebral disks** because of the pronounced lumbar curvature and the considerable body mass superior to this region.

- The **anterior** and **posterior longitudinal ligaments** reinforce the underlying annulus fibrosus but do not meet posterolaterally, resulting in a weak area predisposed to intervertebral disk herniation.
- **Lumbar puncture** and intrathecal anesthesia should be introduced below the third lumbar vertebra as the spinal cord usually terminates between the first and second lumbar vertebrae.
- **Posterolateral disk prolapse** impinges on the spinal nerve of the next lower vertebral level, causing symptoms associated with the dermatomic and myotomal distributions of that nerve.

HERNIATED DISK INVOLVEMENT, SIGNS, AND REFLEX TEST

Hernia	Involvement	Signs	Reflex Test
C3–C4	C4 (Phrenic, C3–C5)	Weak diaphramatic respiration	
C4–C5	C5 (Suprascapular, C4–C6)	Weak arm abduction	
C5–C6	C6 (Musculocutaneous, C5–C6)	Weak forearm flexion	Biceps
C6–C7	C7 (Radial, C6–C8)	Weak forearm extension	Triceps
C7–C8	C8 (Ulnar, C7–T1)	Weak thumb adduction	
L1–L2	L2 (Genitofemoral, L1–L2)	Weak hip flexion	Cremaster
L2–L3	L3 (Obturator, L2–L4)	Weak hip adduction	
L3–L4	L4 (Femoral, L1–L4)	Weak leg extension	Knee jerk
L4–L5	L5 (Fibular, L4–S1)	Weak dorsiflexion	
L5–S1	S1 (Tibial, L5–S2)	Weak plantar flexion	Ankle jerk

LOWER EXTREMITY

NEUROVASCULAR CONTENTS OF THE BUTTOCK

Quadrant	Contents	Symptoms
Upper lateral	No major vessels or nerves; A preferred location for intramuscular injection	
Upper medial	Superior gluteal neurovascular bundle	Abductor lurch
Lower lateral	Inferior gluteal neurovascular bundle	Difficulty climbing stairs or rising from a chair
Lower medial	Sciatic nerve	Foot-drop

- **Intracapsular fractures** of the femoral neck or hip dislocations tear the retinacular arteries that supply the proximal fragment; avascular necrosis may result.

- The **femoral triangle** is bounded by the inguinal ligament, the sartorius muscle, and the adductor longus muscle. A **femoral pulse** is palpable high within the femoral triangle just inferior to the inguinal ligament. The femoral vein, lying just medial to the femoral pulse, is a preferred site for insertion of venous lines.

- The **anterior cruciate ligament** is a key stabilizer of the knee joint, preventing posterior movement of the femur on the tibial plateau.

- The **medial meniscus**, being more mobile and attached to the medial collateral ligament, is most likely to be injured. Twisting movements that combine lateral displacement with lateral rotation pull the medial meniscus toward the center of the joint where it may be trapped and crushed by the medial femoral condyle.

- The **adductor canal**, the location of popliteal aneurysms, contains the femoral artery, femoral vein, and saphenous nerve.

- The **deep fibular nerve** innervates the muscles of the anterior compartment (dorsiflexors of the foot and pedal digits). The **superficial fibular nerve** innervates the lateral crural compartment (plantar flexors and everters of the foot). The **tibial nerve** innervates the posterior crural muscles, which plantarflex and invert the foot.

- The **posterior tibial artery** descends posteriorly to the medial malleolus where the **posterior tibial pulse** is normally palpable.

- **Inversion sprains,** the most common ankle injury, involve the **lateral collateral ligaments.**

- The **plantar calcaneonavicular (spring) ligament** supports the head of the talus and thereby maintains the longitudinal plantar arch. Laxity of this ligament results in fallen arches or "**flat feet.**"

- **Sensory distribution of the anterior leg:** the web space between the first and second toes is specific for the fibular nerve (L5) (see following figure).

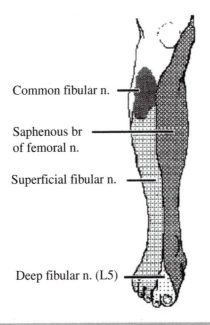

Common fibular n.

Saphenous br
of femoral n.

Superficial fibular n.

Deep fibular n. (L5)

NERVE FUNCTION, TESTS, AND DYSFUNCTION

Nerve	Muscle Group	Reflex	Sign or Functional Deficit
Genito-femoral	Cremaster	Cremasteric (L2–L3)	Cremaster paralysis
Femoral	Anterior thigh	Patellar (L4)	Weakness of hip flexion and loss of knee extension
Obturator	Medial thigh		Loss of thigh adduction
Superior gluteal	Gluteus medius and minimus		Abductor lurch (inability to keep pelvis level when contralateral foot is raised)
Inferior gluteal	Gluteus maximus		Difficulty rising from seated position and difficulty climbing stairs
Sciatic	Hamstrings	Hamstring (L5)	Weakness of hip extension and knee flexion
Fibular	Anterior and lateral crural compartments		Foot slap, inability to stand back on heels
Tibial	Posterior crural compartment	Achilles (S1)	Inability to stand on tip-toes

THORAX

Thoracic Cage and Lungs

RESPIRATORY MUSCULATURE	
Function	**Muscles**
Inspiration	**External intercostals,** interchondral portion of internal intercostals, and the **diaphragm**
Expiration	**Internal intercostals** proper, transverse thoracic, and **abdominal muscles**

- The **anterior border** of the **left pleural cavity** deviates laterally between the fourth and sixth ribs to form the cardiac notch—a preferred route for needle insertion into the pericardial cavity.
- When upright, excess fluid tends to collect in the **costodiaphragmatic recess.**
- Introduction of air into the pleural space results in **pneumothorax** with loss of lung ventilation. Fluid or blood produces hydrothorax and hemothorax, both of which limit expansion of the lung with reduced ventilation/perfusion ratio.
- The **right mainstem bronchus** is wider, shorter, and more vertical than the left mainstem bronchus, and therefore, is where large aspirated objects commonly lodge.
- The **right lower lobar bronchus** is most vertical, most nearly continues the direction of the trachea, and is larger in diameter than the left, and therefore, is where small aspirated objects commonly lodge, causing segmental atelectasis.
- A **bronchopulmonary segment** is defined by a segmental bronchus and accompanying segmental artery that lie centrally, as well as by intersegmental veins that form a peripheral venous plexus.
- Because the **superior segmental bronchi** of the lower lobes are the most posterior, and therefore dependent, when the patient is supine, they are most frequently involved in gastric acid aspiration pneumonia (Mendelson syndrome).

Heart

- The transverse cardiac diameter varies with inspiration and expiration but normally should not exceed one-half the diameter of the chest.

- An **apical pulse** is palpable at the point of maximal impulse (PMI) in **the fifth intercostal space just beneath the nipple.**
- **Ventricular coronary flow** occurs during ventricular diastole when a pressure differential occurs between the left ventricle and the aorta.

CARDIAC FEATURES		
Landmark	**Location**	**Contents**
Coronary sulcus	Between atria and ventricles; nearly vertical behind sternum; marks the annulus fibrosus that supports the valves	Right side contains the right coronary artery, and small cardiac vein; crossed by anterior cardiac veins
		Left side contains circumflex branch of the left coronary artery and coronary sinus
Anterior interventricular sulcus	Between left and right ventricles; marks the interventricular septum	Contains the anterior interventricular branch of the left coronary artery and the great cardiac vein
Posterior interventricular sulcus	Delineates the interventricular septum, posteriorly	Contains the posterior interventricular branch of the right coronary artery and the middle cardiac vein

- The **papillary muscles** take up the slack in the chordae tendineae to maintain the competence of the valvular closure as ventricular volume is reduced during blood ejection. The valves close passively.
- A **ventricular septal defect** produces a serious **right-to-left shunt** with cyanosis-"**blue-baby**" syndrome-because left ventricular pressure exceeds that in the right ventricle. A large VSD is the principal factor in **tetralogy of Fallot.**

		HEART VALVES	
Valve	**Auscultation**		**Comment**
Aortic	Right of sternum over second intercostal space		**Stenosis** will tend to be auscultated as a high-pitched systolic murmur with possible radiation to the carotid arteries
Pulmonary	Left of sternum over second intercostal space		
Tricuspid	Left of sternum in fifth intercostal space		
Mitral	Apex of heart in fifth intercostal space in left midclavicular line		**Insufficiency** produces a low-pitched, late systolic blowing murmur

Note: Left and right are the patient's left and right. As you "read" from left to right and down the patient's chest the valves order is the same as, "All Physicians Take Money."

• The **atrioventricular bundle** passes through the annulus fibrosus and descends along the posterior border of the membranous part of the interventricular septum to enter the muscular portion of the septum. It transmits electrical activity to the ventricles.

	CARDIAC NODAL TISSUE		
Node	**Location**	**Function**	**Vasculature**
Sinoatrial	In myocardium between crista terminalis and opening of superior vena cava	Initiates contractile event with electrical depolarization spreading throughout atrial musculature	Nodal branch of the right coronary artery
Atrioventricular	In right atrial floor in the interatrial septum near the opening of the coronary sinus	Stimulated by atrial depolarization; it leads into the atrioventricular (A-V) bundle to synchronize ventricular depolarization	Branch of right coronary artery near the posterior interventricular branch

• **Autonomic pathways** consist of two motor neurons, a myelinated preganglionic (presynaptic) neuron and an unmyelinated postganglionic (postsynaptic) neuron.

SUMMARY OF AUTONOMIC PATHWAYS

Division	Presynaptic Pathway	Postsynaptic Pathway	Effect
Sympathetic	From spinal levels T1–L2 along the ventral root; Reach the chain of sympathetic ganglia via white rami communicantes	1. Fibers that synapse return to the spinal nerve via a gray ramus to mediate cutaneous piloerection, vasoconstriction, and sudomotor (sweat gland) activity 2. Fibers that do not synapse pass through the chain as splanchnic nerves to synapse in prevertebral ganglia; from these ganglia, postsynaptic neurons run in perivascular plexuses to innervate visceral target tissues	Adrenergic neurotransmission increases heart rate, increases stroke volume, dilates coronary and pulmonary arteries
Para-sympathetic	Presynaptic cell bodies are located in the dorsal vagal nuclei of the brain; The myelinated synaptic axons form cranial nerve X, the vagus nerve	Postganglionic cell bodies lie in numerous ganglia close to the target organ	Cholinergic neurotransmission decreases heart rate, decreases stroke volume, and produces bronchoconstriction

PAIN REFERRAL FROM THORACIC VISCERA

Organ	Referral Area	Pathway
Pericardial cavity	T1–T5: upper and midthorax	Intercostal nerves T1–T5
Heart	T1–T4: upper thorax, postaxial brachium	Cervical and thoracic splanchnic nerves
Thoracic esophagus	T1–T5: thorax and epigastric region	Thoracic splanchnic nerves
Diaphragm		
Central	C3–C5: neck and shoulder	Phrenic nerve
Marginal	T5–T10: thorax	Intercostal nerves

ABDOMEN

Abdominal Wall

DERMATOMAL LANDMARKS	
Dermatome	**Region**
T4	Nipple
T7	Xiphoid process
T10	Umbilicus
L1	Inguinal ligament

- The **abdominal musculature** has three distinct layers that take three different directions. The external oblique muscle, internal oblique muscle, and transverse abdominis muscle may be sequentially split and retracted so that extensive suturing is unnecessary to provide a strong repair (McBurney's incision).
- Because the **linea alba** is relatively avascular, incisions may not heal well and predispose to epigastric herniation.
- **Above the arcuate line,** the anterior leaf of the **rectus sheath** is formed by fusion of the external oblique and internal oblique aponeuroses; the posterior leaf is formed by fusion of the internal oblique and transverse abdominis aponeuroses.
- **Below the arcuate line,** the anterior leaf of the rectus sheath is formed by fusion of all three aponeuroses and there is no posterior leaf.
- The **inferior epigastric artery** passes into the rectus sheath at the arcuate line. This is a potential site for spigelian herniation into the rectus sheath.

HERNIA CHARACTERISTICS	
Hernia	**Pathway**
Direct inguinal	Through the inguinal triangle bounded by inguinal ligament, inferior epigastric artery, and rectus abdominis—therefore, medial to the inferior epigastric artery. Exits through the superficial inguinal ring generally adjacent to the spermatic cord. Usually acquired
Indirect inguinal	Through the deep inguinal ring and along the inguinal canal—therefore, lateral to the inferior epigastric artery. Exits through the superficial ring within the spermatic cord. Usually congenital
Femoral	Passes inferior to the inguinal ligament through the femoral ring into the thigh. More prevalent in women

GI Tract

CHARACTERIZATION OF ABDOMINAL STRUCTURES BY LOCATION AND SUPPORT	
Characterization	**Organ**
Peritoneal (supported by mesentery)	Abdominal esophagus, stomach, superior duodenum, liver, pancreatic tail, jejunum, ileum, a variable portion of the cecum, appendix, transverse colon, and sigmoid colon
Secondarily retroperitoneal (adherent)	Descending and inferior duodenum, pancreatic head and body, ascending colon, and descending colon. These may be surgically mobilized with an intact blood supply
Extra/retroperitoneal	Thoracic esophagus, rectum, kidneys, ureters, and adrenal glands

- **Peptic ulceration** of the lower esophagus, stomach, or superior duodenum is referred along the greater splanchnic nerve to the fifth and sixth dermatomes, which include the epigastric region.
- The **hepatic triangle,** bounded by the cystic duct, gallbladder, and common hepatic duct, contains the cystic arteries and right hepatic artery with potential for extensive variation.
- The **duodenal papilla** usually contains the hepatopancreatic ampulla, formed by the joining of the common bile duct and the pancreatic duct. If blocked by a stone, pancreatitis may develop.
- The **tail of the pancreas** contains most of the pancreatic islets (of Langerhans), a consideration in pancreatic resection.
- **Ileal (Meckel's) diverticulum** is found in about 2% of the population, located within 2 ft of the ileocecal junction (on the anti-mesenteric side of the ileum), and usually about 2 in. long. Often contain two types of ectopic tissue (cardiac and pancreatic). Peptic ulceration of adjacent ileal mucosa and volvulus are complications.
- The **hepatic portal vein** directs venous return from the gastrointestinal tract to the liver.
- Because the **hepatic portal system has no valves,** blood need not flow toward the liver. Liver disease (such as cirrhosis) or compression of a vein (as in pregnancy or constipation) results in blood shunting through the anastomotic connections to the systemic venous system.

ABDOMINAL ORGANIZATION BASED ON EMBRYOLOGY

Structures	Foregut	Midgut	Hindgut
Organs	esophagus, stomach, liver, gall bladder, pancreas, 1/2 of duodenum	1/2 of duodenum, jejunum, ileum, cecum, ascending colon, 2/3 of transverse colon	1/3 of transverse colon, descending and sigmoid colon, rectum, and 2/3 of anal canal
Arteries & branches	**Celiac** splenic, left gastric, short gastric, common hepatic, right gastric, gastroduodenal	**Superior Mesenteric** inferior pancreaticoduodenal, intestinal middle colic, right colic, ileocolic	**Inferior Mesenteric** left colic, superior rectal
Veins	Portal vein	Portal vein	Portal vein
Lymph	Celiac nodes (supracolic compartment)	Superior Mesenteric nodes (infracolic compartment)	Inferior Mesenteric Nodes (infracolic compartment)
Nerves:			
Parasympathetic	Vagus	Vagus	Pelvic Splanchnic, (S 2,3,4)
Sympathetic	Greater thoracic splanchnic (T 5–9)	Lesser thoracic splanchnic (T 10,11)	Least thoracic splanchnic (T12), Upper lumbar splanchnic (L1.2)
Pain refers to:	**Epigastric region**	**Umbilical region**	**Suprapubic region**

Modified, with permission, after a table by Joseph D. Bast, Ph. D. Department of Anatomy and Cell Biology, University of Kansas Medical Center.

PORTAL-SYSTEMIC ANASTOMOSES OCCUR IN SEVERAL AREAS

Location	Anastomotic Connections	Signs and Symptoms
Esophagus	Azygos veins with left gastric and short gastric veins	Esophageal varices, intractable hematemesis
Umbilicus	Paraumbilical veins with superior and inferior epigastric veins	Caput medusae
Rectum	Superior rectal vein with middle and inferior rectal veins	Internal and external hemorrhoids

Kidneys, Ureters, and Adrenal Glands

- The **renal fascia** (the false capsule or **Gerota's fascia**) is a discrete fascial layer that surrounds each kidney. Paranephric fat outside this capsule and perinephric fat inside this fascial layer support the kidney.
- **Minor calyces** receive one or two pyramids before fusing into major calyces. Two to four minor calyces join to form **major calyces** that coalesce to form the renal pelvis.
- The **ureters** narrow at three points—at the renal pelvis, at the pelvic brim, and at the bladder. Kidney stones may lodge at these locations with pain referred, respectively, to the subcostal, inguinal, and perineal regions.
- **Adrenal arteries** arise from the inferior phrenic arteries, the aorta, and the renal arteries. The right adrenal vein usually drains medially into the inferior vena cava; the left adrenal vein usually drains inferiorly into the left renal vein.

PAIN REFERRAL FROM ABDOMINAL VISCERA		
Organ	**Referral Area**	**Pathway**
Diaphragm		
Central	C3–C5: neck and shoulder	Phrenic nerve
Marginal	T5–T10: thorax	Intercostal nerves
Forgut:		
Stomach, gallbladder, liver, bile duct, superior duodenum	T5–T9: lower thorax, **epigastric region**	Celiac plexus to greater splanchnic nerve
Midgut:		
Inferior duodenum, jejunum, ileum, appendix, ascending colon, transverse colon	T10–T11: **umbilical region**	Superior mesenteric plexus to lesser splanchnic nerve
(Kidney, upper ureters, gonads)	T12–L1: lumbar and ipsilateral inguinal	Aorticorenal plexus to least splanchnic nerve regions
Hindgut:		
Descending colon, sigmoid colon, mid-ureters	L1–L2: **suprapubic** and inguinal regions, anterior scrotum or labia, anterior thigh	Aortic plexus to lumbar splanchnic nerves

PELVIS

Perineum

- The **external anal sphincter,** innervated by the pudendal nerve, provides the brief voluntary contraction necessary to counter the passage of a peristaltic wave.
- The **rectal submucosal venous plexus** forms anastomotic connections between the middle rectal veins that drain directly into the internal iliac veins and the superior rectal veins that drain into the hepatic portal system. This is a site for varices (hemorrhoids).
- The **internal pudendal arteries** are the sole vascular supply of both male and female erectile tissue.
- The **deep dorsal vein** provides venous return from the penis or clitoris by passing through the urogenital diaphragm and draining into the prostatic or vesicle venous plexus, respectively.
- The **cremaster muscle** of the spermatic cord is innervated by the genital branch of the genitofemoral nerve. This provides the efferent limb for the cremaster reflex (L1–L2), the elevation of the testes within the scrotum when the inner thigh is scratched.
- The cavity of **tunica vaginalis** is a potential space that represents the detached portion of the peritoneal cavity that surrounds the testis except posteriorly. The testis is "retroperitoneal" even in the scrotum.
- Because the superficial perineal space is limited by superficial fascial attachment to the deep transverse perineal muscle, extravasations of blood or urine will not pass into the anal triangle.
- The superficial perineal space contains "sexually pleasurable structures" (thanks to Dr. L. Wetzel. M.D.) and is superficial to the perineal membrane and limited by Scarpa's and Colles' superficial fascia in females and Scarpa's, dartos and Colles' superficial fascia in males. Scarpa's superficial fascials attached to deep investing fascia of external oblique and rectus abdominis half way up to the umbilicus and laterally at the inguinal ligament. Colles' superficial fascials attached to ischiopubic ramus and inferior edge of perineal membrane.

CONTENTS OF THE PERINEAL SPACES ARE GENDER SPECIFIC		
Gender	Superficial Perineal Space	Deep Perineal Space
Male	Testes, crura of penis, bulb of penis, penile urethra, superficial transverse perineal muscles	Deep transverse perineal external urethral sphincter, bulbourethral glands, membranous urethra
Female	Crura of the clitoris, vestibular bulbs, superficial transverse perineal muscles, greater vestibular glands	Deep transverse perineal muscle, external urethral sphincter, urethra

- The **male external urethral sphincter** is formed by two muscles: sphincter urethra and compressor urethrae muscles, both in the deep perineal space. The female external urethral sphincter is formed by 3 muscles: sphincter urethra, compressor urethrae, and urethrovaginalis muscles
- A **pudendal block** can be effected by injecting an anesthetic into the vicinity of the pudendal nerve in the pudendal (Alcock's) canal close to the ischial spine.

PELVIC AUTONOMIC FUNCTION			
Function	Sympathetic	Parasympathetic	Somatic
Erection		hypogastric plexus, pelvic plexus, cavernous plexus (S2–S4)	
Emission	L1–L2: lumbar splanchnic nerves		
Ejaculation	(some pelvic splanchnic nerves)		Pudendal nerve, S3–S5

Pelvic viscera

- The **female pelvis** is less massive, the subpubic angle is greater (almost 90°), and the pelvic inlet more ovoid than the male pelvis.
- The **obstetric conjugate** is the least anteroposterior diameter of the pelvic inlet from the sacral promontory to a point a few millimeters below the superior margin of the pubic symphysis.

- The **transverse midplane diameter**, measured between the ischial spines, is the smallest dimension of the pelvic outlet.
- The **levator ani muscle** forms most of the pelvic floor and its puborectalis portion (rectal sling) is the principal mechanism for maintenance of fecal continence when the rectum is full.
- The **rectum** is usually empty because feces are stored in the sigmoid colon. Movement of feces into the rectal ampulla generates the urge to defecate.
- **Metastatic carcinoma of the rectum** may be widely disseminated within the abdomen, pelvis, and inguinal region. The upper rectum drains along the superior rectal lymphatics. The mid-rectum drains along middle rectal lymphatics. The lower rectum drains along the inferior rectal lymphatics and then along both internal and external pudendal lymphatic channels. The lower part of the anus drains to superficial inguinal nodes.

URINARY BLADDER INNERVATION IS BY BOTH SYMPATHETIC AND PARASYMPATHETIC ROUTES	
Function	**Pathway**
Afferent limb of the detrusor (bladder-emptying) reflex	Pelvic plexus and pelvic splanchnic nerves (parasympathetic pathways) to spinal segments S2–S4
Efferent limb of the detrusor reflex	Pelvic splanchnic nerves (parasympathetic pathways) from S2–S4

- **Urinary continence** of the partially full to full urinary bladder is a function of the external urethral sphincter.
- A **patent urachus** (rare) allows reflux of urine through the umbilicus.
- The **testes** develop as retroperitoneal structures and remain so in the scrotum. Testicular torsion has high potential for testicular ischemia and necrosis.
- The testicular **pampiniform plexus** functions as a countercurrent heat exchanger that maintains testicular temperature a few degrees below core body temperature.
- The superior mesenteric artery may compress the left renal vein, which receives the left testicular vein. The result may be **varices of the pampiniform plexus** on the left side with reduced fertility.

- In the **male**, palpable during a **digital rectal exam** are posterior and lateral lobes of the **prostate gland**, seminal vesicles if enlarged, and bladder when filling.
- Each **uterine artery** crosses immediately **superior to a ureter** in the transverse cervical ligament—an important surgical consideration.
- Normal uterine position is anteflexed (uterus bent forward on itself at the level of the internal os) and anteverted (angled approximately 90° anterior to the vagina), lying on the urinary bladder.
- In the **female, palpable per vagina** are the cervix and ostium of the uterus, the body of the uterus if retroverted, the rectouterine fossa, and variably the ovary and uterine tubes.
- The **lymphatic drainage from the vagina** is by three routes: the external and internal iliac nodes from the upper portion of the vagina; and the internal iliac nodes as well as the superficial inguinal nodes from the lowest third.

PAIN REFERRAL FROM PELVIC VISCERA		
Organ	**Referral Area**	**Pathway**
Testes and ovaries	T10–T12: umbilical and pubic regions	Gonadal nerves to aortic plexus and then to lesser and least splanchnic nerves
Middle ureters, urinary bladder, uterine body, uterine tubes	L1–L2: pubic and inguinal regions, anterior scrotum or labia, anterior thigh	Hypogastric plexus to aortic plexus and then to lumbar splanchnic nerves
Rectum, superior anal canal, pelvic ureters, cervix, epididymis, vas deferens, seminal vesicles, prostate gland	S3–S5: perineum and posterior thigh	Pelvic plexus to pelvic splanchnic nerves

PELVIC VISCERAL AFFERENT INNERVATION			
Organ	**Afferent Pathway**	**Level**	**Referral areas**
Kidneys Renal pelvis Upper ureters	Aorticorenal plexus, least splanchnic nerve, white ramus of T12, subcostal nerve	T12	Subcostal and pubic regions
Descending colon Sigmoid colon Mid-ureters Urinary bladder Oviducts Uterine body	Aortic plexus, lumbar splanchnic nerves, white rami of L1–L2, spinal nerves L1–L2	L1–L2	Lumbar and inguinal regions, anterior mons and labia, anterior scrotum, anterior thigh
None	No white rami between L3–S1	L3–S1	No visceral pain refers to dermatomes L3–S1
Cervix Pelvic ureters Epididymis Vas deferens Seminal vesicles Prostate gland Rectum Proximal anal canal	Pelvic plexus, pelvic splanchnic nerves, spinal nerves S2–S4	S2–S4	Perineum, thigh, lateral leg and foot

HEAD AND NECK

Somatic Portions

- **The scalp layer of loose connective tissue** between the epicranial aponeurosis and the periosteum forms the subaponeurotic or "danger" space. Emissary veins connect with the dural sinuses with potential for vascular spread of infection through the calvaria.
- **Cranial fractures** preferentially pass through cranial foramina injuring the contained nerves.

PRINCIPAL FORAMINA OF THE ANTERIOR CRANIAL FOSSA		
Foramen	**Contents**	**Result of Injury**
Olfactory	Olfactory nerves	Anosmia
Foramen cecum	An emissary vein	

PRINCIPAL FORAMINA OF THE MIDDLE CRANIAL FOSSA		
Foramen	**Contents**	**Result of Injury**
Optic canal	CN II	Unilateral blindness
	Ophthalmic artery	Ischemic unilateral blindness
Superior orbital fissure	CN III	Ophthalmoplegia
	CN IV	Inability to look down and out
	CN V_1	Unilateral loss of blink reflex
	CN VI	Inability to abduct eye
	Superior ophthalmic vein	Retinal engorgement
Foramen rotundum	CN V_2	Loss of sensation under eye
Foramen ovale	CN V_3	Masticatory paralysis, loss of jaw-jerk reflex
Foramen spinosum	Middle meningeal artery	
Foramen lacerum	Nothing (except occasionally the greater superficial petrosal nerve)	
Hiatus of the facial canal	Gr. superficial petrosal n.	Dry eye, loss of submandibular and sublingual secretion

PRINCIPAL FORAMINA OF THE POSTERIOR CRANIAL FOSSA		
Foramen	**Contents**	**Result of Injury**
Internal auditory meatus	CN VII	Facial paralysis
	CN VIII	Auditory and vestibular deficits
Jugular foramen	CN IX	Loss of gag and carotid reflexes
	CN X	Loss of cough reflex; paralysis of laryngeal muscles and some palatine muscles
	CN XI	Inability to shrug shoulders
	Internal jugular vein	
Hypoglossal canal	CN XII	Paralysis of tongue muscles; lingual deviation toward side of injury upon protrusion

CSF IS PRODUCED BY THE CHOROID PLEXUSES THAT PROJECT INTO THE VENTRICLES OF THE BRAIN		
CSF Production	**Through**	**Into**
Lateral ventricles	Foramina of Monro	Third ventricle (interventricular)
Third ventricle	Cerebral aqueduct	Fourth ventricle
Fourth ventricle	Foramina of Magendie and Luschka	Cisterna magna of subarachnoid space
From	**Through**	**CSF Uptake**
Subarachnoid space	Arachnoid villi	Superior sagittal venous sinus

- The cerebral aqueduct is prone to occlusion, leading to hydrocephalus.

CRANIAL AND CEREBRAL HEMATOMAS			
Hematoma	**Prognosis**	**Location**	**Cause**
Epicranial	Resolves	Subaponeurotic space	Superficial vessels
Epidural	Life-threatening	Epidural space	Torn middle meningeal artery
Subdural	Serious	Subdural space	Torn cerebral vein (usually)
Subarachnoid	Lethal	Subarachnoid space	Torn cerebral artery, cerebral aneurysm
Subpial	Usually resolves	Cerebrum	Cerebral contusion

- **Regions of the orbit** that are prone to fracture include the ethmoid lamina papyracea and the maxilla near the infraorbital groove.
- Contraction of the **orbicularis oculi muscle, innervated by the facial nerve,** produces the blink.

GANGLIA ASSOCIATED WITH CRANIAL NERVES		
Nerve (Classification)	**Ganglion**	**Function**
Optic (SSA)	Bipolar cells	Vision
Oculomotor (GVE)	Ciliary	Pupillary constriction, accommodation
Trigeminal (GSA)	Semilunar (trigeminal)	General sensation from the face, nasal and oral cavities, including afferent limbs of blink, sneeze, and jaw-jerk reflexes
Facial (GSA)	Geniculate	General sensation from external ear
(SVA)	Geniculate	Taste from anterior 2/3 of tongue
(GVE)	Pterygopalatine	Secretomotor for lacrimal, nasal, and palatine glands
(GVE)	Submandibular	Secretomotor for sublingual and submandibular glands
Vestibulocochlear (SSA)	Vestibular and Spiral	Balance, audition
Glossopharyngeal (GSA)	Jugular (superior)	General sensation from external auditory meatus
(GVA)	Petrosal (inferior)	Visceral sensation from posterior 1/3 of tongue and pharynx; afferent limb of gag and carotid reflexes
(SVA)	Petrosal (inferior)	Taste from posterior 1/3 of tongue
(GVE)	Otic	Secretomotor for parotid gland
Vagus (GSA)	Jugular (superior)	General sensation from external auditory meatus
(GVA)	Petrosal (inferior)	Visceral sensation from larynx; afferent limb of cough and aortic body reflexes
(SVA)	Nodose (inferior)	Taste from epiglottis
(GVE)	Distal ganglia	Visceral smooth muscle and gland control

GSA: general somatic afferent; GVA: general visceral afferent; GVE: general visceral efferent; SSA: special somatic afferent; SVA: special visceral afferent.

COURSE, DISTRIBUTION & PRINCIPAL FUNCTION OF CRANIAL NERVES

CN	Foramen	Distribution	Function
I	Cribriform plate	Nasal mucosa	Olfaction
II	Optic canal	Retina	Vision
III	Superior orbital fissure	Levator palpebrae superioris, superior rectus, medial rectus, inferior rectus, inferior oblique muscles	Ocular elevation, depression, adduction, pupillary constriction, accommodation
IV		Superior oblique muscle	Ocular depression and abduction
V_1	Superior orbital fissure	Forehead, conjunctiva	Sensation, afferent limb of blink reflex
V_2	Foramen rotundum, infraorbital foramen	Mid-face	Sensation, afferent limb of sneeze reflex
V_3	Foramen ovale, mandibular foramen, mental foramen	Jaw, lateral face, anterior tongue	Sensation, afferent limb of jaw-jerk reflex, anterior tongue sensation Motor to muscles of mastication
VI	Superior orbital fissure	Lateral rectus muscle	Ocular abduction
VII	Internal acoustic meatus, facial canal, stylomastoid foramen	Face, lacrimal, nasal, sublingual, and submaxillary glands	Motor to muscles of facial expression and efferent limb of blink reflex; secretomotor for lacrimation, nasal and anterior oral secretion Taste from anterior part of tongue
VIII	Internal acoustic meatus	Cochlear and vestibular apparatus	Audition and balance

(Continued)

COURSE, DISTRIBUTION & PRINCIPAL FUNCTION OF CRANIAL NERVES

CN	Foramen	Distribution	Function
IX	Jugular foramen	Oropharynx	Sensation to posterior tongue and pharynx, afferent limb of gag reflex; taste from posterior part of tongue, carotid reflex. Motor to stylopharyngeus muscle
X	Jugular foramen	Pharynx, larynx	Laryngeal sensation, afferent limb of cough reflex; epiglottic taste. Motor to palatine and laryngeal muscles
XI	Foramen magnum, jugular foramen	Sternomastoid and trapezius muscles	Motor to sternomastoid and trapezius muscles
XII	Anterior condylar canal	Tongue	Motor to all intrinsic and most extrinsic tongue muscles

ORBITAL MUSCLE FUNCTION AND INNERVATION

Muscle	Primary Function	Secondary Functions (normally balance)	Innervation
Pupil	Constriction		CN III parasympathetic
	Dilation		Sympathetic chain
Ciliary muscle	Accommodation		CN III parasympathetic
Superior tarsal muscle	Augment levator palpebrae superioris		Sympathetic chain
Levator palpebrae superioris	Elevate eyelid		CN III (Oculomotor)
Medial rectus	Adduction		CN III (Oculomotor)
Superior rectus	Elevation	Adduction, intorsion	CN III (Oculomotor)
Inferior oblique	Elevation	Abduction, extorsion	CN III (Oculomotor)
Inferior rectus	Depression	Adduction, extorsion	CN III (Oculomotor)
Superior oblique	Depression	Abduction, intorsion	CN IV (Trochlear)
Lateral rectus	Abduction		CN VI (Abducens)

- Clinically the function of the extraocular eye muscles is tested using the "H" test with the medial rectus tested by horizontally crossing one's eyes and the lateral rectus tested by moving the eye laterally (abducing). From either full adduction or abduction the the eye is then moved in a second direction. When fully adducted, gazing below the horizon tests the superior oblique muscle. Remember "SO" look like the edge of the nose "S" forming the ala and "O" the nostril). When fully adducted raising the eye above the horizon tests the inferior oblique muscle. When fully abduced, gazing below the horizon tests the inferior rectus muscles. When fully abduced, raising the eye above the horizon tests the superior rectus muscle. See the "H" below patient's left eye.

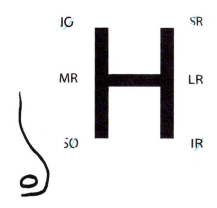

- **Parasympathetic innervation** to the pupil originates in the Edinger-Westphal nucleus and travels with the oculomotor nerve. Temporal lobe herniation (from tumor, hematoma, or edema) compresses the oculomotor nerve within the tentorial notch, causing a dilated pupil that is unresponsive to light.

SPECIAL SENSORY TESTS AND DYSFUNCTION			
Nerve	**Foramen**	**Dysfunction**	**Test**
CN I (olfactory)	Cribriform plate	Anosmia	Whiff of clove
CN II (optic)	Optic canal	Blindness	Optic field tests
CN VIII			
Cochlear	Internal auditory meatus	Deafness	Hearing threshold
Vestibular	Internal auditory meatus	Balance	Nystagmus

- Paralysis of the stapedius muscle, as a result of facial nerve palsy, produces hyperacusis.

Visceral Portions

- The **infrahyoid muscles,** innervated by the ansa cervicalis (C1–C3), stabilize the hyoid bone and larynx during deglutition and phonation.
- The **pretracheal space,** deep to the pretracheal fascia, surrounds the trachea and thyroid gland. Infection in this space may migrate into the superior mediastinum.
- The **retropharyngeal (retrovisceral) space** lies posterior to the oropharynx and esophagus and is defined by septa from the pretracheal fascia. Infection within this space may migrate into the posterior mediastinum.
- The **mandibular neurovascular bundle** enters the mandibular foramen adjacent to the lingula, the point of minimal movement. It may be anesthetized by directing a needle posteriorly through the buccal wall just lateral to the pterygomandibular raphe.
- The **deep cervical nodes** receive lymph from the anteroinferior portion of the face, the nasal cavities, and the oral cavity.
- The **nasal vestibule** (the most common site for nosebleeds) receives vascular branches from internal and external carotid arteries.
- The **palatine tonsil** receives vascular branches from the maxillary, facial, and lingual arteries.
- **Abduction of the vocal cords** is a function of the posterior cricoarytenoid muscle only, innervated by the recurrent laryngeal nerve.

BRANCHIOMERIC NERVE FUNCTIONS AND TESTS				
Nerve	**Course**	**Sensory**	**Motor**	**Test**
CN V (trigeminal)				
V1	Superior orbital fissure, supraorbital notch	Forehead	None	Blink reflex (afferent)
V2	Foramen rotundum, maxillary foramen	Mid-face	None	Sneeze reflex

(Continued)

Nerve	Course	Sensory	Motor	Test
V3	Foramen ovale, mandibular foramen, mental foramen	Anterior pinna, jaw 2/3 of tongue	Muscles of mylohyoid ant. belly of digastric, tensor palatini and tensor tympani	Jaw jerk
CN VII (facial)	Internal auditory meatus, facial canal, stylomastoid foramen	Concha of ear, taste anterior 2/3 of tongue via chorda tympani	Muscles of facial expression, stylohyoid, post. belly of digastric, tensor tympani tensor palati parasympathetic to lacrimal, nasal, palatine, lingual and submandibular glands via gr. superficial petrosal nerve	Blink reflex (efferent)
CN IX (glosso-pharyngeal)	Jugular foramen	External auditory, meatus, oropharynx, carotid body and sinus, taste posterior 1/3 of tongue	Stylopharyngeus muscle, parasym-pathetic to parotid gland via tympanic and lesser super-ficial petrosal nerves	Gag reflex, Carotid reflex
CN X (vagus)	Jugular foramen	External auditory meatus, larynx, taste from epiglottis, aortic body	Palatine muscles, pharyngeal muscles, laryngeal muscles	Phonation

NERVE FUNCTIONS AND TESTS				
Nerve	**Foramen**	**Sensory**	**Motor**	**Test**
CN XI (spinal accessory)	Foramen magnum, jugular foramen	None	Sternocleidomastoid Upper trapezius	Turn head to opposite side
CN XII (hypoglossal)	Hypoglossal canal	None	Intrinsic and 3/4 of extrinsic tongue muscles	Protrudes straight

- **Sensory innervation of the face** is by the trigeminal nerve (see figure below).

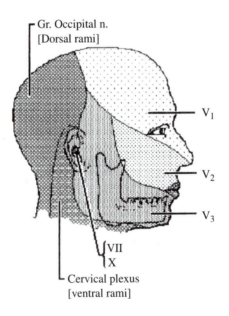

Embryology: Early and General

Questions

DIRECTIONS: Each item below contains a question or incomplete statement followed by suggested responses. Select the **one best** response to each question.

1. A 29-year-old woman (gravida 3, para 2) gave birth to a healthy baby after 38 weeks of gestation and delivered the intact placenta spontaneously. The pregnancy was complicated by preeclampsia, but fetal monitoring and ultrasound were normal throughout gestation. The predominant structures shown in the accompanying photomicrograph of the placenta are derived from which of the following?

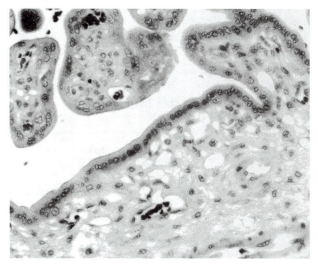

a. A combination of fetal and maternal tissues
b. Endometrial glands
c. Endometrial stroma
d. Fetal tissues
e. Maternal blood vessels

2. A married couple, with diagnosed 6-year-long infertility, presents to the fertility clinic. A spermocytogram, confirmed by electron microscopy, reveals that the husband produces all spermatozoa with rounded heads, a condition known as globozoospermia. The missing sperm structure is associated with which of the following?

a. Loss of decapacitation factors
b. Retention of the developing spermatids from Sertoli cells
c. Maturation of lytic enzymes
d. Mitotic activity
e. Meiotic divisions

3. A 38-year-old (gravida 0, para 0) woman is recently married and pregnant. The zygote is a result of a haploid ovum fertilized by her husband's sperm. Which of the following is required for continuation of the second meiotic division to produce the haploid ovum?

a. Elevation of progesterone titers
b. Expulsion from the mature follicle
c. The environment of the oviduct and uterus
d. Fertilization by a spermatozoon
e. The presence of human chorionic gonadotropin (hCG)

4. A married couple, diagnosed with infertility present to the fertility clinic. The husband's semen contains only 40 million sperm total with a forward motility index slightly below normal. A hamster egg penetration assay was performed in which hamster eggs are collected and their zona pellucidae are enzymatically removed prior to mixing with sperm. The husband's sperm have normal morphology, but his penetration assay results are 3.7% (normal, 10%). The hamster egg penetration assay requires which of the following?

a. Sperm formation, maturation and penetration
b. Addition of cholesterol to the sperm plasma membrane
c. A decrease in the fluidity of the sperm plasma membrane
d. Sequestration of acrosomal enzymes
e. Capacitation, acrosome reaction and penetration

5. A 23-year-old woman with a natural menstrual cycle is nearing ovulation. The oocyte of a mature follicle will be induced to undergo the first meiotic division as a result of which of the following hormonal stimuli?

a. The cessation of progesterone secretion
b. The gradual elevation of follicle-stimulating hormone (FSH) titers
c. The low estrogen titers associated with the maturing follicle
d. The slow elevation of progesterone produced by luteal cells
e. The surge of luteinizing hormone (LH) initiated by high estrogen titers

6. A couple is trying to conceive a child. Following intercourse, which of the following is responsible for the prevention of polyspermy?

a. Resumption of the first meiotic division
b. Resumption of the second meiotic division
c. Capacitation
d. The zona reaction
e. The release of enzymes from the sperm acrosome

7. Oogonia reach their maximum number at which of the following stages of human development?

a. Five months of fetal life
b. Birth
c. Puberty (12 to 14 years of age)
d. Adolescence (16 to 20 years of age)
e. Early adulthood (21 to 26 years of age)

8. A 26-year-old man contracted viral influenza with an unremitting fever of 39.5°C (103°F) for 3 days. Because spermatogenesis cannot occur above a scrotal temperature of 35.5°C (96°F), he was left with no viable sperm after his recovery. Approximately how much time is required for the return of viable sperm to the epididymis?

a. 3 days
b. 1 week
c. 5 weeks
d. 2 months
e. 4 months

9. Implantation of the conceptus at which site in the accompanying diagram of the female reproductive system is most likely to result in excessive, perhaps fatal, vaginal bleeding immediately prior to parturition?

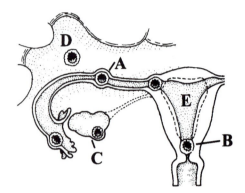

a. A
b. B
c. C
d. D
e. E

10. Cells that form the three primitive germ layers are derived from which of the following?

a. Cytotrophoblast
b. Epiblast
c. Syncytiotrophoblast
d. Hypoblast
e. Yolk sac

11. In the developing human embryo/fetus, most of the internal organs begin to form in which month?

a. First
b. Second
c. Fourth
d. Sixth
e. Ninth

12. The primitive uteroplacental circulation is functionally established during which period of embryonic/fetal development?

a. First week
b. Second week
c. Third week
d. End of first month
e. Second trimester

13. The ectoderm is derived directly from which of the following?

a. Hypoblast
b. Epiblastic cells that undergo gastrulation
c. Mesoderm
d. Endoderm
e. Nongastrulated epiblast

14. Fetal blood from the placenta is about 80% oxygenated. However, mixture with unoxygenated blood at various points reduces the oxygen content. Which of the following fetal vessels contains blood with the highest oxygen content?

a. Abdominal aorta
b. Common carotid arteries
c. Ductus arteriosus
d. Pulmonary artery
e. Pulmonary vein

15. A female infant is born approximately 10 weeks prematurely (at 30 weeks) and weighs 1710 g. She has respiratory distress syndrome and is treated with endogenous surfactant. She is intubated endotracheally with mechanical ventilation immediately after birth. Over the first 4 days after birth the ventilator pressure and the fraction of inspired oxygen are reduced. Beginning on the fifth day after birth, she has brief desaturations that become more persistent. She needs increased ventilator and oxygen support on the seventh day after birth. She becomes cyanotic. Further examination, echocardiogram, and x-rays reveal left atrial enlargement, an enlarged pulmonary artery, increased pulmonary vasculature, and a continuous machine-like murmur. Which of the following is the most likely diagnosis?

a. Persistent foramen ovale
b. Patent ductus arteriosus
c. Ventricular septal defect
d. Pulmonary stenosis
e. Coarctation of the aorta

16. Which of the following hematopoietic tissues or organs develops from endoderm?

a. Thymus
b. Tonsils
c. Bone marrow
d. Spleen
e. Blood islands

17. Which of the following processes places the developing heart in the presumptive thoracic region cranial to the septum transversum?

a. Gastrulation
b. Lateral folding
c. Cranial folding
d. Neurulation
e. Fusion of the endocardial heart tubes

18. Which of the following is in direct contact with maternal blood in lacunae of the placenta?

a. Cells of the cytotrophoblast
b. Extraembryonic mesoderm
c. Fetal blood vessels
d. Cells of the syncytiotrophoblast
e. Amniotic cells

19. A dental hygienist is concerned about the effects of radiation on the *in utero* development of her baby. During which of the following periods is the embryo most susceptible to environmental influences that could induce the formation of nonlethal congenital malformations?

a. Fertilization to 1 week of fetal life
b. The second week of fetal life
c. The third through eighth weeks of fetal life
d. The third month of fetal life
e. The third trimester of fetal life

20. During a visit to her gynecologist, a patient reports she received vitamin A treatment for her acne unknowingly during the first 2 months of an undetected pregnancy. Which of the following organ systems in the developing fetus is most likely to be affected?

a. The digestive system
b. The endocrine organs
c. The respiratory system
d. The urinary and reproductive systems
e. The skeletal and central nervous systems

21. A 32-year-old (gravida 2, para 1) female presents to her obstetrician with abdominal discomfort, increased back pain, shortness of breath, and swelling in her feet and ankles. Ultrasound reveals an amniotic fluid index (AFI) of 27 cm (normal 5 to 24 cm). The condition is caused by which of the following?

a. Duodenal or esophageal atresia
b. Bilateral agenesis of the kidneys
c. Precocious development of the swallowing reflex in the fetus
d. Hypoplasia of the lungs
e. Obstructive uropathy

22. The neural plate forms directly from which of the following?

a. Ectoderm
b. Endoderm
c. Somatopleuric mesoderm
d. Splanchnopleuric mesoderm
e. Hypoblast

23. Which of the following forms from paraxial mesoderm?

a. Adrenal cortex
b. Adrenal medulla
c. Humerus
d. Biceps brachii
e. Masseter

24. The cerebral cortex forms from which of the following?

a. Telencephalon
b. Myelencephalon
c. Metencephalon
d. Mesencephalon
e. Diencephalon

25. The primordial germ cells that eventually form the oogonia and spermatogonia originate in which of the following?

a. Dorsal mesentery of the hindgut
b. Gonadal ridge
c. Endodermal lining of the yolk sac
d. Primary sex cords of the developing gonad
e. Chorion

26. The structure labeled F in the following diagram is important in embryonic development of humans as which of the following?

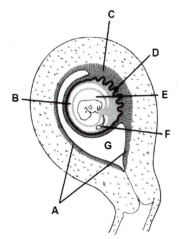

(Modified, with permission, from Sweeney L. Basic Concepts in Embryology. New York, NY: McGraw-Hill, 1998.)

a. The major site of yolk storage
b. Transfer of nutrients after the uteroplacental circulation has been established
c. The origin of the ligamentum teres hepatis
d. The source of the amniotic fluid
e. The initial site of hematopoiesis

27. Monozygotic twins arise by means of which of the following?

a. Fusion of the embryonic blastomeres from two zygotes
b. Fertilization of two oocytes by two sperm
c. Fertilization of one oocyte by two sperm
d. Division of the inner cell mass (embryoblast) into two embryonic primordia
e. Extra cleavage divisions of the zygote induced by the presence of a double chorion

28. In the developing embryo, the edge of the ectoderm is continuous with which of the following?

a. Chorion
b. Amniotic membrane
c. Yolk sac lining
d. Extraembryonic mesoderm
e. Adventitia of the umbilical vessels

29. Which of the following processes is responsible for fusion of the paired dorsal aortae?

a. Lateral folding
b. Craniocaudal folding
c. Looping of the heart tube
d. Neurulation
e. Gastrulation

Embryology:
Early and General

Answers

1. The answer is d. (*Sadler, pp 95–100. Moore and Persaud, Developing, pp 47–50.*) The placental structures shown in the photomicrograph are chorionic villi that are fetal tissues. The mother's contribution to the placenta **(answers a and e)** is the blood that flows past the chorionic villi. A fertilized ovum reaches the uterus about 4 days after fertilization. At that time, it has developed into a multicellular, hollow sphere referred to as a blastocyst. The blastocyst soon adheres to the secretory endometrium and differentiates into an inner cell mass that will develop into the embryo and a layer of primitive trophoblast. The expanding trophoblast penetrates the surface endometrium **(answers b and c)** and erodes into maternal blood vessels. Eventually, it develops two layers, an inner cytotrophoblast and an outer syncytiotrophoblast. Solid cords of trophoblast form the chorionic villi, which then are invaded by fetal blood vessels.

2. The answer is c. (*Alberts, pp 1051–1052. Junqueira, pp 423–426. Moore and Persaud, Developing, pp 20–21.*) The husband in the scenario has sperm, which lack the acrosome (globozoospermia) and therefore the enzymes necessary for penetration of the ovum are missing. The formation of the acrosome, a specialized secretory granule, is one of many maturation events occurring during spermiogenesis (the process by which mature sperm are formed from the spermatids). Acrosome formation involves lytic enzyme maturation and occurs after division of secondary spermatocytes. It involves no mitotic or meiotic activity **(answers d and e)**. The acrosome develops from Golgi vesicles just like any other secretory granules. It contains acrosin, a serine protease, hyaluronidase, and neuraminidase, responsible for the penetration ability of the sperm. The developing cells are in contact with Sertoli cells for all of the stages of spermiogenesis. At the end of spermiogenesis, spermatids are released by Sertoli cells in a process called spermiation **(answer b)**. Decapacitation factors are not involved in acrosomal maturation **(answer a)**.

3. The answer is d. (*Alberts, pp 1151–1152. Junqueira, pp 435, 439–440, 443.*) The secondary oocyte enters the second meiotic division just before ovulation and arrests at metaphase. Fertilization by a spermatozoon provides the stimulation for the division of chromatin to the haploid number. By the time the fertilized ovum reaches the uterus, the progesterone (**answer a**) produced by the corpus luteum has initiated the secretory phase in the endometrium. Once implantation occurs and the chorion develops, human chorionic gonadotropin (hCG) is synthesized and the corpus luteum is maintained (**answer e**). Expulsion from the follicle (**answer b**) and the environment of the oviduct and uterus (**answer c**) do *not* induce the second meiotic division.

4. The answer is e. (*Junqueira, p 443. Moore and Persaud, Developing, pp 31–33. Gilbert, pp 194–195. Sadler, p 35.*) Capacitation, the acrosome reaction and penetration are required for the hamster sperm penetration assay (SPA). Capacitation prepares the sperm for fertilization and requires an increase in fluidity of the sperm plasma membrane. Sperm must reside in the female reproductive tract or under appropriate *in vitro* conditions for about 1 hour for capacitation to occur. During capacitation there is a loss of decapacitation factors that have been added to the sperm by epididymal cells and accessory male reproductive organs. Cholesterol is removed (not added, **answer b**) from the sperm plasma membrane during this period, which results in the increased fluidity (not a decrease, **answer c**) of this membrane that is required for the fusion of the acrosomal membrane with the sperm plasma membrane. Next, there is release of the acrosomal enzymes (not sequestration, **answer d**), which are required for the breakdown of the corona radiata and the zona pellucida of the oocyte to facilitate sperm penetration. Sperm formation and maturation occur in the testis and epididymis (**answer a**) and thus are not directly tested in a hamster egg penetration assay.

5. The answer is e. (*Sadler, pp 22–25. Ross and Pawlina, p 774.*) Primary oocytes have developed by the time of birth. From puberty to menopause, these germ cells remain suspended in meiotic prophase I (diplotene or dictyate stage). A midcycle surge of LH triggers the resumption of meiosis and causes the FSH-primed follicle to rupture and discharge the ovum. Under the influence of LH, the ruptured follicle is transformed into a corpus luteum, which produces progesterone. FSH and LH produced in the adenohypophysis result in growth and maturation of the ovarian follicle. Under FSH stimulation, the theca cells proliferate, hypertrophy, and begin to produce estrogen.

6. The answer is d. (*Sadler, pp 34–37.*) On fusion of the first sperm with the oocyte cell membrane, the contents of secretory granules stored just beneath the oocyte membrane (cortical granules) are released (the zona reaction). Enzymes stored in those granules cause biochemical and electrical changes in the zona pellucida and the oocyte membrane that prevent the binding of additional sperm. Primitive female germ cells (oogonia) enter the first meiotic division during fetal development **(answer a).** This process becomes arrested in prophase I until individual primary oocytes are hormonally induced to resume the first meiotic division during puberty and early adulthood (menarche to menopause). Fusion of the sperm and oocyte membranes initiates the resumption of the second meiotic division, resulting in the formation of a haploid pronucleus in the oocyte and extrusion of the second polar body **(answer b).** Capacitation **(answer c)** is a process by which enzymatic secretions of the uterus and oviducts strip glycoproteins from the sperm cell membrane. This is required for penetration of the layer of cells surrounding the oocyte (corona radiata). The release of enzymes **(answer e)** from the sperm acrosomal cap (an enlarged lysosome) results in digestion of the zona pellucida surrounding the oocyte, allowing penetration by sperm.

7. The answer is a. (*Moore and Persaud, Developing, pp 17–21. Sadler, pp 22–25.*) The maximum number of oogonia occurs at about the fifth month of development. Primordial germ cells arrive in the embryonic gonad of a genetic female during the 7th to 12th week where they differentiate into oogonia. After undergoing a number of mitotic divisions, those fetal cells form clusters in the cortical part of the ovary. Some of those oogonia differentiate into the larger primary oocytes (*not* to be confused with primary follicles). The primary oocytes begin meiosis. At the same time, the number of oogonia continues to increase to about 6,000,000 by the fifth month. At this time, most of the surviving oogonia and some of the oocytes become atretic **(answers b and c).** However, the surviving primary oocytes (400,000 to 1,000,000) become surrounded by epithelial cells and form the primordial follicles by the seventh month. During childhood **(answers d and e)** there is continued atresia, so that by puberty only about 40,000 primary oocytes remain.

8. The answer is d. (*Moore and Persaud, Developing, pp 16–21.*) In man, the time required for the progression from spermatogonium to motile spermatozoon is about 2 months (61 to 64 days). Spermatogenesis, the process by which spermatogonia undergo mitotic division to produce primary spermatocytes, occurs at 1°C (2°F) below normal body temperature. Subsequent meiotic divisions produce secondary spermatocytes with a bivalent haploid chromosome number and then spermatids with a monovalent haploid chromosome number. Spermiogenesis, the maturation of the spermatid, results in spermatozoa. Morphologically, adult spermatozoa are moved to the epididymis, where they become fully motile.

9. The answer is b. (*Moore and Persaud, Developing, pp 47–51, 52–54. Sadler, pp 41, 42, 49–52.*) Implantation of the conceptus low on the uterine wall near the cervical opening (os) could result in growth of the placenta between the embryo and the cervical os (placenta previa). The placenta could become dislodged from the uterine wall before, as well as during delivery, resulting in rapidly fatal hemorrhage. Implantation at site A (the uterine tube or oviduct) results in rupture of the oviduct wall, whereas implantation on the ovary (C) would result in destruction of that organ. Implantation could also occur in the wall of the peritoneal cavity (D). Implantation normally occurs in the superior posterior or posterolateral walls of the uterus (E).

10. The answer is b. (*Moore and Persaud, Developing, pp 44–46. Sadler, pp 39–40, 45–46, 48, 55–56, 58.*) Cells of the inner cell mass (embryoblast) of the blastocyst differentiate into the epiblast and hypoblast. Cells of the epiblast migrate toward the primitive streak during the second week and become internalized, forming the mesodermal and endodermal germ layers. Remaining cells of the epiblast become the ectodermal germ layer. Cells of the hypoblast **(answer d)** will contribute to the yolk sac. Cells of the outer cell mass of the blastocyst will differentiate into the cytotrophoblast and syncytiotrophoblast **(answers a and c)**, which will contribute to formation of the placenta. The yolk sac **(answer e)** is incorporated into the embryo as the primitive gut during embryonic folding.

11. The answer is b. (*Moore and Persaud, Developing, pp 88–90, 520.*) Formation of most internal organs occurs during the second month, the period of organogenesis. The first month **(answer a)** of embryonic development generally is concerned with cleavage, formation of the germ layers, and establishment of the embryonic body. The period from the ninth week to the end of intrauterine life **(answers c, d and e)**, known as the fetal period, is characterized by maturation of tissues and rapid growth of the fetal body.

12. The answer is d. (*Moore and Persaud, Developing, pp 46–50, 74. Sadler, pp 45–47, 63–64.*) During the second week of fetal development, lacunar spaces develop between cells of the syncytiotrophoblast, particularly in the region of the embryonic pole as the conceptus invades the endometrium. Endometrial capillaries in this region become dilated and engorged with blood to form sinusoids. The syncytial cells direct erosion of the endothelium of the maternal capillaries, allowing maternal blood to enter the lacunae and bathe the syncytial cells. During the second week, primary villi consist of projections of syncytial cells surrounding a core of cytotrophoblast cells **(answer b)**. During the third week **(answer c)**, the villus core is invaded by mesodermal cells to form a secondary villus. Cells of the mesodermal core will then differentiate to form capillaries and blood cells by the end of the third week (tertiary villus). Those vessels become connected to the fetal circulation early in the fourth week establishing the functional uteroplacental circulation.

13. The answer is e. (*Sadler, pp 45–46, 48, 55–56, 58. Moore and Persaud, Developing, pp 63–64.*) The nongastrulating cells of the epiblast form the ectoderm (epidermis, epidermal appendages, and the nervous system). During the second week of development, the embryoblast gives rise to two primitive germ layers, the epiblast and the underlying hypoblast **(answer a)**. At the beginning of the third week, cells from the epiblast **(answer b)** migrate toward the midline (primitive streak) and move inward (gastrulation). The migrating epiblast cells displace the hypoblast cells to the periphery to form the endodermal lining **(answer d)** of the digestive tract and form an intermediate layer of mesoderm **(answer c)** that will give rise to muscle, bone, and cartilaginous structures.

14. The answer is b. (*Moore and Persaud, Developing, pp 372–373. Sadler, pp 189–192.*) Blood from the placenta in the umbilical cord is about 80% oxygenated. Mixture with unoxygenated blood from the vitelline veins and the inferior vena cava reduces the oxygen content somewhat. However, this stream with relatively high oxygen content is directed by the valve of the inferior vena cava directly through the foramen ovale into the left atrium. This prevents admixture with oxygen-depleted blood entering the right atrium from the superior vena cava. Thus, the oxygen-saturated blood entering the left ventricle and pumped into the aortic arch, subclavian arteries, and common carotid arteries has the highest oxygen content. The oxygen-depleted blood from the superior vena cava is directed into the right ventricle and then to the pulmonary trunk. Although a small portion of this flow passes through the lungs (where any residual oxygen is extracted by the tissue of the non-respiring lung), most is shunted into the thoracic aorta via the ductus arteriosus and thereby lowers the oxygen content of that vessel. This occurs distal to the origins of the carotid arteries and ensures that the rapidly developing brain has the best oxygen supply. The pattern of blood supply in the fetus and the changes that occur at birth are shown in the following figures.

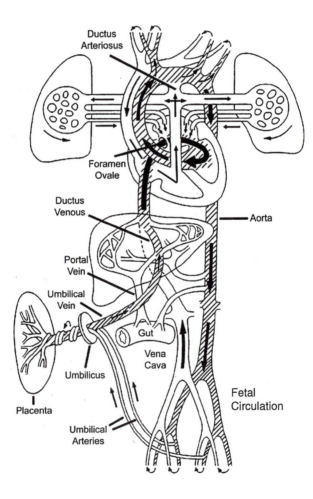

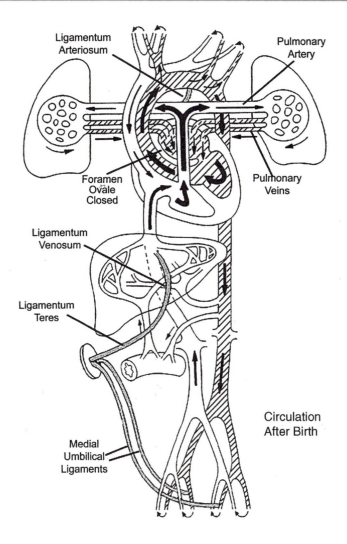

Ligamentum Arteriosum

Pulmonary Artery

Foramen Ovale Closed

Pulmonary Veins

Ligamentum Venosum

Ligamentum Teres

Circulation After Birth

Medial Umbilical Ligaments

15. The answer is b. *(Sadler, pp 169–172. Moore and Persaud, Developing, pp 354–355, 372–373. See diagram provided after the answer for question 14.)* The presence of a murmur could be indicative of any of the conditions. The presence of a continuous machine-like murmur is indicative of a patent ductus arteriosus (PDA). Usually, as in this case, the premature baby with PDA does not acutely become cyanotic and ill, although brief desaturations can occur that become more persistent. The ventilator requirements are increased due to increasing pCO_2 (as the lungs become "wet," the pCO_2 increases). The diastolic blood pressure usually drops and there is a widened pulse pressure (usually greater than 20). The PDA was always there, it is just that her pulmonary vascular resistance relaxed enough to allow more left-to-right shunting and more blood flow to the lungs (less to the body). An atrial septal defect (ASD), such as a persistent foramen ovale, could be eliminated from the diagnosis because the murmur would be heard as an abnormal splitting of the second sound during expiration **(answer a)**. A patent foramen ovale is a common echo finding in premature babies and is usually not followed up unless it appears remarkable to the pediatric cardiologist or there is a persistent murmur. A patent foramen ovale might result in only minimal or intermittent cyanosis during crying or straining to pass stool. A murmur caused by a ventricular septal defect (VSD, **answer c)**, occurs between the first and second heart sounds (S_1 and S_2) and is described as holosystolic (pansystolic) because the amplitude is high throughout systole. Pulmonary stenosis would be heard as a harsh systolic ejection murmur **(answer d)**. Coarctation of the aorta **(answer e)** would result in a systolic murmur. PDA refers to the maintenance of the ductus arteriosus, a normal fetal structure. In the fetus, the ductus arteriosus allows blood to bypass the pulmonary circulation, since the lungs are not involved in CO_2/O_2 exchange until after birth. The placenta subserves the function of gas exchange during fetal development. The ductus arteriosus shunts flow from the left pulmonary artery to the aorta. High oxygen levels after birth and the absence of prostaglandins from the placenta cause the ductus arteriosus to close in most cases within 24 hours. A PDA most often corrects itself within several months of birth, but may require infusion of indomethacin (a prostaglandin inhibitor) as a treatment, insertion of surgical plugs during catheterization, or actual surgical ligation.

16. The answer is a. (*Moore and Persaud, Developing, pp 210–211. Sadler, pp 77–78, 263–264.*) The thymic parenchyma (epithelial cells) develops from endoderm of the third pharyngeal (branchial) pouches. The thymic rudiment is invaded by bone marrow–derived lymphocyte precursors early in the third month of development. The tonsils **(answer b)** develop as partially encapsulated lymph nodules. Their parenchymal framework is derived from pharyngeal mesoderm. Bones, of course, whether formed by intramembranous or endochondral ossification, are derived from mesoderm. Their forming marrow cavities are populated by hematopoietic stem cells **(answer c)** beginning in the second month of fetal life. The connective tissue capsule and skeletal framework of the spleen develop from splanchnic lateral plate mesoderm during the fifth week and are quickly invaded by hematopoietic cells of the myeloid lineage **(answer d)**. It remains an active hematopoietic organ until at least the seventh month *in utero*. Blood islands develop by differentiation of mesodermal cells in the extraembryonic mesoderm lining the yolk sac during the third week of fetal development **(answer e)**. They give rise to vitelline vessels and are the major site of red blood cell formation in the early embryo.

17. The answer is c. (*Moore and Persaud, Developing, pp 78, 80–81. Sadler, pp 79–80, 159–162.*) Cranial folding is responsible for the placement of the developing heart in the presumptive thoracic region of the embryo. Initially, the developing cranial portion of the neural tube lies dorsal and caudal to the oropharyngeal membrane. However, overgrowth of the forebrain causes it to extend past the oropharyngeal membrane and overhang the cardiogenic area. Subsequent growth of the forebrain pushes the developing heart ventrally and caudally to a position in the presumptive thoracic region caudal to the oropharyngeal membrane and cranial to the septum transversum that will form the central tendon of the diaphragm. Gastrulation **(answer a)** is the process by which epiblast cells migrate to the primitive streak and become internalized to form the mesodermal and endodermal germ layers. Lateral folding **(answer b)** of the embryo forms the endoderm tube and surrounding concentric layering of mesoderm and ectoderm. Neurulation refers to formation of the neural tube from surface ectoderm **(answer d)**. The fusion of the two endocardial heart tubes **(answer e)** occurs as lateral folding occurs. The fused tube will form the endocardium surrounded by the primordial myocardium derived from splanchnic mesoderm that will form the heart muscle (myocardium).

18. The answer is d. (*Moore and Persaud, Developing, pp 45–49,126. Sadler, pp 45–49.*) In the developing fetus, the maternal blood is in direct contact with the syncytiotrophoblast. During implantation, the syncytiotrophoblast invades the endometrium and erodes the maternal blood vessels. Maternal blood and nutrient glandular secretions fill the lacunae and bathe the projections of syncytiotrophoblast. Primary villi consist of syncytiotrophoblast with a core of cytotrophoblast cells. In secondary villi, the cytotrophoblast core is invaded by mesoderm and subsequently by umbilical blood vessels in tertiary villi.

19. The answer is c. *(Sadler, pp 112–117. Moore and Persaud, Developing, pp 171–185.)* Exposure of the embryo to harmful environmental factors (teratogens), such as chemicals, viruses, and/or radiation, can occur at any time. During the third through eighth weeks of embryonic life, organ systems are developing and are most susceptible to teratogens. During that time, each organ system has its own specific period of peak susceptibility. Exposure of the embryo to teratogens during the first 2 weeks of fetal life **(answers a and b)** generally induces spontaneous abortion and is, therefore, lethal. After the eighth week of intrauterine development **(answers d and e)**, teratogenic exposure generally results in retardation of organ growth rather than in new structural or functional changes.

20. The answer is e. *(Sadler, pp 67, 75, 135, 136, 305. Moore and Persaud, Developing, pp 171–172, 178, 439.)* Vitamin A is a member of the retinoic acid family. Retinoic acid directs the polarity of development in the central nervous system, the axial skeleton (vertebral column), and probably the appendicular skeleton. Retinoic acid induces transcription of various combinations of homeobox genes, depending on tissue type and location (distance and direction from the source of retinoic acid). Exogenous sources of retinoic acid may induce the wrong sequence or combination of homeobox genes, leading to structural abnormalities in nervous and skeletal systems. The other organ systems listed are not as susceptible to vitamin A **(answers a, b, c, and d)**.

21. The answer is a. *(Sadler, pp 104, 195, 206. Moore and Persaud, Developing, pp 139–141, 143, 158, 184, 196, 251, 295, 421.)* An amniotic fluid index of 27 cm is indicative of polyhydramnios. Duodenal and/or esophageal atresia result in an inability of the fetus to swallow amniotic fluid **(answer c)**. The result is that normal recirculation of amniotic fluid through the embryo is greatly reduced or eliminated, causing an excess of amniotic fluid. Excess amniotic fluid is defined as greater than 2000 mL in the third trimester. Low volumes of amniotic fluid (oligohydramnios) are caused by rupture of the fetal membranes, bilateral agenesis of the kidneys **(answer b)**, or obstructive uropathy **(answer e,** blockage of the calyces or ureters), which prevents urine from being added to the amniotic fluid. Hypoplasia of the lungs **(answer d)** and compression of the umbilical cord are associated with oligohydramnios, but do not cause it. The presence of adequate fluid in the uninflated lungs is essential for lung maturation, and growth factors in the amniotic fluid may also be important. Low levels of amniotic fluid severely inhibit lung development. The formula for understanding the relationship between urine and amniotic fluid is:

Less urine output = less amniotic fluid; less swallowing = more amniotic fluid.

22. The answer is a. *(Sadler, pp 67–71, 267. Moore and Persaud, Developing, pp 67–69. Alberts, pp 1086–1087, 1233.)* The first stage of neural tube formation is the induction by notochord and prechordal plate mesoderm of the neural plate that forms from ectoderm. This is known as primary induction and is accompanied by molecular changes in cell adhesion molecules [restriction to neural cell adhesion molecule (N-CAM)]. This first stage of neural tube development is followed by a reshaping phase, neurulation, and neural tube closure. Endoderm **(answer b)** is responsible for the formation of the GI tract and respiratory system. The somatopleuric mesoderm **(answer c)** makes important contributions to the skin (dermis) and nonmuscle portions of the limbs. The splanchnopleuric mesoderm **(answer d)** forms the heart and the muscles of the GI tract and urinary system. The hypoblast **(answer e)** is the thin layer of cells ventral to the epiblast; it is displaced by the epiblast cells, which form endoderm.

23. The answer is d. *(Sadler, pp 143–147.)* The muscles of the extremities form from the somites that are derived from paraxial mesoderm; the bones, tendons, and connective tissue of the extremities are derived from somatopleuric mesoderm. The intermediate mesoderm is the origin of the urogenital systems and the adrenal cortex **(answer a).** The adrenal medulla **(answer b)** forms from the neural crest. The humerus **(answer c)** forms from somatopleuric mesoderm, but the muscles attached to it are of somite origin. The masseter **(answer e)** is a muscle of mastication formed from the first branchial arch and innervated by branchial visceral efferent (special visceral efferent) fibers from the nucleus ambiguus compared with the general somatic efferent innervation of the biceps and other muscles, not of branchial arch origin.

24. The answer is a. *(Sadler, pp 300–303. Moore and Persaud, Developing, pp 432, 448–450, 473.)* The cerebral cortex forms from the telencephalon. The cortex develops in waves of proliferation, forming layers I to VI with the innermost layers forming first and the more superficial layers later. The wall of the developing CNS contains three layers: ventricular, mantle (intermediate), and marginal zones. The cortex, peripheral areas of gray matter, is formed through the migration of cells from the mantle zone to the marginal zone. Segmentation of the cranial neural tube forms the brain vesicles listed in the table below.

Primary Brain Vesicle	Secondary Brain Vesicle	Adult Brain Derivative
Prosencephalon (forebrain)	Telencephalon	Cerebral cortex, corpus striatum
	Diencephalon	Hypothalamus, thalamus
Mesencephalon (midbrain)	Mesencephalon	Superior and inferior colliculi
Rhombencephalon (hindbrain)	Metencephalon	Pons and cerebellum
	Myelencephalon	Medulla

25. The answer is c. (*Sadler, pp 11–12 .Moore and Persaud, Developing, pp 143, 304, 306, 308, 326.*) The primordial germ cells are first seen in the endodermal lining of the wall of the yolk sac (derived from the hypoblast) at the end of the third or beginning of the fourth week in the region of the allantois. During embryonic folding, the dorsal part of the yolk sac is incorporated into the embryo as the primitive gut. The primordial germ cells subsequently migrate along the dorsal mesentery of the hindgut **(answer a)** and into the gonadal (genital) ridge by week 6 **(answer b)**. The primary sex cords grow into the mesenchyme underlying the ridge, and the primordial germ cells become incorporated into the primary sex cords **(answer d)**. The chorion **(answer e)** is the outermost fetal membrane and is composed of extraembryonic somatic mesoderm, cytotrophoblast, and the syncytiotrophoblast. It is divided into the chorion frondosum, where the villi form and proliferate, and the smooth chorion, also known as the chorion laevae. The following diagram illustrates the arrangement of the fetal membranes.

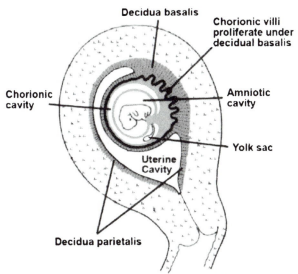

(Modified, with permission, from Sweeney L. Basic Concepts in Embryology. New York, NY: McGraw-Hill, 1998.)

26. The answer is e. *(Sadler, pp 12, 55–56, 58–59, 101, 203–206. Moore and Persaud, Developing, pp 44–49, 142–143.)* The yolk sac is important as a source of blood until the fetal liver replaces this function in about the sixth week of development. The yolk sac produces predominantly hematocytoblasts (stem cells) and primitive erythroblasts. Vasculogenesis is also initiated in the yolk sac. The endoderm of the yolk sac is incorporated into the embryo as part of the primitive gut during embryonic folding and is home to the primordial germ cells before they migrate to the hindgut. There is no yolk storage in human embryos **(answer a)**. The transfer of nutrients is an important function of the yolk sac early in development, but once the uteroplacental circulation is established, the placenta takes over that role **(answer b)**. The umbilical vein forms the ligamentum teres hepatis **(answer c)**. The cells of the amnion **(answer d)** form the amniotic fluid with eventual addition of urine from the developing kidneys. The diagram above illustrates the location of the yolk sac and other embryonic structures.

27. The answer is d. *(Sadler, pp 104–107. Moore and Persaud, Developing, pp 144–150. Alberts, p 1153.)* Monozygotic (MZ) twins arise from divisions of the embryoblast to form two embryos. MZ twins also form from early separation of the blastomeres. Basically, MZ twins can arise anywhere from the two-cell (blastomere) to the morula stage. MZ twins may have fused or separate placentae, separate or fused dichorionic sacs or one chorionic sac, and diamniotic sacs. Dizygotic (DZ) twins arise from fertilization of two oocytes by two sperm **(answer b)** and are merely "womb mates." They differ in genotype and, therefore, may be different sexes. Fertilization of one oocyte by two sperm **(answer c)** cannot occur because of the Ca^{2+}-dependent block to polyspermy (see question 6). That egg cortical reaction affects the zona pellucida in two ways: (1) hydrolysis of carbohydrate prevents sperm binding and (2) proteolytic activity hardens it.

28. The answer is b. (*Sadler, pp 63–72, 80. Moore and Persaud, Developing, pp 125–142.*) Each of the embryonic germ layers is continuous with an extraembryonic structure (see figure below). Ectoderm is continuous with the amniotic membrane, endoderm with the lining of the yolk sac **(answer c)**, and embryonic mesoderm with the extraembryonic mesoderm **(answer d)**. The chorion **(answer a)** consists of two parts, smooth (laeve) and villous (frondosum; see figure in feedback to question 25.) The villous chorion attaches to the decidua basalis of the placenta. There is no tunica adventitia in the umbilical vessels **(answer e)**.

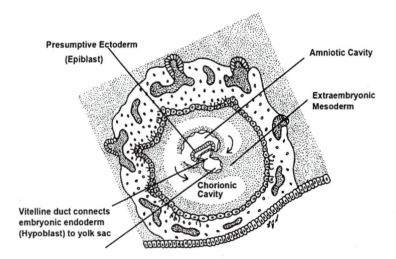

Presumptive Ectoderm (Epiblast)

Amniotic Cavity

Extraembryonic Mesoderm

Chorionic Cavity

Vitelline duct connects embryonic endoderm (Hypoblast) to yolk sac

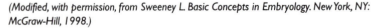

(*Modified, with permission, from Sweeney L. Basic Concepts in Embryology. New York, NY: McGraw-Hill, 1998.*)

29. The answer is a. *(Sadler, pp 157–162. Moore and Persaud, Developing, pp 60–69, 80–81, 336–338.)* The fusion of the dorsal aortae occurs through lateral folding. Fusion of the endocardial heart tube and incorporation of the yolk sac into the primitive gut also occurs as a result of lateral folding. Craniocaudal folding **(answer b)** establishes the definitive head and tail regions of the embryo. Fusion is already complete at the time that looping of the heart tube occurs **(answer c)**. Gastrulation **(answer d)** establishes the three germ layers (trilaminar disk), and neurulation establishes the neural groove with two neural folds. Neurulation is the formation of the neural tube **(answer e)**.

Cell Biology: Membranes

Questions

DIRECTIONS: Each item below contains a question or incomplete statement followed by suggested responses. Select the **one best** response to each question.

30. The region labeled with the arrow in the accompanying electron micrograph of the plasma membrane is responsible for which of the following functions?

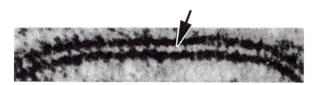

a. Creation of a barrier to water-soluble molecules
b. Specific cellular receptors for ligands
c. Catalyzing membrane-associated activities
d. Transport of small ions
e. Connections to the cytoskeleton

31. A 14-month-old boy presents with a fever of 102°F. The child has a longstanding history of recurrent lower respiratory tract infections including bronchitis and pneumonia. Chronic diarrhea is a longstanding problem. His mother reports that she had numerous upper respiratory infections and chronic diarrhea as a young child. A complete blood count, lung function tests, and urinalysis values are all within normal range. Serum immunoglobulin levels are normal for IgG and IgM, but IgA was 25 mg/dL (normal = 40–60 mg/dL). There are numerous neutrophils and other white cells in the stool sample and the stool is cultured for specific bacteria. IgA coats pathogens facilitating repulsion of the negative charge on the cell membrane. That negative charge on the cell membrane is primarily caused by which of the following?

a. Free saccharide groups
b. Glycoprotein
c. Cholesterol
d. Peripheral membrane protein
e. Integrins

32. The face labeled by asterisks in the freeze-fracture preparation shown below may be characterized as which of the following?

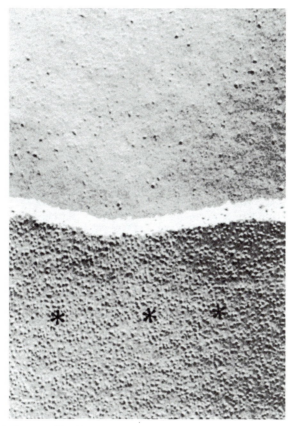

(Micrograph Courtesy of Dr. Giuseppina Raviola.)

a. Containing primarily glycoproteins and glycolipids
b. Facing away from the cytoplasm
c. In direct contact with the cytoplasm
d. Backed by the extracellular space
e. Generally possessing a paucity of intramembranous particles

33. Band 3 protein exists as a 95-kDa multipass membrane protein that functions as the primary anion exchanger in erythrocytes. Within the red blood cell (RBC) membrane, band 3 binds to spectrin dimers and tetramers indirectly through ankyrin. The spectrin tetramers are bound together by actin and band 4.1 protein, which also binds to band 3 and glycophorin. Null mutations in band 3 occur in the human population. Which of the following is most likely to decrease in the absence of band 3 protein?

a. Osmotic fragility
b. Destruction of RBCs in the spleen
c. Bile production
d. Erythroid production in the bone marrow
e. Blood pH

34. A 56-year-old man who drinks a six-pack of beer a day, with higher alcoholic intake on weekends, holidays, and "special days," presents to the internal medicine clinic. He has an abnormal plasma lipoprotein profile. It is known that erythrocyte fluidity is altered in liver disease. Which of the following would increase membrane fluidity in the hepatocytes of this patient's liver?

a. Restriction of rotational movement of proteins and lipids in the membrane
b. Transbilayer movement of phospholipids in the plasma membrane
c. Increased cholesterol/phospholipids ratio in the plasma membrane
d. Binding of integral membrane proteins with cytoskeletal elements
e. Binding of an antibody to a cell-surface receptor

35. The asymmetry of the cell membrane is established primarily by which of the following?

a. Membrane synthesis in the endoplasmic reticulum
b. Membrane modification in the Golgi apparatus
c. Presence of carbohydrates on the cytoplasmic surface
d. The distribution of cholesterol
e. Flipping proteins between the leaflets of the lipid bilayer

36. A 44-year-old African-American woman calls 911. When the MedAct unit arrives they find a patient with acute shortness of breath and audible wheezing. A physical exam reveals: pulse 115 (normal 60–100), RR 42 (normal 15–20) with signs of accessory muscle use. She is coughing up mucus. Auscultation reveals decreased breath sounds with wheezing on inspiration and expiration. The patient has taken her prescribed medications with no relief of symptoms prior to her 911 call. Her current medication is albuterol, a moderately selective β_2-receptor agonist. Which of the following is true regarding those receptors:

a. They possess a single hydrophobic transmembrane segment in the form of an α-helix.

b. They can activate plasma membrane–bound enzymes or ion channels

c. They possess an intracellular ligand-binding domain

d. They possess intrinsic enzyme activity

e. They are arranged so that both the amino- and the carboxy-terminals are located intracellularly

Cell Biology: Membranes

Answers

30. The answer is a. *(Ross and Pawlina, pp 28, 30. Alberts, pp 583–585.)* The hydrophobic layer of the cell (plasma) membrane is labeled with the arrow. It is responsible for the fundamental structure of the membrane and provides the barrier to water-soluble molecules in the external milieu. It also provides a two-dimensional solvent for membrane proteins. Other membrane functions are performed primarily by proteins that function as receptors, enzymes (catalysis of membrane-associated activities), and transporters **(answers b, c, and d)**. Connection to the cytoskeleton **(answer e)** is performed by members of the spectrin family of proteins reinforcing the membrane on the cytosolic side.

The membrane consists of a bilayer of phospholipids with the nonpolar, hydrophobic layer in the central portion of the membrane and the hydrophilic polar regions of the phospholipids in contact with the aqueous components at the intra- or extracellular surfaces of the membrane. Proteins are generally dispersed within the lipid bilayer. The polar head groups of the lipid bilayer react with osmium to create the trilaminar appearance observed in electron micrographs of the plasma membrane. Cell membranes range in thickness from 7 to 10 nm [$1 nm = 10^{-9} m$, $1 \mu m = 10^{-6} m$; the diameter of a red blood cell (erythrocyte) is 7 μm].

31. The answer is b. *(Alberts, pp 584, 612, 613. Junqueira, pp 23–25. Ross and Pawlina, pp 23–25. Kasper, pp 1943–1944.)* The child in the scenario suffers from IgA deficiency, the most common immunoglobulin deficiency. IgA functions in several ways, one of which is to coat pathogens with a negative charge that repels the polyanionic charge on the cell surface. In IgA deficiency, pathogens can more easily attach to the cell surface leading to persistent infections. The carbohydrate of biological membranes is found in the form of glycoproteins and glycolipids rather than as free saccharide groups **(answer a)**. The polyanionic charge of the membrane is produced by the sugar side chains on the glycoproteins and glycolipids. Glycoproteins often terminate in sialic acid side chains, which impart a negative (polyanionic) charge to the membrane. Similarly, the glycolipids (also called glycosphingolipids), particularly the gangliosides, terminate in sialic acid residues with a strong negative charge. Cholesterol **(answer c)** alters membrane fluidity (see figure below and question 34) and is amphipathic (hydrophilic and hydrophobic properties). It reduces the packing of lipid acyl groups through its steroid ring structure and hydrocarbon tail and cements hydrophilic regions of the membrane through interactions with its hydroxyl (OH⁻) region. Peripheral membrane proteins **(answer d)** are found primarily on the cytosolic leaflet of the membrane bilayer. Integrins **(answer e)** are heterodimeric receptors that bind with extracellular matrix (ECM) molecules such as laminin and fibronectin.

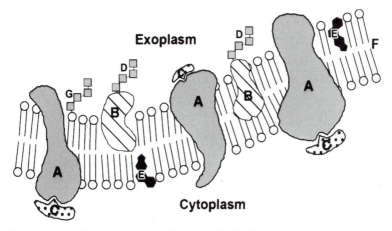

A = Integral membrane protein, B = Glycoprotein, C = Peripheral membrane protein (more abundant on cytosolic surface), D = sugar, E = cholesterol, F = hydrophobic fatty acid chains (hydrophilic polar head groups are not labeled), G = glycolipid

32. The answer is b. *(Alberts, p 567. Ross and Pawlina, p 30.)* The P face of a cell-membrane freeze fracture is labeled with the asterisks and faces away from the cytoplasm. Freeze fracture is a procedure in which the tissue is rapidly frozen and fractured with a knife. The fracture plane occurs through the hydrophobic central plane of membranes, which is the plane of least resistance to the cleavage force. The two faces are essentially the two interior faces of the membrane. They are described as the extracellular face (E face) and the protoplasmic face (P face). The cytoplasm is the backing for the P face, which in general contains numerous intramembranous particles (mostly protein). The E face is backed by the extracellular space and in general contains a paucity of intramembranous particles (see upper part of figure) compared with the P face (labeled with asterisks).

33. The answer is e. *(Alberts, pp 604–605. Rubin, p 1039. Kumar, pp 625–626. Kasper, pp 608–609.)* In its anion exchanger role, band 3 protein exchanges bicarbonate ion for chloride ion. Bicarbonate is transported by band 3 out of the RBC in exchange for chloride, permitting the highly efficient transport of CO_2 to the lungs as bicarbonate. In the absence of band 3 protein, the bicarbonate buffering of the blood is reduced, leading to acidosis or lowering of blood pH. The result is reduced capacity to carry CO_2. In addition to its functional, bidirectional anion exchanger role, band 3 plays a key membrane structural role, since the cytoplasmic domain of the protein interacts with spectrin through an ankyrin bridge. Spectrin exists as dimers and trimers; the trimers are bound together by actin, thus providing a connection to the cytoskeleton maintaining the shape and stability of the RBC. The result of a null mutation in band 3 is the formation of erythrocytes that are small and round instead of biconcave (spherocytosis). Spherocytes are osmotically fragile because of their decreased surface area per unit volume **(answer a)**. The defective RBCs do not readily pass through the small sinusoids of the spleen, resulting in destruction and further membrane conditioning, which leads to accelerated destruction **(answer b)** and, eventually, enlargement of the spleen (splenomegaly). The accelerated hemolysis leads to increased bile production **(answer c)** and jaundice. Hemoglobin production is also increased, as exemplified by an increase in mean corpuscular hemoglobin concentration (MCHC) by about 35 to 40%. The bone marrow compensates for the increased destruction of RBCs with hyperplasia of erythroid precursors in the bone marrow **(answer d)** and increase in the number of reticulocytes (polychromasia).

34. The answer is e. *(Alberts, pp 584–592, 608–612.)* The patient in the scenario is suffering from cirrhosis in which there are alterations in plasma lipoproteins. Binding of an antibody to a cell surface receptor results in lateral diffusion of protein in the lipid bilayer, resulting in increased membrane fluidity—patching and capping. Rotational and lateral movements of both proteins and lipids contribute to membrane fluidity. Restriction reduces membrane fluidity **(answer a)**. Phospholipids are capable of lateral diffusion, rapid rotation around their long axis, and flexion of their hydrocarbon (fatty acyl) tails. They undergo transbilayer movement **(answer b)**, known as "flip-flop," between bilayers in the endoplasmic reticulum; however, in general this does not occur in the plasma membrane. Other factors reduce membrane fluidity. An increase in the amount of cholesterol relative to phospholipid **(answer c)** has been shown by a variety of physicochemical techniques to decrease fluidity in both biological and artificial membranes by interacting with the hydrophobic regions near the polar head groups and stiffening this region of the membrane. Association or binding of integral membrane proteins with cytoskeletal elements **(answer d)** on the interior of the cell and peripheral membrane proteins on the extracellular surface limit membrane mobility and fluidity.

35. The answer is a. *(Alberts, pp 588–589.)* Asymmetry of the lipid bilayer is established during membrane synthesis in the endoplasmic reticulum **(answer a)** before reaching the Golgi apparatus **(answer b)**. Carbohydrates are associated with the N terminals of transmembrane proteins that extend from the extracellular surface, not the cytoplasmic surface **(answer c)**. Cholesterol is different from proteins and phospholipids that are asymmetrically distributed within the bilayer **(answer d)**. Cholesterol is found on both sides of the bilayer. The small polar head group structure of cholesterol allows it to flip-flop from leaflet to leaflet and respond to changes in shape. In contrast to cholesterol, most proteins and phospholipids are capable of only rare flip-flop **(answer e)**. For example, transbilayer movement of phospholipid is limited mostly to the endoplasmic reticulum.

36. The answer is b. *(Alberts, pp 595–596, 868–870. Junqueira, pp 28–30.)* Albuterol binds to β-receptors, which are multipass G-protein-linked receptors. Binding to G-protein-linked receptors activates or inactivates enzymes bound to the plasma membrane (adenylyl cyclase or phospholipase C) or opens or closes ion channels using G proteins. A table of G proteins and their functions appears below. The β-receptors, as well as muscarinic cholinergic receptors and rhodopsin, are multipass transmembrane **(answer a)** proteins consisting specifically of seven hydrophobic spanning segments of the single polypeptide chain. The peptide bonds of the spanning segments are polar. In the hydrophobic environment of the lipid bilayer, in the absence of water, they form hydrogen bonds with each other. There is a remarkable homology between the cell-surface receptors linked to the G proteins. Ligand binding occurs on the extracellular surface **(answer c)**. Receptors with intrinsic enzyme activity belong to a separate class of single-pass transmembrane proteins (**answer d**). All of these transmembrane proteins show a carboxyl terminus on the cytosolic side and N-linked glycosylation sites on the extracellular surface (**answer e**).

TRIMERIC G PROTEINS AND THEIR FUNCTIONS	
G Protein	**Function**
G_s	Adenylyl cyclase
G_{olf}	Adenylyl cyclase (in olfactory neurons)
G_i	Adenylyl cyclase
G_o	Phospholipase C; K^+ and Ca^{2+} channels
G_t (transducin)	cGMP (specific to rod photoreceptors)
G_q	Phospholipase C

Cell Biology: Cytoplasm

Questions

DIRECTIONS: Each item below contains a question or incomplete statement followed by suggested responses. Select the **one best** response to each question.

37. A patient is diagnosed with a pleomorphic adenoma of the submandibular gland. The pathologist uses anti-vimentin antibodies with immunocytochemistry to stain the biopsy tissue. One would expect to find vimentin staining in which of the following structures?

a. Fibrous stromal connective tissue
b. Parasympathetic ganglia
c. Serous acini
d. Mucous acini
e. Striated ducts

38. Which of the following is the function of the large subunit of the ribosome?

a. Bind messenger RNA (mRNA)
b. Bind transfer RNA (tRNA)
c. Catalyze peptide bond formation
d. Link adjacent ribosomes in a polyribosome
e. Initiate protein synthesis

39. The stability and arrangement of actin filaments as well as their properties and functions depend on which of the following?

a. The structure of the actin filaments
b. Microtubules
c. Intermediate filament proteins
d. Actin-binding proteins
e. Motor molecules, such as kinesin

40. A 47-year-old man presents with fatigue and over the next few years became progressively weaker, eventually becoming paralyzed. He encounters severe problems with speech and swallowing. Weakness and paralysis of the thoracic muscles leads to progressive respiratory insufficiency and death. At autopsy transmission electron microscopy reveals fragmentation of the structures delineated by the arrows within motoneurons. Which of the following correctly characterizes these structures?

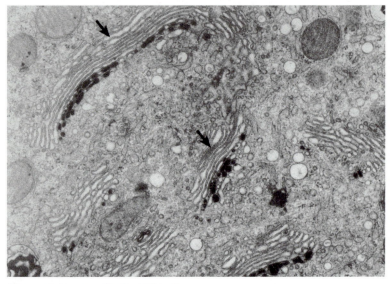

(Micrograph Courtesy of Dr. Doniel Friend.)

a. There is no functional, topological specialization within the stacks
b. They present an entry face associated with granule formation
c. They present a *trans* face associated with COP-II-coated transport vesicles
d. They are biochemically compartmentalized
e. They receive proteins but not lipids

41. The primary function of intermediate filaments is which of the following?

a. Generate movement
b. Provide mechanical stability
c. Carry out nucleation of microtubules
d. Stabilize microtubules against disassembly
e. Transport organelles within the cell

42. A 20-year-old man arrives in the emergency room by ambulance. He has taken an overdose of "goof balls" (Phenobarbital) he obtained from a drug dealer on the street. In a hepatocyte from this patient, what is occurring in the organelle labeled with arrows in the accompanying transmission electron micrograph?

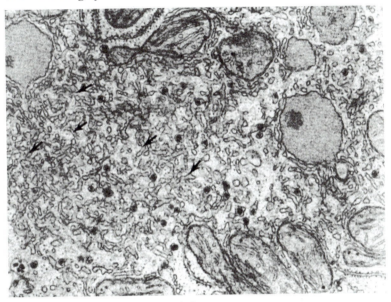

(Micrograph Courtesy of Dr. Robert Bolender.)

  a. Oxidative demethylation
  b. Decreased P450 expression
  c. Decreased solubility of the phenobarbital
  d. Increased synthesis of enzymes for detoxification
  e. Destruction of the phenobarbital by acid hydrolases

43. Which of the following mechanisms is used to establish the mitochondrial electrochemical gradient?

  a. The action of ATP synthase
  b. Transfer of electrons from NADH to O_2 in the intermembrane space
  c. Pumping of protons into the mitochondrial matrix by respiratory chain activity
  d. Proton-translocating activity in the inner membrane
  e. Transport of ATP out of the matrix compartment by a specific transporter

44. A 15-month-old girl is referred for ophthalmologic and neurologic follow-up by her pediatrician. The child has shown a failure to thrive, is microcephalic, exhibits myoclonic jerks, delayed psychomotor development, visual disturbance and seizures. Analysis of fibroblasts from the skin by electron microscopy confirms the presence of fingerprint inclusion bodies. Elevated levels of dolichol are found in the urine. Normally, dolichol is associated with which cellular process:

a. Sulfation in the *trans* compartment of the Golgi
b. O-linked glycosylation in the medial compartment of the Golgi
c. O-linked glycosylation in the *cis* compartment of the Golgi
d. N-linked glycosylation in the endoplasmic reticulum
e. Sorting of proteins to the lysosome from the TGN

45. A boy is born with epicanthal folds, a high forehead, hypoplastic supraorbital ridges, and upslanting palpebral fissures. He shows growth retardation following birth, he feels like a rag doll when held, and he exhibits neonatal seizures. He also has a ventricular septal defect, glaucoma, cataracts, elevated iron and copper levels in his blood, and hepatomegaly. A liver biopsy is prepared for electron microscopy and shows the presence of empty peroxisomes. The pathologist describes them as peroxisome "ghosts." Which of the following cellular activities should be decreased in the hepatocytes from this patient?

a. Energy production
b. Plasmalogen synthesis
c. Exocytosis
d. Detoxification by the smooth endoplasmic reticulum
e. Lysosomal enzyme synthesis

46. Inhibition of actin assembly by cytochalasins would interfere primarily with which of the following?

a. Separation of chromosomes in anaphase of the cell cycle
b. Vesicular transport between the Golgi apparatus and cell membrane
c. Ciliary movement
d. Phagocytic activity by macrophages
e. The structure of centrioles

47. Chloroquine is a weak base that neutralizes acidic organelles. In a pancreatic beta cell, which of the following would be a direct effect of chloroquine treatment?

a. Increased proinsulin content in secretory vesicles
b. Increased release of C peptide
c. Increased number of amylase-containing secretory vesicles
d. Reduced translation of glucagon mRNA
e. Increased stability of insulin mRNA

48. A 6 month-old boy is brought to the pediatric neurology clinic as a referral from a pediatrician concerned about the child's developmental delay, ataxia, hyperventilation, and repeated episodes of vomiting. The parents report one "seizure-like event." Your examination reveals hypotonia, some spasticity, and deafness. You note mild choreoathetosis when the boy is attempting to move. Laboratory results show high lactate in the cerebrospinal fluid, a muscle biopsy shows normal histology, but tests reveal a deficiency in Cytochrome C Oxidase, complex IV. In the electron micrograph below, where would you expect to find that enzyme localized?

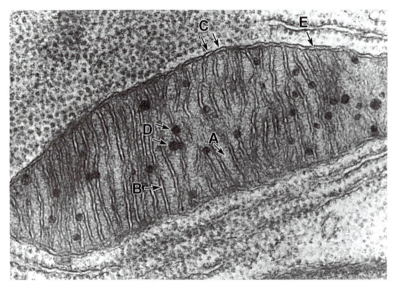

(Reproduced, with permission, from Fawcett DW: The Cell, 2/e. Philadelphia: WB Saunders, 1981.)

a. A
b. B
c. C
d. D
e. E

49. A 22-year-old woman presents at the ophthalmology clinic. She describes an initial inability to drive at night because of what she describes as "night blindness." She says that the deterioration of her vision has continued and she is having difficulty seeing objects on the periphery of her vision. Visual acuity, color, visual field, dark adaptation, and ERG testing is completed. The tests show rod degeneration with limited peripheral vision. She has pigment deposits in the mid-peripheral retina known as "bone spicules" She also has attenuated vessels in the retina and paleness of the optic nerves. An electroretinogram (ERG) is reduced in amplitude. The cause may be related to a failure of opsin and other protein vesicle transport. This transport would occur along which of the following?

a. Microfilaments (thin filaments)
b. Thick filaments
c. Microtubules
b. Intermediate filaments
e. Spectrin heterodimers

50. Which of the following molecules forms the coating of vesicles involved in transport of secretory vesicles from the *trans*-Golgi network (TGN) to targets?

a. Clathrin
b. Spectrin
c. Ankyrin
d. Actin
e. Vimentin
f. COP I
g. COP II

51. A girl to parents of eastern Mediterranean Jewish descent is brought to the pediatric neurology clinic. She appeared normal at birth and is now 6 months of age. There is a loss of peripheral vision and an abnormal startle response to auditory stimuli. She has suddenly shown a loss of coordination and has lost some responsiveness to her environment. She has a cherry-red spot on her macula. Treatments to cure this disease might focus on developing therapies that would do which of the following?

a. Stimulate ganglioside GM2 production
b. Stimulate synthesis of GM2 by the rough endoplasmic reticulum
c. Stimulate hexosaminidase production
d. Stimulate transport of ganglioside GM2 to the lysosome
e. Remove mannose-6-phosphate from hexosaminidase

52. A 14-year-old boy presents with hepatic failure, slurred speech, tremors in the hands and feet, and Kayser-Fleischer rings. A 24 hour urine copper test is 120 micrograms (μg)/24 hours (normal below 100 μg/24 hours) and ceruloplasmin of 15 mg/dL (normal 25 to 50 mg/dL). Liver biopsy reveals 295 μg/g (normal <250 μg/g) dry weight of copper with microscopic changes including glycogen nuclei, microvesicular and macrovesicular fatty changes, steatosis and fibrosis. Genetic studies reveal mutations in the ATP7B gene which has been localized to the late endosome. Such mutations may alter the transport of cargo within late endosomes to which of the following?

a. Lysosome for degradation
b. Clathrin-coated pits and vesicles
c. Multivesicular bodies
d. Cell surface to recycle receptors
e. TGN for further processing

53. A 72-year-old woman is brought to the office of her family medicine physician by her daughter. Her daughter indicates that mom has abrupt mood swings and uncharacteristic moments of anger and aggressiveness. Recently, she drove to her daughter's house for her granddaughter's birthday party and "got lost" returning to her own apartment, eventually completing the 2 mile drive in 2 hours. The patient has recently been unwilling or unable to bathe or brush her teeth regularly and her hair is unkempt. There are grease stains on her blouse. She has lost 15 pounds since her last visit to her physician a year ago. While the patient denies any problems with memory or cognitive ability her daughter reports episodes of forgetfulness and loss of concentration. The pathogenesis of the disease from which this patient suffers, involves the organelles labeled with asterisks in the accompanying electron micrograph. Which of the following processes occurs abnormally in that structure during the progression of this patient's illness?

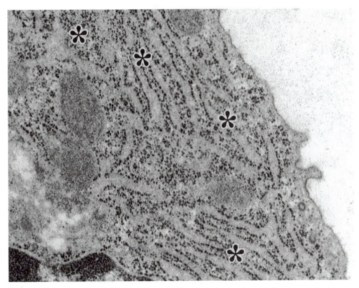

(Micrograph Courtesy of Dr. Kuen-Shan Hang.)

a. O-linked glycosylation
b. Sorting of tau proteins
c. Sulfation of amyloid precursor protein
d. Conformational changes and folding
e. Glycogenolysis

Cell Biology: Cytoplasm

Answers

37. The answer is a. (*Alberts, pp 923–929.*) Anti-vimentin is specific for mesenchymal cells such as fibroblasts, macrophages, endothelial cells, and smooth muscle of the vasculature. In the salivary glands fibrous stromal tissue is derived from mesenchyme. The acini and ducts (**answers c, d, and e**) are derived from epithelium. The parasympathetic ganglia will stain with pan-neuronal markers such as peripherin (**answer b**). The type of intermediate filament protein is relatively specific for cells derived from the three embryonic germ layers. Antibodies to intermediate filament proteins have been used by pathologists to determine the origin of tumors. Intermediate filament proteins have a structural role but also are involved in the anchorage of the proteins that form ion channels. Cytokeratins (also known as keratins) are specific for epithelial cells. Neurofilament proteins (NFL, NFM, and NFH) are found in neurons. In Alzheimer's disease, extensive plaques of neurofilament proteins occur. Desmin is found in striated and most smooth muscle, except vascular smooth muscle. Glial fibrillary acidic protein, GFAP, is specific for astrocytes, not microglia or oligodendrocytes.

38. The answer is c. (*Alberts, pp 343–346. Ross and Pawlina, p 46.*) The large subunit of the ribosome catalyzes peptide bond formation by activation of peptidyl transferase. The small ribosomal subunit contains the peptidyl-tRNA-binding (P) site that binds the tRNA molecule (**answer a**) attached to the carboxyl end of the growing end of the polypeptide chain. The small subunit also contains the aminoacyl-tRNA-binding (A) site that holds the incoming tRNA and amino acid. The initiation factors are loaded on the small ribosomal subunit that must locate the AUG (start) codon to initiate protein synthesis. This occurs before binding of the large subunit. In addition, the initiator tRNA containing methionine provides the amino acid necessary to start protein synthesis. The initiator tRNA is also located on the small subunit. It resides at the P site (the normal peptidyl site) even though it is an aminoacyl-tRNA. This occurs before binding to the mRNA (**answer b**). Therefore, the initiation phase of protein synthesis is regulated by the small subunit of the ribosome **(answer d)**. Ribosomes are composed of both protein and RNA (predominantly rRNA, but also mRNA and tRNA). Single ribosomes are involved in synthesis of cytosolic proteins. Polyribosomes, linked by mRNA **(answer e)**, synthesize proteins that are translocated into the cisternal space of the rough endoplasmic reticulum (RER) and destined for export or specific organelles.

39. The answer is d. *(Alberts, pp 923, 936, 940–944.)* The stability, arrangement, and functions of actin filaments depend on the actin-binding proteins. The fundamental structure of the actin molecule is the same no matter what the function or arrangement in a cell. Actin-binding proteins have a variety of functions: (1) tropomyosin strengthens actin filaments, (2) fibrin and villin are actin-bundling proteins, (3) filamin and gelsolin regulate transformation from the sol to the gel state, (4) members of the myosin II family are responsible for sliding filaments, (5) myosin I (minimyosin) is responsible for movement of vesicles on filaments, and (6) spectrin cross-links the sides of actin filaments to the plasma membrane.

40. The answer is d. *(Alberts, pp 736–738. Ross and Pawlina, pp 48–51. Junqueira, pp 35–37.)* The biochemically compartmentalized organelle, labeled with the arrows in the electron micrograph, is the Golgi apparatus. There is a specific organization to the Golgi stacks related to the function of specific enzymes. Histochemical stains, such as acid phosphatase and nucleoside diphosphates, show that the Golgi apparatus is topologically compartmentalized **(answer a)**. It presents two faces: a *cis* face, which is the point of entry of transport vesicles (COP-II-coated, see question 50 feedback) in transit from the rough endoplasmic reticulum (RER) to the Golgi **(answer b)**, and a *trans* face, which is the exit point associated with granule formation and the maturation of proteins **(answer c)**. Both proteins and lipids are transported from the transitional elements of the ER to the Golgi apparatus **(answer e)**. Packaging is not the sole function of the Golgi. This organelle is also involved in the processing of proteins (e.g., addition and trimming of oligosaccharide chains) that was initiated in the RER as well as sulfation.

41. The answer is b. *(Alberts, pp 801–803, 952–953. Ross and Pawlina, pp 57–58.)* There are differences in the way that intermediate filaments interact with microtubules and microfilaments within the cytoplasm; however, their ropelike arrangement is well suited to providing mechanical stability to the cell and resisting stretch, allowing the cell to respond to tension. The different types of intermediate filaments all have a similar structural pattern: nonhelical head and tail segments with a helical arrangement in the center of the intermediate filament structure. Movement is generated by motor proteins (**answer a**) such as myosin, dynein, and kinesin. There is a good mnemonic device for remembering the direction of movement directed by kinesin and dynein. Kinesin kicks the molecules out; dynein drags them in; also, the plus end of the microtubule is oriented toward the plasma membrane, so minus end toward nucleus. This works for fibroblasts as well as neurons, to be discussed in a later chapter. Nucleation of microtubules is conducted by centrosomes (**answer c**); microtubule-associated proteins (MAPs) stabilize or destabilize microtubules (**answer d**). Microtubules function in organellar transport—for example, axonal transport (**answer e**).

42. The answer is a. (*Alberts, pp 691–693. Ross and Pawlina, pp 47–48.*) Oxidative metabolism by cytochrome p450 enzymes in hepatocytes is a primary mechanism for drug metabolism. Barbiturates are modified in the liver by oxidative demethylation through the P450 oxidase system found in the smooth endoplasmic reticulum (SER) (the structure shown in the electron micrograph). The SER in hepatocytes responds to Phenobarbital ingestion by increasing its volume. The proliferation (hypertrophy) of the SER facilitates metabolism of drugs. There is a concomitant increase in enzymatic activity, however, the synthesis of those enzymes occurs in the rough endoplasmic reticulum (RER) not in the SER (**answer d**). The purpose of drug metabolism is to make drugs more water soluble (**answer c**) so they can be more easily excreted from the liver through the bile. Increase in enzymatic activity following Phenobarbital ingestion catalyzes reactions that increase the solubility of various xenobiotics including toxins, alcohol, steroids, eicosanoids, carcinogens, insecticides, and other environmental pollutants. Lysosomes not the SER contain acid hydrolases (**answer e**). The P450 system and the SER are involved in drug interactions. Hepatocytes adapted to metabolize one drug may develop increased capability to metabolize other drugs. For example, if patients taking Phenobarbital for epilepsy increase their alcohol intake they may be ingesting subtherapeutic levels of the antiseizure medication because of induction of smooth ER in response to the alcohol.

43. The answer is d. (*Alberts, pp 769–783. Junqueira, pp 29–30, 32. Ross and Pawlina, pp 52–54.*) The mitochondrial electrochemical gradient is established by a proton pump. The pump is located in the inner membrane, associated with the respiratory chain and ATP synthase. The impermeability of the inner membrane to protons causes an osmotic and electrochemical gradient to develop. Mitochondria produce energy that the cell uses in transport and other energy-dependent processes. Cellular energy is stored as ATP, which is synthesized by the phosphorylation of ADP by ATP synthase **(answer a)**. Mitochondria use the electron-transport (respiratory) chain that transfers energy from NADH to O_2 **(answer b)**. As electrons released by oxidation of substrate in the matrix flow down the respiratory chain, hydrogen ions are pumped into the intermembrane space **(answer c)**. Protons in the matrix drive ATP synthase in a mechanism similar to that of a waterwheel. ATP synthase, therefore, couples oxidative transport through the electron-transport (respiratory) chain with energy storage (ATP). ATP is not transported out of the matrix compartment by a specific transporter **(answer e)**.

44. The answer is d. (*Alberts, pp 702–703. Mole, pp 70–76.*) The patient is suffering from the infantile form of Batten's disease, neuronal ceroid lipofuscinoses, in which there is a build-up of lipofuscin because of the absence of specific lysosomal enzymes. Dolichol is normally associated with N-linked glycosylation in the rough endoplasmic reticulum (RER) an *en bloc* method in which dolichol is added to the protein. O-linked glycosylation occurs in the Golgi, by a mechanism involving oligosaccharide (glycosyl) transferases rather than *en bloc* with dolichol **(answers b and c)**. N-linked oligosaccharides are the most common oligosaccharides found in glycoproteins and contain sugar residues linked to the NH_2 amide nitrogen of asparagine. O-linked oligosaccharides have sugar residues linked to hydroxyl groups on the side chains of serine and threonine. The diversity in oligosaccharides is produced by selective removal of glucose and mannose from the core oligosaccharide. This trimming process begins in the RER before reaching the Golgi, where the final mannose-residue trimming occurs. Sulfation **(answer a)** and protein sorting **(answer e)** are carried out in the Golgi apparatus, but do *not* involve dolichol.

45. The answer is b. (*Alberts, pp 687–688. Ross and Pawlina, p 55. Junquiera, p 40.*) The child suffers from Zellweger syndrome, in which peroxisomes are empty. Peroxisomes are the sole site of plasmalogen synthesis. Plasmalogen is a group of glycerol-based phospholipids in which the aliphatic side chains are not attached by ester linkages. They have a widespread distribution with highest concentrations in the brain, spinal cord, liver, and kidney. Energy production (**answer a**), exocytosis (**answer c**), detoxification (**answer d**), and the synthesis of lysosomal enzymes (**answer e**) would not be affected in that disease. In Zellweger syndrome, peroxisomes are empty because of the failure of the signal system that sorts protein to the peroxisome. Because the peroxisome lacks a genome (DNA) or synthetic machinery (ribosomes), it must import all proteins. The defect appears to be in the peroxisomal membrane (peroxins), but errors or absence of the peroxisomal signal sequence would result in the same symptoms. Peroxisomes have only a single membrane around them and contain catalase. Peroxisomes carry out oxidation reactions to protect the cell. Those oxidation reactions remove hydrogen atoms from molecules like alcohol and phenols to form hydrogen peroxide. In the peroxidative reaction, catalase breaks down hydrogen peroxide to water and oxygen. Most of the alcohol humans consume is broken down by the ADH (alcohol dehydrogenase) and MEOS (microsomal ethanol-oxidizing system, that is, P450 cytochrome) pathways in the hepatocyte (liver cell) cytoplasm; the remaining small percentage is broken down by oxidation in the peroxisomes of hepatocytes using catalase. See "High-Yield Facts" page 30 for more information on alcohol metabolism.

46. The answer is d. (*Alberts, pp 928, 966–968, 976, 1041–1042.*) Cytochalasins are potent inhibitors of cell motility and other cellular events that depend on actin assembly: cytokinesis, which is conducted by the actin-containing contractile ring; phagocytosis; and formation of lamellipodia. Cytochalasins bind to the plus end of actin filaments and prevent further polymerization. The movement of chromosomes in anaphase of the cell cycle depends on disassembly of microtubules at the kinetochore in anaphase A and addition at the plus end of the polar microtubules in anaphase B (**answer a**). Ciliary movement, vesicular transport, and the structure of centrioles depend on microtubules (**answers b, c, and e**).

47. The answer is a. (*Alberts, pp 758–761.*) Chloroquine neutralizes acidic compartments such as the secretory vesicles. Chloroquine treatment inhibits the conversion of proinsulin to insulin, resulting in decreased formation of insulin within secretory vesicles. Acidification causes concentration of the contents of secretory vesicles, facilitates breakdown of the contents of phagosomes and lysosomes, and is involved in the cleavage of prohormones to their active forms (e.g., proinsulin to insulin). The acidification process functions through a vacuolar H^+ (proton) pump that is present in the membranes of most endocytic and exocytic vesicles, including those of the phagosomes, lysosomes, secretory vesicles, and some compartments of the Golgi. Ribosomes are not dependent on a proton pump mechanism and are, therefore, less sensitive to chloroquine. Note that pancreatic beta cells synthesize insulin. Proinsulin is split into C-peptide + insulin in secretory vesicles **(answer b)**. *In vivo*, C-peptide release can be used to measure production of insulin by a patient's pancreatic beta cells. This is particularly useful in patients who are receiving insulin. Glucagon is synthesized by alpha cells **(answer d)**, and amylase is an exocrine pancreatic product produced by the acinar cells **(answer e)**. Gene and message expression and message stability are also *not* targets for chloroquine **(answers d and e)**.

48. The answer is b. *(Alberts, pp 770–774. Junqueira, pp 30–33.)* The structure labeled B is the inner membrane of the mitochondrion, which is highly impermeable to small ions because of the presence of cardiolipin. The inner membrane contains the proteins required for the oxidative reactions of the respiratory transport chain; it is the location of the cytochromes, dehydrogenases, and flavoproteins including cytochrome C as well as the transmembrane complex (ATP synthase) that is responsible for ATP synthesis. The inner membrane is folded into convolutions called cristae. The number of cristae is directly related to the metabolic activity of the cell. The elementary particles that have been identified on the cristae are composed primarily of ATP synthase complexes. The patient in the vignette is suffering from Leigh's Disease (Subacute Necrotizing Encephalomyelopathy), a generalized (systemic) form of Cytochrome C oxidase (COX) Deficiency, characterized by progressive degeneration of the brain and dysfunction of the heart, kidneys, muscles, and liver. Symptoms include loss of acquired motor skills and loss of appetite, vomiting, irritability, and/or seizure activity. As Leigh's Disease progresses, symptoms include generalized weakness; loss of muscle tone (hypotonia); and/or episodes of lactic acidosis with lactate higher in the CSF than the blood. The region labeled **A** in the electron micrograph of the mitochondrion is the mitochondrial matrix, or intercristal space. The matrix contains the circular DNA of the mitochondrial genome. Most mitochondrial proteins are encoded for by nuclear DNA, but small proportions are encoded within the mitochondrial DNA and are synthesized on mitochondrial ribosomes. The matrix also contains the enzymes responsible for the Krebs (citric acid) cycle. The outer mitochondrial membrane, labeled **C**, is highly permeable to molecules 10,000 Da or less because of the presence of porin, a channel-forming protein. This membrane contains enzymes involved in lipid synthesis and lipid metabolism. Matrix granules represent accumulations of calcium ions (**D**). The outer membrane also mediates the movement of fatty acids into the mitochondria for use in the formation of acetyl CoA. The intermembrane space (**E**) is the site of cytochrome b and other unique proteins.

49. The answer is c. (*Alberts, pp 923–927, 952–953, 966–968. Rubin, pp 1518, 1519. Kumar, p 172. Junqueira, pp 464–465.*) The woman in the scenario suffers from retinitis pigmentosa. Vesicles and organelles move unidirectionally along microtubules from the inner segment to the outer segment of the photoreceptor. Opsin, which is needed to sense light, is transported to sites of utilization in the disks of the outer segment. Transport occurs through the connecting, non-motile cilium, driven by the microtubule motor, kinesin, an ATPase. Microtubules are composed of tubulin and are involved in motility as the principal protein in the composition of the axoneme (the core of the cilium or flagellum). Microfilaments (thin filaments) are composed of actin, the most abundant protein in cells of eukaryotes (**answer a**). They are involved in cell motility and changes in cell shape. Myosin is the main constituent of the thick filament (**answer b**) that binds to actin and functions as an ATPase activated by actin. Intermediate filaments (**answer d**) that are "intermediate" in diameter (8 to 10 nm) between thin and thick filaments are of five different types. Type I and type II are the acidic and basic keratins (cytokeratins) respectively and are found specifically in epithelial cells. Type III intermediate filaments are composed of vimentin, desmin, and glial fibrillary acidic protein (GFAP). Vimentin is found in cells of mesenchymal origin, desmin in muscle cells, and glial fibrillary acidic protein in astrocytes. Type IV intermediate filaments are neurofilament proteins found in neurons. Type V intermediate filaments include the nuclear lamins A, B, and C and are associated with nuclear lamina of all cells. Spectrin heterodimers stabilize the plasma membrane and connect the membrane to actin (**answer e**).

50. The answer is a. (*Alberts, pp 601–602, 713, 716–719, 908–909, 923–927.*) Clathrin is an important protein that forms the coating of: secretory vesicles transported from the TGN to targets and coated pits and vesicles involved in endocytosis. It is involved in the retrieval of membrane following exocytosis. Spectrin heterodimers **(answer b)** form tetramers that interact with actin and provide flexibility and support for the membrane. The protein ankyrin **(answer c)** "anchors" the band 3 protein to the spectrin-membrane skeleton indirectly binding band 3 protein to the cytoskeleton (spectrin tetramers) of the red blood cell (RBC). The band 3 protein is known to be an anion transport protein of the RBC. Actin **(answer d)** is the protein found in thin filaments in the RBC cytoplasm. Intermediate filaments are important cytoskeletal elements with specificity that depends on the origin of the cells in question. Vimentin **(answer e)** is specific for cells derived from mesenchyme, e.g., fibroblasts and chondrocytes. COP-I (COat Protein-I) coats vesicles involved in retrograde transport from Golgi→RER **(answer f)**. COP-II is the coat protein for vesicles transported in an anterograde direction from the RER→Golgi **(answer g)**.

51. The answer is c. (*Ross and Pawlina, p 44. Kasper, p 2318. Kumar, pp 160–161. Rubin, pp 254–255.*) The child in the scenario suffers from Tay-Sachs disease, a lysosomal storage disease. Lysosomes contain an array of specific hydrolases. In Tay-Sachs disease, hexosaminidase A is deficient, resulting in the buildup of GM2 ganglioside and leading to mental retardation, blindness, and mortality. A pharmacological approach would target reducing GM2 ganglioside levels by increasing hexosaminidase A activity **(answer c)**. Increase in GM2 levels **(answers a and b)** or increased transport **(answer d)** to a lysosome deficient in hexosaminidase would worsen the disease. The table on page 124 summarizes the enzyme deficiencies and resulting effects in some of the more prominent lysosomal disorders. Mannose-6-phosphate and its receptor are involved in the trafficking of proteins to the lysosomal compartment. Removal of mannose 6-phosphate **(answer e)**, as occurs in inclusion-cell (I-cell) disease, would result in default of lysosomal enzymes to the secretory pathway, and the hexosaminidase deficiency would worsen.

LYSOSOMAL STORAGE DISEASES

Disease	Enzyme Deficit	Cellular Site	Accumulation	Organ Most Affected
Tay-Sachs	β-N-hexosaminidase-A	Neurons	Glycolipid	CNS
Gaucher	β-D-glycosidase	Macrophages	Glycolipid	Spleen, liver
Hurler	α-L-iduronidase	Fibroblasts, chondroblasts, osteoblasts	Dermatan sulfate	Skeletal system
Niemann-Pick	Sphingomyelinase	Oligodendrocytes, fibroblasts	Sphingomyelin	CNS
Inclusion (I)–cell	N-acetylglucosamine-phosphotransferase	Fibroblasts, macrophages	Glycoproteins and glycolipids	Nervous and skeletal systems (liver unaffected)

52. The answer is a. *(Alberts, pp 742–743, Fig. 13-35. Rubin, pp 785–787. Kumar, pp 910–911. Kapser, pp 409–410.)* The patient in the scenario suffers from Wilson's disease in which copper accumulates in the tissues. For example, in the liver the mutation in ATP7B prevents translocation of copper from the cytosol to the late endosome blocking biliary copper excretion via lysosomes and resulting in accumulation of copper in the liver. The late endosome is part of the endocytic pathway. Cargo proteins from the late endosome reach the lysosome by development into lysosomes, transport to lysosomes via vesicles, or fusion with lysosomes. Clathrin-coated pits and vesicles **(answer b)** endocytose and subsequently deliver proteins to the early endosome in the first stages of the endocytic process. Multivesicular bodies (MVBs) are the means of transport from early to late endosomes **(answer c).** The CGN (*cis*-Golgi network) receives transitional elements in the form of coatomer-coated vesicles carrying proteins and lipids from the rough endoplasmic reticulum and participates in phosphorylation. The remaining Golgi stacks are the *cis*, medial, *trans*, and TGN (trans-Golgi network). The medial compartment is responsible for the removal of mannose and the addition of N-acetylglucosamine. The *trans* face is responsible for the addition of sialic acid and galactose. The TGN serves as a sorting station for proteins destined for various organelles (e.g., lyosomes), the plasma membrane, and protein for export from the cell **(answer e).** Golgi-derived transport and secretory vesicles bud off from the TGN. Recycling of receptors occurs from early endosomes to the plasma membrane **(answer d).**

53. The answer is d. *(Junqueira, pp 34–35.)* The predominant organelle in the transmission electron micrograph is the rough endoplasmic reticulum (RER). Different proteins display different rates of folding in the ER, and these rates determine the time required for transport to the cell surface. Within the ER there are protein chaperones and mechanisms to prevent aberrant protein folding and to catalyze isomerization of correct covalent bonds. Frequently, changes in the extracellular environment result in aberrant protein folding in the ER as occurs in Alzheimer disease from which the patient in the vignette suffers. O-linked glycosylation, sorting of proteins and sulfation **(answers a, b and c)** occur in the Golgi apparatus and glycogenolysis **(answer e)** occurs in the smooth endoplasmic reticulum.

Cell Biology: Intracellular Trafficking

Questions

DIRECTIONS: Each item below contains a question or incomplete statement followed by suggested responses. Select the **one best** response to each question.

54. Endocytosis of low-density lipoprotein (LDL) differs from phagocytosis of damaged cells in which of the following?

a. Use of membrane-enclosed vesicles in the uptake process
b. Coupling with the lysosomal system
c. Dependence on acidification
d. Use of clathrin-coated pits
e. Use of hydrolases

55. In the signal hypothesis, which of the following is the function of the signal recognition particle (SRP)?

a. Binds the N-terminal sequence of the newly synthesized peptide to the ribosome
b. Induces an immediate increase in the translation rate
c. Prevents degradation of newly synthesized peptides by proteases
d. Binds the docking protein to the ER membrane
e. Enzymatically cleaves the newly synthesized peptide from the signal sequence

56. A 65-year-old man presents to the neurology clinic with a several year history in which he has less and less energy and spontaneity, memory loss (especially recent events), and mood swings. He is described by his wife as uncharacteristically slow to learn and react and shying away from anything new, preferring the familiar, confused, getting lost easily, and exercising poor judgment. He scores poorly on the mini-mental status examination (MMSE). This disease is believed to be caused by protein misfolding. Chaperonins regulate protein folding in which of the following ways?

a. Stimulating aggregation of proteins
b. Contributing folding information to the native protein
c. Controlling the docking of the signal peptide with its receptor on the rough endoplasmic reticulum
d. Inhibiting proteolytic activity of misfolded proteins
e. Using their ATPase activity to bind and release themselves from hydrophobic regions of the protein

57. A 23-year-old man who is allergic to peanuts has a plain vanilla ice cream cone at a local ice cream store. Unfortunately, the server did not sufficiently clean the scoop after serving a cup of peanut brittle ice cream. The young man begins to have an allergic reaction and reaches for his inhalator filled with albuterol, a beta-adrenergic drug that binds to beta receptors in the cells of the respiratory airways. The diagram below shows the mechanism involved in binding of albuterol to its receptor. Which of the following statements regarding the molecule labeled "B" in the diagram is true?

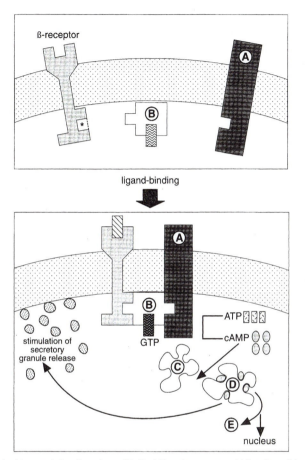

(Modified, with permission, from Avery JK: Oral Development and Histology, *3/e. New York:Thieme Medical, 2001).*

a. It is the inactive cAMP kinase
b. It lacks GTPase activity
c. It inactivates adenylate cyclase
d. It is bound to GTP in the inactive state
e. It is the stimulatory G protein (G$_s$)

58. A 32-year-old (gravida 2, para 2) woman who gave birth to a baby girl 24 hours before is having difficulty urinating and is retaining urine in her bladder. She is given bethanechol, a muscarinic agonist, which is the ligand shown in the diagram below. Which of the following is the function of molecule A?

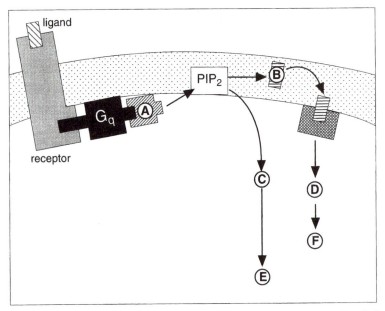

(Modified, with permission, from Avery JK: Oral Development and Histology, 3/e. New York: Thieme Medical, 2001.)

a. Directly activates protein kinase C
b. Binds to the endoplasmic reticulum
c. Hydrolysis of PIP_2 to form DAG and IP_3
d. Stimulation of G_i activity through phosphorylation of PIP_2
e. Stimulation of G_S activity through phosphorylation of PIP_2

59. The two major secretory pathways A → B → C → D (pathway I) and C → E (pathway II) are illustrated in the diagram. Albumin secretion by hepatocytes occurs by pathway II. In a patient with cirrhosis, the serum levels of albumin are reduced. The reduced secretion of albumin most likely occurs through:

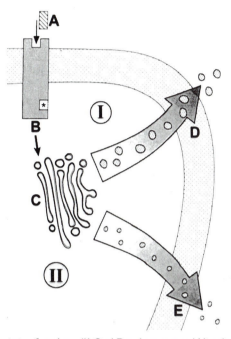

(Modified, with permission, from Avery JK: Oral Development and Histology, 3/e. New York: Thieme Medical, 2001.)

a. Reduced binding of "A" to receptors
b. Reduced numbers of functional hepatocytes
c. Down-regulation of "B" on hepatocytes
d. Reduced activity of the cAMP-activated signal transduction system
e. Increased cyclic AMP levels

60. A 6-month-old boy is brought into the pediatric clinic. He weighs 12 lb, 2 oz and is 22 in. tall. Neither his height nor his weight is on the growth chart for his age; mean weight and height for a 6-month-old are 17 lb, 4 oz and 26.5 in., respectively. Through functional tests, you determine that he is suffering from an inherited condition known as I-cell disease and is missing UDP N-acetylglucosamine: lysosomal enzyme N-acetylglucosamine-1-phosphotransferase, which is more conveniently referred to as phosphotransferase. You recall from your cell biology that the phosphotransferase enzymes phosphorylate mannose to form mannose-6-phosphate. Electron microscopy is performed on a biopsy, and blood tests are completed. Which of the following explains the altered cell biological processes in this patient?

a. Lysosomal enzymes missorted back to the Golgi apparatus
b. Peroxisomal proteins missorted to other organelles
c. Abnormal KDEL sequence on vesicles
d. Absence of SNARE proteins on vesicles
e. Secretion of lysosomal enzymes into the blood

Cell Biology: Intracellular Trafficking

Answers

54. The answer is d. (*Alberts, pp 749–751.*) Receptor-mediated endocytosis of ligand-receptor complexes is a selective process that requires invagination of the cell membrane to form clathrin-coated pits and vesicles. Clathrin is not involved in phagocytosis. Phagocytosis of damaged cells occurs by evagination to engulf the IgG-coated surface of the target. Both processes use acidification of compartments and hydrolases to uncouple receptor and ligand (receptor-mediated endocytosis) or destroy engulfed material (phagocytosis). Both processes use membrane-enclosed vesicles and are associated with lysosomal activity (**answers a, b, c, and e**).

Low-density lipoprotein (LDL) is the form in which most cholesterol is transported in the blood; cellular uptake of LDL is the classic example of receptor-mediated endocytosis. The receptors are bound to clathrin-coated pits, but the ligand is only directly bound to its cell surface receptor. The LDL-LDL receptor (ligand-receptor) complexes are incorporated into the cell in coated vesicles. The acidic environment of the endosome results in the cleavage of the ligand from its receptor (i.e., LDL from its receptor). The LDL receptors are recycled to the membrane for additional exposure to LDL, and the LDL in the endosome is transferred to lysosomes, where it is broken down to cholesterol.

Other ligands differ in subtle ways from LDL in their endocytic pathways.

55. The answer is c. (*Alberts, pp 693–694.*) The SRP prevents degradation of newly synthesized peptides because translocation across the ER membrane protects the nascent peptide from proteases. The signal hypothesis is the basis of the targeting of transmembrane, lysosomal, and exportable proteins across the ER membrane. It is the key event in the segregation of noncytosolic proteins in the ER cisternae. The result of SRP activity is attachment of ribosomes translating the secretory protein to the ER membrane and the translocation of the protein across the ER membrane. The SRP binds to the N terminus of the signal peptide (**answer a**) as the peptide emerges from the ribosome and induces an immediate delay (**answer b**) in translation until the ribosome interacts with a docking protein (**answer d**), also known as an SRP receptor, in the ER membrane. In the function of the RER, a presequence on the 3'-end of the AUG initiation codon is translated as an N-(amino)-terminal presequence [amino-terminal signal leader (prepeptide) sequence] that recognizes the ER membrane and leads to the translocation of the peptide across the ER membrane. This recognition is accomplished through the SRP, which cycles between the ER membrane and the cytosol. After the SRP-bound ribosome attaches to the ER membrane via the docking protein, translation continues with displacement of the SRP for subsequent recycling and translocation of the peptide across the ER membrane. Enzymatic cleavage (**answer e**) of the signal sequence releases the newly synthesized peptide.

56. The answer is e. (*Alberts, pp 355–357.*) The patient in the scenario suffers from Alzheimer disease which is related to protein misfolding leading to neurofibrillary tangles. Three-dimensional folding is required for functional activity of proteins. Native folding of a protein is encoded in its amino acid sequence; however, protein folding inside cells requires molecular chaperones binding and releasing themselves from hydrophobic regions of the newly synthesized protein and ATP to reach their native folded state. Various chaperones protect nonnative protein chains from misfolding and aggregation (**answer a**), but do not contribute conformational information to the folding process (**answer b**). Many chaperones are also stress- or heat-shock proteins (HSPs) that stabilize preproteins for membrane translocation, present misfolded proteins for proteolysis (**answer d**), and regulate the conformation of signaling molecules. The underlying principle in all these functions is the recognition by chaperones of proteins in their nonnative states. Chaperones also inhibit the formation of partially folded intermediates. Chaperones in conjunction with calreticulin monitor the progress of folding and ensure that only properly folded proteins are secreted from the cell or shipped to lysosomes. It is hypothesized that this level of ER "quality control" is absent in Alzheimer and other neurodegenerative diseases. Chaperones assist with translocation of proteins across internal membranes (e.g., mitochondria) by maintaining precursor proteins in their unfolded state during membrane trafficking. They do *not* function in the docking of the signal peptide (**answer c**).

57. The answer is e. *(Alberts, pp 868–870. Junqueira, pp 28–30.)* Albuterol binds to the β-receptor initiating a cyclic AMP (cAMP) signal transduction cascade. The structure labeled B is the stimulatory G protein (G_S). The figure illustrates the response of the β-adrenergic receptor to ligand binding. β-receptors mediate the tissue effects of epinephrine and norepinephrine and respond to pharmacological agents such as albuterol, a β-adrenergic agonist. Signal transduction following ligand binding involves a specific G protein [shorthand for guanosine-triphosphate (GTP)–binding regulatory protein]. G proteins associated with increasing cAMP levels in the cell are known as stimulatory G proteins (G_S) because of their role in enzyme activation. In the inactive state, G_S is bound to GDP. After ligand binding, a G_S binding site is exposed and the G_S protein (B in the figure) binds to the β receptor. The resulting complex is capable of binding GTP in exchange for GDP, activating the G protein. The α subunit of the activated G_S protein exchanges GDP for GTP and activates adenylate cyclase (**A** in the figure). Intrinsic GTPase activity of the α-subunit is increased resulting in a short activation time for the complex and recycling of the subunits to the inactive state. The inactive cAMP-dependent kinase is labeled **C** in the figure. It is the phosphorylating action of cAMP-dependent protein kinase (kinase A), stimulated by increased intracellular cAMP concentration, that affects many aspects of intracellular metabolism and function. Phosphorylation **(E)** stimulates exocytosis and induces nuclear changes, including transcriptional events. The star in the figure delineates the site of ligand-binding-induced conformational change, exposing the G_S-binding site. (See table in the answer for question 36.)

58. The answer is c. *(Alberts, pp 859–860.)* Bethanechol binds to muscarinic receptors, Molecule A in the figure is phospholipase C that catalyzes the formation of diacylglycerol (DAG) and inositol triphosphate (IP_3) from phosphatidylinositol 4,5–bisphosphate (PIP_2). The phosphoinositide (PI) cycle illustrated in the figure is based on the formation of PIP_2 in the inner leaflet of the plasma membrane. Breakdown of PIP_2 leads to the formation of the key functional agents of the PI cycle. Binding of a ligand to its G protein–linked receptor on the cell surface (Gq) activates a phosphoinositide-specific phospholipase C. PI-specific phospholipase C hydrolyzes PIP_2 to form DAG and IP_3. Those two molecules function differently to regulate intracellular function. IP_3 functions in the mobilization of calcium, while DAG activates protein kinase C **(answer a)**, leading to multiple phosphorylations of cytosolic proteins. DAG (**B** in the figure) activates protein kinase C (so called because of its Ca^{2+}-dependency), which is labeled **D**. The protein kinase C phosphorylates (**F**) specific serine and threonine residues and may alter gene transcription. In contrast, IP_3 functions to mobilize Ca^{2+} by binding to IP_3-gated channels in the ER membrane (**answer b**). The two intracellular messenger pathways do interact in that elevated Ca^{2+} translocates protein kinase C from the cytosol to the inner leaflet of the plasma membrane. G_i (**answer d**) is the inhibitory G protein that leads to 5'-AMP production through the action of phosphodiesterase instead of cAMP. G_s is involved in adenylate cyclase signal transduction (**answer e**).

59. The answer is b. (*Alberts, pp 757–758.*) Cirrhosis damages hepatocytes leading to a reduction in synthesis of serum proteins. The pathway labeled in the figure as II (C → E) is the constitutive (default) pathway, which is followed by proteoglycans, fibronectin, and collagen synthesized by fibroblasts, serum proteins synthesized by hepatocytes (albumin, transferrin and lipoprotein), and immunoglobulins produced by lymphocytes. The pathway labeled as I (A → D) differs from constitutive secretion (C → E) in several ways. The most important difference is the requirement for a secretagogue (substance that induces secretion from cells) in the regulated pathway (**answers a and c**), which binds to a cell-surface receptor. Secretion in the constitutive pathway is not regulated at the level of second messengers (**answers d and e**). Regulated secretion (process I) shows the recognition of a receptor (**B**) for its ligand (**A**), resulting in the release of secretion in response to the stimulus of secretagogue-receptor binding. The synthetic processes in the two pathways are then identical until the Golgi. The vesicles that bud from the Golgi (**D**) in the regulated pathway are clathrin-coated and contain a receptor involved in the concentration of secretory product that normally occurs before release. The constitutive pathway shuttles proteins such as integral membrane proteins and lipids in vesicles to the apical and basolateral membranes. The vesicles are nonclathrin-coated in the constitutive pathway. Exocytosis requires vesicle fusion with the membrane in both regulated and constitutive pathways. Ras-superfamily GTPases, members of the protein kinase D family and tethering complexes such as the exocyst are involved in constitutive secretion.

60. The answer is e. (*Alberts, pp 720–722, 724, 729–730, 744–745. Junqueira, pp 39, 50.*) The child is suffering from inclusion (I)–cell disease.

There is an absence or deficiency of N-acetylglucosamine phosphotransferase and an absence of mannose-6-phosphate (M6P) on the lysosomal enzymes. The failure to add M6P in the cis-Golgi results in inappropriate vesicular segregation by M6P receptors in the trans–Golgi network (TGN). The default pathway is transport to the cell membrane and secretion from the cell by exocytosis for proteins lacking M6P. Lysosomal enzymes are secreted into the bloodstream, and undigested substrates build up within the cells. There is no missorting back to the Golgi **(answer a)**. Peroxisomal enzymes, which are sorted by the presence of three specific amino acids located at the C-terminus: Ser–Lys–Leu–COO⁻, are not affected **(answer b)**. KDEL **(answer c)** is the signal used for retrieval of proteins from the Golgi back to the endoplasmic reticulum. SNAREs [soluble-N-ethylemalemide sensitive factor (NSF) attachment protein receptors] are the receptors for SNAPs [soluble-N-ethylemalemide sensitive factor (NSF) attachment proteins] and bind vesicles to membranes **(answer d)**. Trafficking to other structures, such as the nucleus and mitochondria, is regulated by nuclear localization signals (NLSs) or an N-terminal signal peptide, respectively.

Cell Biology: Nucleus

Questions

DIRECTIONS: Each item below contains a question or incomplete statement followed by suggested responses. Select the **one best** response to each question.

61. A newborn boy is born with first arch congenital malformations classified as Treacher-Collins syndrome, which is an autosomal dominant inherited disorder. The Treacher Collins-Franceschetti syndrome 1 (TCOF) gene encodes the protein treacle. Treacle is localized to the structure labeled with the arrows in the accompanying transmission electron micrograph. Treacle is most likely involved in which of the following?

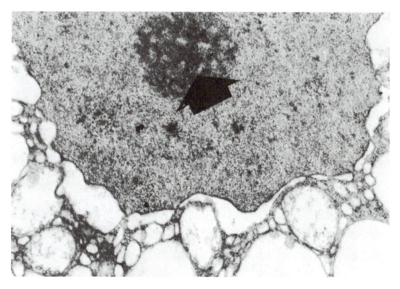

a. Assembly of ribosomal subunits into mature ribosomes
b. Translation of cytosolic proteins
c. Transcription of nuclear proteins
d. Transcription of ribosomal proteins
e. Organelle degradation

62. Which of the following is true for the process that the dividing cell shown in the electron micrograph below is undergoing?

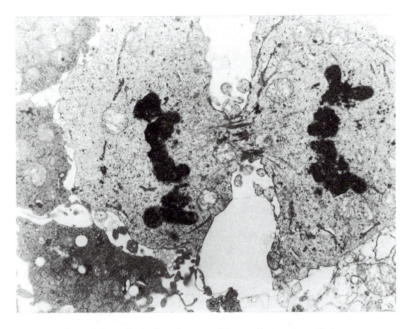

a. It is achieved through the lengthening of kinetochore microtubules
b. It is accomplished by the contraction of a ring composed of cytoskeletal elements
c. It is achieved through the shortening of polar microtubules
d. It is regulated by M-cdk complex (MPF)
e. It is blocked by anti-tubulin antibodies

63. A 29-year-old woman presents with a 101°F fever, pericardial effusions and Libman-Sacks endocarditis, arthralgias, rash across the malar region of the face ("butterfly rash") that is accentuated by sun exposure; creatinine is 1.7 mg/dL (normal 0.5 to 1.1 mg/dL). Laboratory tests show high titers of antinuclear autoantibodies (ANA), Smith antigen and antinucleosome antibodies in the serum. Which of the following is most likely to be directly affected by the disruption of nucleosomes in this patient.

a. Packaging of genetic material in a condensed form
b. Transcribing DNA
c. Forming pores for bilateral nuclear-to-cytoplasmic transport
d. Forming the nuclear matrix
e. Holding together adjacent chromatids

64. A G_1-phase and an M-phase cell are fused together with a Sendai virus. The result is that the chromosomes in the G_1-phase cell condense. Which of the following would be a possible cell biological explanation?

a. Lamins will be phosphorylated in the G_1 cell
b. The S-phase activator will be expressed in the M-phase cell
c. The M-phase cell will reduplicate its DNA
d. The G_1/S-cdk complex will be activated in the M-phase cell
e. A re-replication block will occur in the G_1-phase cell.

65. A middle aged anatomy professor went to the hottest Indianapolis 500 race in decades and sat with the sun facing him; there was no breeze. He had a history of borderline high uric acid. When he became dehydrated at the race, it triggered the uric acid crystal formation in his foot. The foot became sore, red, hot and swollen; he could not walk on that foot or even fit into a regular pair of shoes. The race was great and he drank about 2 L of water and soda at the race and another couple of liters when he arrived home. Evidently that was not enough fluid because he was anuric for about 10–12 hours. His physician prescribes colchicine as an anti-inflammatory. A metaphase-blocking dose of colchicine functions through which of the following mechanisms?

a. Depolymerization of actin
b. Depolymerization of myosin
c. Enhancement of tubulin polymerization
d. Inhibition of tubulin polymerization
e. Binding to and stabilizing microtubules

66. The structure labeled A in the accompanying electron micrograph is which of the following?

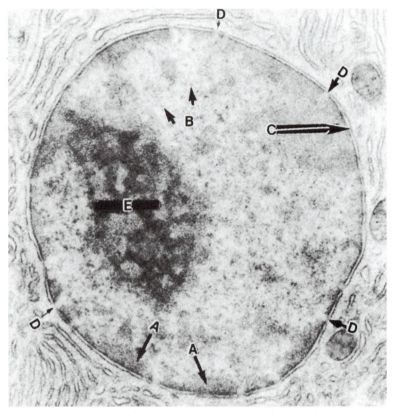

(Reproduced, with permission, from Fawcett DW: A Textbook of Histology, 11th ed. Philadelphia: WB Saunders, 1986.)

a. The site of translation of messenger RNA
b. Chromatin that is transcriptionally inactive during interphase
c. The site of ribosomal protein synthesis
d. A shield between the nucleus and cytoplasm in eukaryotic cells
e. The site of aqueous channels for the passage of molecules between the nucleoplasm and the cytoplasm

67. A 55-year-old man with difficulty urinating, blood in the urine, burning during urination and accelerating prostate-specific antigen (PSA) has a radical prostatectomy. The diagnosis is prostate carcinoma with a Gleason score of 7. Rb, p53, and bcl-2 genes are involved in the development of prostate carcinoma. Which of the following mechanisms may be involved in the loss of cell cycle control that occurs in prostate carcinoma?

a. Increased CdkI activity
b. Decreased transcription of G_1/S cyclin
c. Decreased expression of bcl-2
d. Increased transcription of gene regulatory proteins such as E2F
e. Dephosphorylation of Rb

68. Decreased recombination is associated with the production of aneuploid sperm in humans. Meiotic crossover occurs in which of the following stages?

a. Leptotene
b. Zygotene
c. Pachytene
d. Diplotene
e. Diakinesis

69. An obese 18-year-old man presents with small firm testes, a small penis, little axillary and facial hair, azoospermia, gynecomastia, and elevated levels of plasma gonadotropins. He has had difficulty in social adjustment throughout high school, but this has worsened and he has been referred for genetic and endocrine screening. The karyotype from peripheral blood leukocytes would most likely show how many Barr body/bodies?

a. None
b. One
c. Two
d. Three
e. Four

70. A 20-month-old boy is diagnosed with Hutchinson-Gilford progerial syndrome (HGPS), a severe form of early-onset premature aging. He experienced normal fetal and early postnatal development, but now shows severe failure to thrive, some lipoatrophy, bony abnormalities, a small, beaked nose and receding mandible, hair loss, and speckled hypopigmentation with some areas of tight hard skin. His neurological and cognitive tests are normal. Genetic analysis shows a single spontaneous mutation in codon 608 of the *LMNA* gene, which encodes both lamin A and lamin C.

Which of the following would you most likely expect to be directly affected in cells obtained in a biopsy from this patient?

a.   Increased heterochromatin
b.   Interference with microtubule treadmilling
c.   Increased synthesis of rRNA in the nucleolus
d.   Loss of ability to adhere to the basement membrane through integrins
e.   Aberrations in nuclear architecture

71. A newborn boy is diagnosed with Apert syndrome. He has craniosynostosis, hypoplasia of the middle part of his face with retrusion of the eyes, and syndactyly that includes fusion of the skin, connective tissue, and muscle of the first, middle, and ring fingers with moderate fusion of the bones of those digits. There is very limited joint mobility past the first joint. Which of the following were most likely *decreased* in cells in the inter-digital region of the developing hand of this newborn child?

a.   Random DNA degradation
b.   Inflammation
c.   Cell swelling
d.   bcl-2
e.   DNA degradation by endonucleases

72. A 25-year-old man presents with Triple A (Allgrove) syndrome including the clinical triad of adrenal failure, achalasia, and alacrima. The patient shows progressive neurological impairments involving cranial nerves IX, X, XI, and XII, optic atrophy, upper and lower limb muscle weakness, and Horner's syndrome. Causative mutations for the disease have been identified in a gene that encodes the protein ALADIN, a component of the structure labeled with the arrows in the transmission electron micrograph. Which of the following would be directly affected by the mutation?

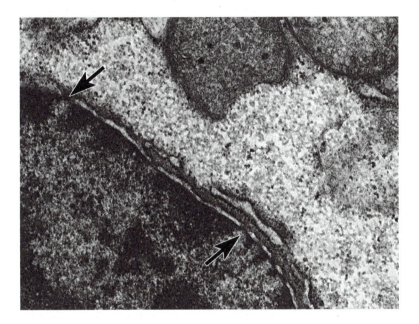

a. Import of macromolecules to the nucleus
b. Reconstitution of the nuclear envelope in telophase
c. Breakdown of the nuclear envelope in prometaphase
d. Condensation of chromatin
e. RNA synthesis

Cell Biology: Nucleus

Answers

61. The answer is d. (*Junqueira, pp 52, 56–57. Ross and Pawlina, pp 71, 74–75.*) The TCOF1 gene encodes treacle. Expression of treacle is critical during early embryonic development in structures that form bones and other facial structures. Treacle is active in the nucleolus, the structure labeled in the transmission electron micrograph. The nucleolus is the site of ribosomal protein transcription and treacle regulates ribosomal DNA transcription and therefore ribosomal RNA (rRNA) synthesis. The nucleolus is a highly organized, heterogeneous structure within the nucleus, with distinct regions visible by electron microscopy: (1) fibrillar centers, which represent the nucleolar organizer regions where DNA is not being actively transcribed; (2) dense fibrillar components (*pars fibrosa*) where RNA molecules are being transcribed; and (3) a granular component (*pars granulosa*) where ribosomal subunits undergo maturation. The nucleolar organizer contains clusters of rRNA genes (DNA). The size and number of nucleoli differ with the metabolic activity of cells.

Ribosomal synthesis occurs in the nucleolus, but the complete assembly and maturation of ribosomes requires transport to the cytoplasm (**answer a**). Ribosomal proteins as well as all proteins that function in the nucleus are synthesized in the cytosol and transported into the nucleus (**answer b**). Nuclear proteins are also translated on ribosomes in the cytoplasm (**answer c**) and targeted to the nucleus (traveling through the nuclear pores) by specific nuclear localization signals (NLSs). Cytosolic proteins are synthesized on isolated ribosomes compared with most protein synthesis that occurs on polyribosomes. Nuclear proteins are transcribed on euchromatin (**answer c**). Lysosomes carry out degradation of organelles (**answer e**).

62. The answer is b. (*Alberts, pp 1039–1041, 1046–1051.*) The mitotic cell in the micrograph is undergoing cytokinesis, or the cleavage of the cytoplasm to form two cells. It occurs after completion of nuclear division (i.e., nuclear condensation and separation of the chromosomes that are mediated by microtubules). Cytokinesis requires the action of the contractile ring composed of actin and myosin. The force for cytokinesis is generated by the action of actin and myosin, which may be inhibited by treatment with antimyosin antibodies *in vitro.* The contractile ring pulls the plasma membrane of the telophase cell into the cleavage furrow. Kinetochore microtubules, which attach the kinetochores to the spindle apparatus, shorten and pull the chromatids to opposite poles in anaphase A (**answer a**). Growth of polar microtubules results in the separation of the spindle poles in anaphase B (**answer c**). M-cdk complex (MPF) regulates metaphase events through phosphorylation (**answer d**). Antitubulin antibodies block movement of chromosomes (**answer e**). The events that occur during each stage of the cell cycle are shown in the table below.

Phase of Cell Cycle	Defining Event(s)
Interphase (G_1, S, and G_2 phases)	Duplication of centrioles and DNA synthesis (S phase)
Prophase	Nucleolus disappears
Prometaphase	Nuclear envelope breaks down
Metaphase	Alignment of chromosomes in metaphase plate
Anaphase	Separation of sister chromatids; initiation of cytokinesis
Telophase	Nuclear envelope reforms; completion of cytokinesis

(Reproduced, with permission, from McKenzie JC, Klein, RM: Basic Concepts in Cell Biology and Histology. *New York: McGraw-Hill, 2000.)*

63. The answer is a. (*Alberts, pp 207–211. Junqueira, pp 54–55.*) The patient in the scenario suffers from systemic lupus erythematosus (SLE), a chronic autoimmune disease. Nucleosomes are the basic structural packaging unit of chromatin. Chromatin strands that have been treated to unpack the chromatin structure have the appearance of beads on a string in electron micrographs. The beads are formed by a core of histones as an octamer (i.e., two of each of the four nucleosomal histones: H2A, H2B, H3, and H4) plus two turns of DNA. The nucleosome beads plus the DNA between beads (i.e., linker DNA) constitute the nucleosome. There are additional orders of chromosome packing, including nucleosomal packing. The transcription of DNA is carried out by RNA polymerases I, II, and III, which are responsible for transcription of different types of genes (**answer b**). The nuclear pores are perforations in the nuclear envelope, each composed of a nuclear pore complex (**answer c**). The nuclear matrix is the intranuclear cytoskeleton and forms the scaffolding for nuclear structures (**answer d**). Chromatids are held together at the centromere (**answer e**).

64. The answer is a. *(Alberts, pp 997–1000.)* When a cell in any phase of the cell cycle is fused with a mitotic cell, the mitotic cell dominates. The reason for this is the dominance of M-Cdk complex (formerly called MPF). The G_1-phase cell is quickly pulled or driven into mitosis as the chromosomes condense. The M-Cdk complex will cause the phosphorylation of the lamins. The lamins are a subclass of intermediate filaments including three nuclear proteins: lamins A, B, and C. Phosphorylation of intermediate filaments leads to disassembly, as occurs with the lamins. The disassembly of lamins results in the dissolution of the nuclear envelope in prometaphase of the cell cycle. The S-phase activator cannot be expressed in the M-phase cell, and it also cannot reduplicate its DNA because of the re-replication block (answers **b, c, and d**). A re-replication block cannot occur in the G_1 cell because it has not gone through S **(answer e)**. The lamins differ from other intermediate filament proteins in the presence of a nuclear import signal. The lamins form the core of the nuclear lamina, interact with nuclear envelope proteins, and play a role in the maintenance of the shape of the nucleus. Dephosphorylation of the lamins is associated with the reassembly of the nuclear envelope in telophase.

65. The answer is d. *(Alberts, pp 927–928.)* At a mitosis-inhibiting dose, colchicine functions by binding specifically and irreversibly to tubulin. The colchicine-tubulin complex is added at the positive end of the kinetochore, but it inhibits further addition of tubulin **(answer c)**. The result is a biochemical capping of the tubulin at the growth end, preventing further tubulin addition. Cells are blocked in metaphase and cannot escape because microtubule motors are unable to function in generating the forces required for anaphase. At higher doses of colchicine, cytosolic microtubules depolymerize. Actin and myosin are involved in cytokinesis [the division of cytoplasm **(answers a and b)**], whereas tubulin and the microtubules regulate separation of the daughter nuclei and their contents. Taxol, like colchicine, inhibits mitosis, but it uses a different mechanism. Taxol binds and stabilizes microtubules **(answer e)**, causing a disruption of microtubule dynamics and inhibition of mitosis. Taxol and colchicine are similar in binding only to α,β-tubulin dimers and microtubules.

66. The answer is b. *(Junqueira, pp 51–52, 56–57. Alberts, pp 222–229.)* Heterochromatin **(A)** is visible with the light microscope as condensed basophilic clumps and with the electron microscope as compact, electron-dense material within the nucleus. It is transcriptionally inactive during the interphase stage of the cell cycle, when the genetic material is normally duplicated. Heterochromatin is one of two subclassifications of chromatin on a morphologic basis. Euchromatin (**B**) is actively transcribed chromatin and is visible only with the use of electron microscopy. Cells with extensive euchromatin are considered metabolically active.

The nucleolus (**E**) is the site of ribosomal RNA synthesis. ^{3}H-uridine may be localized in the nucleolus by use of autoradiography and is often used as a marker for RNA synthesis because uridine is preferentially incorporated into RNA. RNA is packaged with ribosomal proteins to form ribosomes. The nuclear envelope (**C**) shields the nucleus from the cytoplasm, which allows the sequestration of the genetic material from mechanical cytoplasmic forces. The separate nuclear compartment also allows for separation of the cellular processes of transcription and translation. The nuclear envelope consists of two concentric unit membranes. The outer membrane is continuous with the rough endoplasmic reticulum. The inner nuclear membrane is associated with a lamina of fibrous proteins including intermediate filament proteins, known as lamins, that regulate the assembly and disassembly of the nuclear membrane during mitosis.

Nuclear pores (**D**) are interruptions in the nuclear envelope that function as aqueous channels for the passage of soluble molecules from the nucleus to the cytoplasm (ribosomal subunits) and from the cytoplasm to the nucleus (nuclear proteins synthesized in the cytoplasm and transported to the nucleus). The nuclear envelope is highly selective, with selection based on pore size, the presence of nuclear import signals, and receptor recognition of RNAs. Translation of mRNA occurs in the cytoplasm.

67. The answer is d. (*Alberts, pp 1005, 1335–1336. Kumar p 100. Ross and Pawlina, pp 80–81, 91.*) Increased transcription of the transcription factor, E2F leads to loss of cell cycle control. E2F is regulated through phosphorylation and dephosphorylation of Retinoblastoma protein (Rb), a key "negative" regulator of the cell cycle. Cells that enter G_1 have dephosphorylated Rb protein that is subsequently phosphorylated, allowing passage of cells from G_1 to "S." Dephosphorylated Rb is inhibitory because it sequesters E2F. Upon Rb phosphorylation, E2F is released and induces the expression of various genes associated with the initiation of the cell cycle.

The phosphorylation or absence of Rb facilitates E2F binding to DNA (**answer e**). Bcl-2 is an antiapoptotic gene (**answer c**). Accumulation of bcl-2 has been associated with the increased incidence and severity of prostate carcinoma in African-American males. Cell division kinase inhibitors block activation of cyclin-Cdk [cyclin dependent kinase complexes **(answer b)**] and cell cycle progression **(answer a)**. p53 and Rb are tumor suppressor genes. In the absence of Rb or p53, tumor suppression and normal control are lost. p53 increases in the presence of DNA damage, resulting in the inhibition of cell division. p53 mutations inhibit cell division kinase (Cdk) inhibitors such as p21, resulting in uncontrolled cell division. The absence of p53 also permits proliferation of damaged cells. For more details on the regulation of the cell cycle, see "High-Yield Facts."

68. The answer is c. *(Alberts, pp 1130–1139. Ross and Pawlina, pp 86–87.)* Pachytene begins as soon as the synapsis is complete and includes the period of crossover. The fully formed synaptonemal complex is present during the pachytene stage. At each point where crossover has occurred between two chromatids of the homologous chromosomes, an attachment point known as a chiasma forms. Meiosis is the mechanism used by the reproductive organs to generate gametes—cells with the haploid number of chromosomes. DNA synthesis occurs before meiotic prophase I begins and is followed by a G_2 phase. Cells then enter meiotic prophase I. During meiotic prophase I, maternal and paternal chromosomes are precisely paired, and recombination occurs in each pair of homologous chromosomes. The first meiotic prophase consists of five substages: leptotene, zygotene, pachytene, diplotene, and diakinesis. During metaphase I, there is random segregation of maternal and paternal chromosomes. Homologous chromosomes are aligned on the metaphase plate of the meiotic spindle in metaphase I. The second meiotic division is responsible for the reduction in the chromosome content of the cell by 50%. In meiotic division II, metaphase consists of daughter chromatids of single homologous chromosomes aligned on a metaphase plate (metaphase II). Condensation of the chromatids occurs in leptotene **(answer a)**. In zygotene **(answer b)**, the synaptonemal complex begins to form, which initiates the close association between chromosomes known as synapsis. The bivalent is formed between the two sets of homologous chromosomes (one set maternal and one set paternal equals a pair of maternal chromatids and a pair of paternal chromatids). The four chromatids form a tetrad (bivalent). The formation of chiasmata and desynapsing (separation of the axes of the synaptonemal complex) occurs in the diplotene stage **(answer d)**. Diakinesis **(answer e)**

is an intermediate phase between diplotene and metaphase of the first meiotic division.

69. The answer is b. (*Kasper, p 2215. Sadler, pp 18–19, 251. Moore and Persaud, Developing, p 165.*) Cells from a patient with the most common form of Klinefelter's syndrome (47,XXY genotype) will have one inactive X chromosome and, therefore, one Barr body. The formula is the number of Barr bodies equals the number of X chromosomes minus one. Klinefelter's syndrome occurs at a ratio of about 1:500 males and is due to meiotic nondisjunction of the chromosomes. The nondisjunction is more frequent in oogenesis than in spermatogenesis, and increased occurrence is directly proportional to increasing maternal age. Klinefelter's may occur as 47,XXY, 48,XXYY, 48,XXXY, and 49,XXXXY. A combination of abnormal and normal genotype occurs in mosaic individuals who generally have less severe symptoms. Females have two X chromosomes, one of maternal and the other of paternal origin. Only one of the X chromosomes is active in the somatic, diploid cells of the female; the other X chromosome remains inactive and is visible in appropriately stained interphase cells as a mass of heterochromatin. Detection of the Barr body (sex chromatin) has been an efficient method for the determination of chromosomal sex and abnormalities of X-chromosome number; however, it is not definitive proof of maleness or femaleness. The genotypic sex of Klinefelter's syndrome and XXX individuals would be male and female as determined by the presence or absence of the testis-determining Y chromosome. In Turner's syndrome (XO), no Barr bodies would be present. In comparison, "superfemales" (XXX) would possess two inactive X chromosomes (2 Barr bodies) and one active X chromosome. Buccal scrapings for Barr body analysis are being used less—chromosomal analysis is the standard test now.

70. The answer is e. (*Kasper, p 1382. Rubin, p 37.*) In Hutchinson-Gilford progerial syndrome (HGPS) an abnormal protein, progerin, is generated and has a "dominant negative" effect on the function of lamins. The lamins are intermediate filament proteins that regulate the nuclear envelope, maintain its stability, and are phosphorylated (prometaphase) and dephosphorylated (telophase) during the cell cycle. In HGPS the results are dramatic abnormalities in the architecture of the nucleus, changes in nuclear shape, loss of heterochromatin (unable to attach to lamins), and an altered distribution of nuclear proteins **(answer a)**. Microtubule treadmilling (answer b) and synthesis of ribosomal RNAs in the nucleolus (answer c) should not be directly affected. Laminin binds to integrins on the cell surface to facilitate attachment of cells to the basement membrane (answer d).

71. The answer is e. (*Ross and Pawlina, pp 88–91. Kumar, pp 26–32.*) DNA degradation is the hallmark of programmed cell death (apoptosis). Random DNA degradation, inflammation, and cell and nuclear swelling (answers a → c) are involved in necrosis (the response to cell injury or toxins), not apoptosis. Bax and bcl-2 are members of the bcl-2 family of apoptosis regulatory proteins. Bax is a proapoptotic member of that protein family and inhibits the antiapoptotic actions of bcl-2. Bax would be down-regulated and bcl-2 up-regulated in syndactyly where apoptosis has failed (answer d). Apoptosis works through several different pathways and ultimately through the caspases, which induce DNA degradation by endonucleases.

72. The answer is a. (*Junqueira, pp 51–54. Ross and Pawlina, p 78.*) Triple A syndrome is an autosomal recessive neuroendocrinological disease caused by mutations in a gene that encodes the nucleoporin ALADIN, a component of the nuclear pore complex labeled with the arrows in the electron micrograph. The immediate effect of mutations in the nucleoporins is decreased import of macromolecules from the cytoplasm. Patients with triple A syndrome have adrenocorticotrophic (ACTH)-resistant adrenal failure, achalasia (abnormal esophageal motility most often due to inability of the esophageal sphincter to relax), and alacramia (reduced ability to produce tears). They also demonstrate neurological symptoms affecting the cranial nerves, autonomic nervous system (Horner's syndrome and orthostatic hypotension). Phosphorylation (breakdown) and dephosphorylation (reconstitution) of the lamins regulates nuclear envelope stability during the cell cycle (answers b and c). Condensation of chromosomes would not be directly affected (answer d) and the nucleus is the site of RNA synthesis (answer e).

Epithelium

Questions

DIRECTIONS: Each item below contains a question or incomplete statement followed by suggested responses. Select the **one best** response to each question.

73. A male child is born with an absence of the normal structure labeled between the arrows; inclusions of that structure are found within the cells in the photomicrograph. He presents with refractory diarrhea and is chronically dependent on parenteral nutrition. What is the primary function of the structure labeled between the arrows in the photomicrograph below?

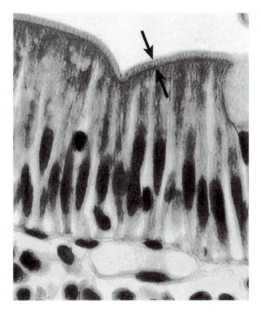

a. Extensive movement of substances over cell surfaces
b. Increase in surface area for absorption
c. Cell motility
d. Transport of intracellular organelles through the cytoplasm
e. Stretch

74. Following a positive α-fetoprotein test a child is born with anencephaly. The development of this open neural tube defect (NTD) is caused by failure of primary neurulation. The mechanism for tube formation as occurs during development of the neural tube could best be explained by which of the following?

a. Contraction of microfilament bundles associated with the zonula adherens
b. Increased condensation of the transmembrane linkers of the desmosomes
c. Expansion of the sealing strands in the zonulae occludentes
d. Condensation of the gap junctions
e. Contraction of tonofilaments associated with desmosomes

75. In the figure below, A is a transmission electron micrograph, and B is a freeze-fracture preparation of a specific cellular structure. Mutations in the proteins that constitute the intramembranous particles labeled in the freeze-fracture image below occur in humans. Which of the following would one expect to occur in the presence of such mutations?

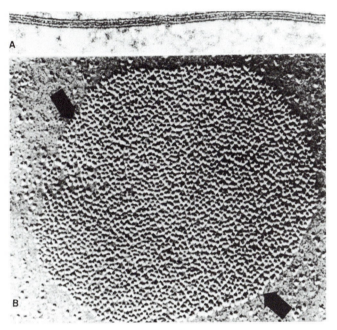

(Micrographs courtesy of Drs. David F. Albertini and Kiyoshi Hama.)

a. Faster conduction of nerve impulses
b. Increased peristalsis in the small intestine
c. Cardiac arrhythmias
d. More rapid mobilization of glycogen to glucose in response to low blood sugar levels
e. Decreased adherence of epithelial cells to the basement membrane

76. Which of the following is a function of the basement membrane?

a. Molecular filtering
b. Contractility
c. Excitability
d. Modification of secreted protein
e. Active ion transport

77. A mother brings her son to the pediatrics clinic. The child rapidly developed extensive blistering of the skin shortly after birth. He has painful erosions of the oral mucosa and has refused ingestion. He has also had a history of recurrent infections, with sepsis, on one occasion. Antigen mapping of a skin biopsy shows a split within the lamina lucida of the epidermal basement membrane, and junctional epidermolysis bullosa (JEB) was the diagnosis. In which specific layer of the accompanying electron micrograph would you expect to see the disruption?

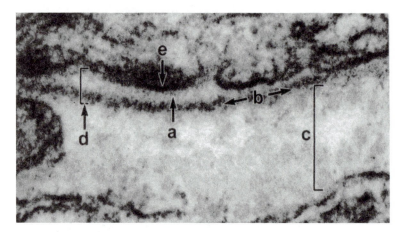

a. a
b. b
c. c
d. d
e. e

78. Which of the following definitively characterizes the basolateral membrane?

a. The presence of hormone receptors
b. Endocytosis
c. Exocytosis
d. The presence of Na$^+$,K$^+$–ATPase
e. The presence of a glycocalyx

79. A 54-year-old woman presents to the oral surgeon on referral by her general dentist. She complains of pain during eating or even thinking about food. The pain lasts for about 2–3 hours after eating. Her dentist observes a firm mass in the anterior right side of the floor of the mouth. Her dentures were made by a denturist to save money and her general dentist indicates they fit very poorly. A calcified density is identified in the transverse CT film (see arrow below). The calcification blocks the submandibular duct leading to atrophy of the acini and ducts with reduced secretory function. One would expect which of the following functional changes to occur in association with the basal folds of the striated duct cells?

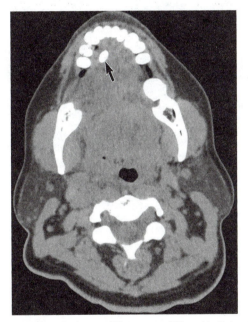

(Radiograph courtesy of Drs. Per-Lennart Westesson and Xiang Liu, University of Rochester, Case #98 http://www.urmc.rochester.edu/smd/Rad/neurocases/Neurocase98.htm.)

a. Increased lipid transport
b. Increased absorption of carbohydrate
c. Decreased active transport
d. Decreased secretion of the primary saliva
e. Decreased lysosomal activity

80. In the electron micrograph below, the structure labeled D primarily does which of the following?

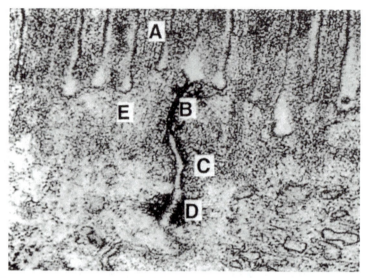

(Reproduced, with permission, from Erlandsen SL, Magney JE: Color Atlas of Histology, St. Louis, MO: CV Mosby, 1992.)

a. Forms a spot weld between cells
b. Interacts with actin in the cytoplasm of the apical cytosol
c. Facilitates communication between adjacent cells
d. Seals membranes between cells
e. Moves microvilli

81. An 11-year-old boy presents with ciliary dyskinesia, sinusitis, and bronchiectasis. He has had persistent infections and otitis media since birth. A PA radiograph shows dextrocardia, and he has a negative saccharin test. In the cross-section of the cilium shown below, which of the following is primarily affected in this disorder?

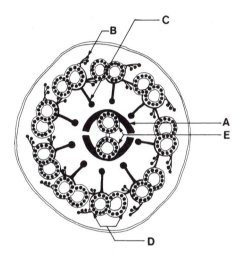

a. Structure A
b. Structure B
c. Structure C
d. Structure D
e. Structure E

82. The conversion of sliding to bending in the cilium is accomplished by which of the following?

a. Restriction of movement by dynein binding of the central microtubules to each other
b. The bending of the basal bodies against the axoneme
c. Sliding of nexin along the adjacent microtubule doublet
d. Sliding of the radial spokes against nexin
e. Restriction of the microtubule doublets by radial spokes, nexin, and basal bodies

83. The structure responsible for the linkage of the intermediate filament network of cells to the basal lamina is which of the following?

a. Macula adherens
b. Zonula adherens
c. Hemidesmosomes
d. Focal contacts
e. Zonula occludens

84. A 42-year-old woman, of Mediterranean descent, presents with multiple oral blisters (see photograph), which she says have been present for several months, and a few cutaneous blisters on her back and buttocks that she just noticed over the past week. The bullae are fairly superficial, with the site of skin disruption clearly in the epidermis. Vesicles are fragile and some have unroofed and led to ulcerated lesions. The Nikolsky's sign is positive. Analysis of her sera indicates autoantibodies to a subfamily of cadherins with the distribution shown in the immunofluorescence image (see photomicrograph). You are asked to review the electron micrographs of the biopsy. Where would you expect to find the lesion?

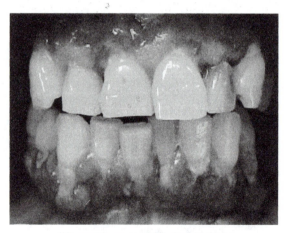

(Micrograph courtesy of Dr. David A. Sirois)

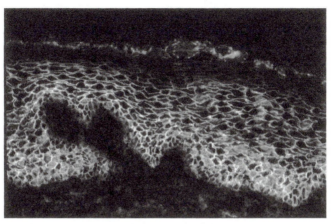

(Micrograph courtesy of Dr. Erik Dabelsteen.)

a. Hemidesmosome
b. Zonula adherens
c. Macula adherens
d. Gap junctions
e. Lamina densa of the basal lamina

85. The triplet arrangement of microtubules is found in which of the following?

a. Centrioles
b. Cytoplasmic microtubules
c. Flagellae
d. Axonemes
e. Stereocilia

Epithelium

Answers

73. The answer is b. *(Young, p 91. Junqueira, pp 68–70, 72.)* The child in the vignette suffers from microvillous inclusion disease (MID) which results in the absence of microvilli in the small intestinal absorptive cell (enterocyte) brush border (apical structure labeled between the arrows in the photomicrograph). MID is associated with an inability to absorb even simple nutrients; the disease presents as refractory diarrhea in the newborn period with chronic dependency on total parenteral nutrition. In MID, microvilli are found as inclusions in the apical enterocyte. Microvilli increase surface area for specialized uptake of molecules by pinocytosis, receptor-mediated endocytosis, and phagocytosis. The microvilli also contain the brush border enzymes such as lactase and alkaline phosphatase. Microvilli are supported by a core of microfilaments and are capable of movement; however, cilia **(answer a)** function in the movement of substances, such as mucus and foreign material, over the surface. Cell movement is controlled by interactions between the cytoskeleton and the extracellular matrix **(answer c)**, while microtubules facilitate organellar movement within the cytoplasm **(answer d)**. Transitional epithelium characteristic of the urinary system facilitates distensibility and stretch **(answer e)**. A table listing functions and locations of epithelia is provided below.

EPITHELIAL TYPES, LOCATION, AND FUNCTION		
Epithelial Type	**Location**	**Function**
Simple		
Simple squamous	Endothelium of blood vessels	Transport, absorption, secretion
Simple cuboidal	Collecting ducts of kidneys	Transport, reabsorption, secretion
Simple columnar	Epithelium of the gut: stomach, intestines	Absorption, protection, lubrication (mucus)
Stratified		
Stratified cuboidal	Sweat ducts	Transport
Stratified columnar	Excretory ducts of salivary glands	Transport

(Continued)

Epithelial Type	Location	Function
Stratified squamous (keratinized)	Epidermis	Protection, water conservation
Stratified squamous (nonkeratinized)	Esophagus, anus, vagina	Protection, lubrication, secretion
Pseudostratified	Respiratory system (trachea with cilia), male reproductive system (no cilia)	Movement of material across epithelial surface
Transitional	Urinary system: ureter, bladder	Stretch, protection

74. The answer is a. (*Alberts, pp 1217–1218.*) Open neural tube defects (NTDs), such as anencephaly, are detected by a positive α-fetoprotein (AFP) test and are attributed to failure of primary neurulation in which the neural folds (plate) form the neural tube. Tubular structures form from flat sheets by contraction of the microfilament bundles associated with the adhesion belt junctions (zonula adherens). In the apical part of the cells, the actin filament bundles contract, narrowing the cells at their apical ends. The position of the zonula adherens, forming a contractile ring around the circumference of the cell, coupled with the contractile nature of the actin microfilament bundles is ideal for regulating morphogenetic changes. Desmosomes (**answers b and e**) are involved in resisting shear forces and are not directly involved in this process. The zonula occludens (**answer c**) prevents leakage between cells. Gap junctions facilitate communication between cells (**answer d**). See table in answer for question 83 for detailed summary of function of components of the junctional complex.

75. The answer is c. (*Young, p 89. Kumar, p 557. Junqueira, pp 27, 68–71.*) The transmission and freeze-fracture electron micrographs illustrate the structure of a nexus, or gap junction. Gap junctions are composed of connexons that traverse the intercellular gap. Gap junctions play an essential role in conduction within cardiac muscle. The action potential is transmitted from cell to cell through the heart, providing the rhythmic contraction of the heartbeat. Abnormalities in the spatial distribution of gap junctions or the proteins (connexins) that compose the connexons will lead to arrhythmias and play a role in obstructive coronary heart disease. Such mutations may also play a role in the racial differences seen in the outcome following myocardial infarction and cardiac disease. For example, alterations in connexin density or distribution may be differentially affected during the development of hypertrophy, thereby increasing the risk of reentrant or nonsustained ventricular tachycardia seen in African-American males.

In the freeze-fracture micrograph, the connexons are seen in circular arrangements on the P face of the membrane. When the connexons of adjacent cells are in alignment, a pore of about 1.5 nm is open, and there is continuity between the interior of the two cells. Gap junctions maintain electrical or chemical coupling, between cells. Rapid nerve conduction in some systems uses gap junctions to avoid the chemical synapse, which requires the release of neurotransmitter. Mutations in connexins would slow down normal nerve impulse conduction **(answer a)**. Normal peristalsis **(answer b)** requires normal gap junctions between smooth muscle in the small intestine and would be slowed down in the absence of normal gap junctions. Not all hepatocytes are innervated. Innervated and noninnervated hepatocytes are connected by gap junctions, which allows for a more coordinated effect of norepinephrine on hepatocytes to facilitate release of blood glucose from stored glycogen in hepatocytes **(answer d)**. Adherence of epithelial cells to the basement membrane **(answer e)** is dependent on integrins and hemidesmosomes, not gap junctions.

76. The answer is a. (*Alberts, pp 1106–1108. Junqueira, pp 67–68.*) Epithelial cells require a basement membrane as a structural support. In most epithelia, the basement membrane prevents penetration from the underlying lamina propria into the epithelium. Basement membranes are a pathway for migrating cells during development and repair processes (e.g., healing of skin wounds). In the kidney, the basement membrane of the renal glomerulus forms a selective barrier for the filtration of the plasma. Contractility and excitability **(answers b and c)** are characteristics that are associated with muscle and nerve, respectively, not with the basement membrane. Active ion transport and modification of secretory proteins **(answers d and e)** are characteristics of the epithelia that are positioned on the basement membrane, not of the basement membrane itself.

77. The answer is a. (*Alberts, pp 1106–1108. Junqueira, pp 67–68.*) The regions labeled in the electron micrograph are **a** (lamina rara, also known as the lamina lucida), **b** (lamina densa), **c** (reticular lamina), **d** (basal lamina), and **e** (basal cell membrane). Junctional epidermolysis bullosa (JEB) represents a disruption between laminin, specifically the beta and gamma chains, with integrins. The split occurs through the lamina lucida of the basal lamina, which contains primarily laminin and its connections with the integrins. At the light microscopic level, a uniform basement membrane is visible under epithelia. Ultrastructurally, basement membranes are composed of one or two electron-lucent areas (laminae rarae) that contain laminin, proteoglycans, and adhesive proteins. Deep to the lamina rara is the lamina densa with its electron-dense type IV collagen. The third layer is the reticular layer that is formed by the underlying connective tissue. This reticular lamina is composed of collagen fibrils formed by the connective tissue below the epithelium (basement membrane = basal lamina + reticular lamina. The table below summarizes the components of the basal lamina.

COMPONENTS OF THE BASEMENT MEMBRANE		
Molecular Component	Component Arrangement	Function
Type IV collagen	3 α-chains	Insoluble structural support
Laminin	3 chains	Bridge between the cells and type IV collagen
Heparan sulfate	Protein core (polypeptide chain) with glycosaminoglycan side chains	Electrostatic charge (anionic sugar side chains repel one another)
Entactin (nidogen)	Single polypeptide chain	Bridge between two networks: laminin and type IV collagen

78. The answer is d. *(Junqueira, pp 84–85.)* The basolateral membrane is characterized by the ubiquitous presence of Na⁺,K⁺–ATPase, responsible for generating the Na⁺, K⁺ gradient of the cell. Na⁺ is pumped out of the cell, and K⁺ is pumped into the cell by this ATP-dependent pump. Ouabain is a specific inhibitor of the Na⁺,K⁺–ATPase. Radioactive forms of this inhibitor are used to label Na⁺,K⁺–ATPase in the basolateral membrane in experimental studies. Hormonal receptors **(answer a)** are found on both apical and basolateral surfaces. Neurotransmitter receptors are more prevalent on the basolateral surfaces. Exocytosis and endocytosis **(answers b and c)** may occur across both apical and basolateral membranes, as does ion transport. The apical surface of cells is covered by a glycocalyx **(answer e)** that consists of oligosaccharides linked to glycoproteins and glycolipids and proteoglycans. The presence of those sugars results in a negative (polyanionic) charge on the luminal surface. Polarity of the epithelial cell is based on these apical and basolateral specializations of the cell membrane and is maintained by the zonula occludens of the junctional complex.

79. The answer is c. *(Junqueira, p 83. Ross and Pawlina, pp 121, 131–132.)* Distal tubule cells of the kidney and striated duct cells of the submandibular glands possess prominent basal infoldings that are observed at the light microscopic level as basal striations. Basal folds are modifications of the basal region of the cell. These deep infoldings of the basal plasma membrane increase surface area and compartmentalize numerous mitochondria that provide energy for ionic and water transport. The primary (isotonic) saliva **(answer d)** is formed by acinar cells and modified by the striated duct cells which resorb Na^+ and excrete K^+. Other activities listed **(answers a, b and e)** are not directly associated with the basal folds.

80. The answer is a. *(Young, pp 86–89. Junqueira, pp 68–70.)* The structure labeled **D** in the transmission electron micrograph is the macula adherens (desmosome). It forms a spot weld or rivet between the adjacent cells and resists shearing forces on the epithelium. The transmission electron micrograph illustrates a junctional complex between two enterocytes in the small intestine. Label **A** represents the microvilli, which constitute the brush border. The brush border is covered by the glycocalyx and in the small intestine contains enzymes involved in the degradation of food in the lumen. The structure labeled **B** is the zonula occludens, which provides a tight seal between the epithelial cells. Label **C** marks the zonula adherens, which interacts with actin which comprises the terminal web (label **E**).

81. The answer is b. *(Alberts, pp 966–968, 1221. Young, p 90. Junqueira, pp 44, 50, 340, 425. Kierszenbaum, pp 7–8, 28–29.)* The patient in the scenario presents with Kartagener's syndrome, also known as immotile cilia syndrome, and has cilia that do not function normally. This leads to chronic infections (otitis media) and infertility (immotile sperm or suboptimal oviductal ciliary function in females). In that disorder, abnormalities occur in the organization of axonemal (ciliary) dynein arms **(answer b)** that bridge the nine outer doublet microtubules **(answer d)** to each other. Dynein is a high-molecular-weight ATPase. When dynein is activated, it produces the sliding motion of the microtubules as it walks along the adjacent doublet. The protein nexin links the outer microtubular doublets, creating a straplike arrangement of paired microtubules around the central microtubule doublet. The radial spokes (**answer c**) restrain the sliding movement of the outer doublets, so those doublets are held in place and sliding is limited lengthwise. The inner sheath (**answer a**) surrounds the central microtubule doublet (**answer e**). The basal body that anchors the microtubules also plays an essential role in converting the sliding of the outer microtubules into the bending of the cilium.

Bronchiectasis is the irreversible, abnormal dilation of one or more bronchi associated with various lung conditions, commonly accompanied by chronic infection. In Kartagener's syndrome it has been found that uncoordinated dyskinesia is more prevalent than immotile cilia. There is therefore a movement in the literature to call this syndrome primary ciliary dyskinesia (PCD), and Kartagener's syndrome would be a subclassification of that group of disorders. Dextrocardia (cardiac apex to the right) occurs in mild cases and *situs inversus* in more severe cases. In *situs inversus*, the morphologic right atrium is on the left, and the morphologic left atrium is on the right. Pulmonary structures (i.e., right and left lungs) as well as abdominal organs may also be reversed in a mirror image of normal. The development of right-left asymmetry is at least partially regulated by ciliary beat at Hensen's node.

The saccharin test is a test of nasal mucociliary clearance. It is carried out by placing a small amount of saccharin behind the anterior end of the inferior turbinate. In the presence of normal mucociliary action, the saccharin will be swept backward to the nasopharynx and a sweet taste perceived. Failure of sweetness to be detected within about 20 minutes indicates delayed mucociliary clearance.

82. The answer is e. (*Kierszenbaum, pp 7–8, 28–29. Alberts, pp 966–968, Junqueira, pp 44, 46. Ross and Pawlina, pp 104–106.*) Nexin, the radial spokes, and the basal body all play a role in restricting the sliding motion and converting it to the bending of the axoneme in relation to the basal body. Dynein is a high-molecular-weight ATPase. When dynein is activated, it produces the sliding motion of the microtubules as it walks along the adjacent doublet (**answer a**). The basal body (**answer b**) anchors the microtubules and also plays an essential role in converting the sliding of the outer microtubules into the bending of the cilium. The basal bodies resist the sliding movement generated by dynein activation. Nexin (**answer c**) links the outer microtubular doublets, creating a strap-like arrangement of paired microtubules around the central microtubule doublet. The radial spokes hold the microtubule doublets in place, and sliding is limited lengthwise. The radial spokes (**answer d**) are rigid and do not slide against nexin.

83. The answer is c. (*Alberts, pp 1066–1078. Young, pp 86–89. Junqueira, p 70. Ross and Pawlina, pp 130–131.*) The hemidesmosome interacts with the extracellular matrix molecules within the basal lamina through intermediate filament proteins. The hemidesmosomes combined with the desmosomes act to distribute tensile forces through the epithelial sheet and the supporting connective tissues. For information on gap junctions see the answer for question 75. Junctional complexes are summarized in the table below.

Classification	Type	Function	Interactions
Occluding	Zonula occludens (tight junction)	Prevents passage of luminal sub-stances; confers epithelial tight-ness or leakiness; maintains apical vs. basolateral polarity	Intramembranous sealing strands occlude the space between cells (# of strands directly proportional to tightness of epithe-lium)
Anchoring	Zonula adherens	Mechanical stability—cohesive function of cell groups, important during embryonic folding; transmits motile forces across epithelial sheets	Link actin filament network be-tween cells, cadherins are transmembrane linkers
	Focal contacts	Attach cells to the ECM	Link actin filament network of cell to integrins in ECM; actin-binding proteins form link
Anchoring	Desmosome (macula adherens)	Spot welds (rivets) provide high tensile strength and resist shearing forces, numerous in stratified squamous epithelia	Link intermediate filaments to transmembrane proteins (cadherins: desmogleins and desmocollins). Linkage through plaque proteins (desmoplakins)

(Continued)

Classification	Type	Function	Interactions
	Hemidesmosome	Increased stability of epithelia on extracellular matrix (ECM)	Link intermediate filaments in the cell to the ECM through integrins rather than cadherins
Communicating	Gap junction (nexus)	Selective communication in the form of diffusible molecules between 1 and 1.5 kD	Connexons in hexameric arrangement with central pores in adjacent cells align

84. The answer is c. *(Kasper, pp 311–312. Junqueira, p 366. Kierszenbaum, pp 16, 35, 307. Alberts, p 1072.)* In pemphigus vulgaris, autoantibodies to desmogleins (a member of the cadherin protein family) result in disruption of the macula adherens (desmosomes). The desmogleins are the transmembrane linker proteins of the desmosome. Specific desmogleins are the target of the autoantibodies in different forms of the disease. Cadherins are Ca^{2+}-dependent transmembrane linker molecules essential for cell-cell contact, so their disruption in pemphigus leads to severe blistering of the skin because of disrupted cell-cell interactions early in the differentiation of the keratinocytes (epidermal cell) and excessive fluid loss. The other parts of the junctional complex: zonula occludens **(answer b)** and gap junctions **(answer d)** are not affected in pemphigus. The connections to the basal lamina, hemidesmosomes **(answer a),** as well as the basal lamina itself, are not part of the etiology of pemphigus. This is in contrast to bullous pemphigoid (BP), where the BP antigen causes the separation of the epithelium from the basal lamina. Cadherins are also critical molecules in the maintenance of the zonula adherens, but the autoantibodies in pemphigus are specific to the desmogleins. Pemphigus vulgaris, which is described in the clinical scenario, often begins as oral lesions and subsequently appears cutaneously. The Nikolsky sign is positive (pressure at the edge of a blister causes extension of the bulla into adjacent normal skin) in pemphigus, while in bullous pemphigoid the Nikolsky sign is negative. For more details on junctional complexes, see the table in the answer for question 83. Also, see questions 197 and 199.

85. The answer is a. *(Junqueira, pp 42–44, 46, 71, 471–474.)* The centriole consists of nine microtubule triplets arranged together by linking proteins to form a cartwheel arrangement. Microtubules are found in different structural patterns within the cell. The basal body is a centriole-like structure associated with the ciliary axoneme. It too has a nine-triplet arrangement of microtubules. Cytoplasmic microtubules **(answer b)** are found in the singlet form and undergo constant association and dissociation of tubulin at their plus ends and minus ends, respectively. Flagella **(answer c)** have the same "9+2" arrangement as cilia, but are limited to one per cell and in adult humans are found only in sperm. The axoneme **(answer d)** has the classic "9+2" arrangement of microtubules. Stereocilia **(answer e)** are large, modified microvilli, found in the epididymis and on hair cells in the organ of Corti, therefore, they are not composed of microtubules.

Connective Tissue

Questions

DIRECTIONS: Each item below contains a question or incomplete statement followed by suggested responses. Select the **one best** response to each question.

86. A 27-year-old, 5-ft-10 in. tall woman presents in the emergency room with a pneumothorax but is afebrile. On physical examination it is noted that she has scoliosis, pectus excavatum, ectopia lentis, and myopia. Her musculoskeletal exam reveals long upper and lower extremities, including the fingers and toes, and an overall gangly, lanky appearance. Her armspan (6 ft 3 in.) noticeably exceeds her height. She has very flexible fingers and a narrow face as well as a narrow mouth with overcrowded teeth. There are stretch marks across her buttocks. Which part of the cardiovascular system would often be adversly affected in this syndrome?

a. Middle cerebral artery
b. Basilar artery
c. Aorta
d. Lymphatic vessels
e. Superior vena cava

87. The extracellular matrix and the cytoskeleton communicate across the cell membrane through which of the following?

a. Proteoglycans
b. Integrins
c. Cadherins
d. Intermediate filaments
e. Microtubules

88. A pregnant 29-year-old woman diagnosed with type I diabetes 2 decades ago, taking Humulin three times per day, is referred to the ophthalmology clinic. She is complaining of "floaters" and difficulty with night-time driving. Dilated indirect ophthalmoscopy coupled with biomicroscopy and fundus photography detect the presence of proliferative diabetic retinopathy with leaky retinal vessels indicative of increased vascular permeability, growth of new, fragile vessels on the retina and posterior surface of the vitreous and macular edema. Overexpression of fibronectin is a histological marker of diabetic microangiopathy. Which of the following is the primary function of fibronectin in the basement membrane?

a. Elasticity
b. Cell attachment and adhesion
c. Binding to selectins
d. Binding to cadherins
e. Binding to actin filaments

89. A 36-year-old man is referred by his family medicine physician to the pulmonary clinic. He complains of shortness of breath following physical activity and a decreased capacity for exercise. He says that strenuous exercise including yard work is impossible without sitting down and resting every few minutes. After he takes several deep breaths during the physical exam he begins to wheeze. He is not a smoker and as an office worker he is not exposed to dust, fumes or other irritants at work. He appears slightly jaundiced. Serum alpha-1 antitrypsin (AAT) concentration is below normal and is followed up with alpha-1 antitrypsin phenotype and DNA testing indicating one copy of S and one of Z (SZ) mutations and 40% abnormal AAT protein production. Desmosine and isodesmosine are elevated in the urine. Desmosine and isodesmosine contribute to the elasticity of the lung by:

a. Cross-linking fibrillin
b. Cross-linking tropoelastin
c. Activating elastase
d. Inactivating AAT
e. Binding type IV collagen to elastin

90. In the synthesis of collagen, the hydroxylation of proline and lysine occurs in which of the following?

a. Golgi apparatus
b. Secretory vesicles
c. Rough endoplasmic reticulum
d. Smooth endoplasmic reticulum
e. Lysosomes

91. Tropocollagen is not assembled in the cell because of which of the following?

a. Action of lysyl oxidase in the Golgi apparatus
b. Acidity of clathrin-coated vesicles
c. Presence of nonhelical registration peptides at the ends of the triple helix
d. Presence of specific collagenases in the RER and Golgi apparatus
e. Presence of specific inhibitors of peptidase activity in the Golgi apparatus

92. The primary function of entactin (also known as nidogen) is to cross-link which of the following?

a. Laminin to collagen
b. Cells to the basal lamina
c. Cells to the extracellular matrix
d. Collagen
e. Actin

93. A 14-year-old boy presents with thin, translucent skin, and a history of easy bruising. Biochemical studies of the patient's dermal fibroblasts cultured from a skin biopsy show abnormal electrophoretic mobility and abnormal secretion of type III procollagen. A mutation in the COL3A1 gene is identified by molecular testing. Which of the following symptoms would be most expected in this patient?

a. Rupture of the intestinal or aortic walls
b. Hyperextensibility of the integument
c. Hypermobility of synovial joints
d. Increased degradation of proteoglycans in articular cartilages
e. Imperfections in dentin formation (dentinogenesis imperfecta)

94. The tissue shown in the photomicrograph differs from white adipose tissue in which of the following ways?

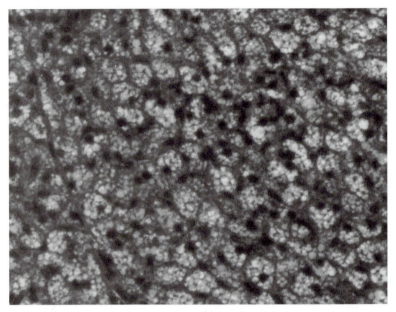

(Micrograph courtesy of Dr. WenFang Wang.)

a. Export of fatty acids
b. Role as a thermal insulator
c. Use of fatty acids to produce heat
d. Activation of the adenylate cyclase system
e. Initiation of shivering

95. Diseases in which there is a loss of function mutation in integrin expression on lymphocytes would most likely result in:

a. Leukopenia
b. Leukocytosis
c. Lymphadenopathy
d. Lymphocyte apoptosis
e. Increased numbers of plasma cells in the blood

96. A 33-year-old homeless woman has been living in an abandoned building eating dried meat, bread from the trash cans outside a bakery. She smokes cigarettes she "bums" from others. She presents at the free clinic with bleeding under the skin particularly around hair follicles with bruises on her arms and legs. She is irritable, clinically depressed, and fatigued with general muscle weakness. Her gums are bleeding, swollen, purple, and spongy. Her incisors and second molars are loose. She has an infected toe, which may be broken. She is afebrile and a glucose finger stick is normal and urine dipstick shows no sugar, protein or ketones. You suspect a vitamin deficiency. What might be the underlying mechanism for the symptoms in this patient?

a. Decreased degradation of collagen
b. Stimulation of prolyl hydroxylase
c. Formation of unstable collagen helices
d. Excessive callus formation in healing fractures
e. Organ fibrosis

97. Which of the following is a major contributor to the tensile strength of collagen?

a. Interactions with the FACIT collagens
b. The double helical arrangement of collagen
c. Electrostatic interactions
d. Intramolecular and intermolecular cross-links
e. Low concentrations of lysine

98. Laminin functions in which of following ways?

a. As an integrin
b. In cell-cell adhesion
c. As the insoluble scaffolding of the basal lamina
d. As the filtration molecule in the basement membrane
e. In adherence of epithelia to the basement membrane

99. A 40-year-old woman is referred to a dermatologist with more than 100 oval or round red-brown macules on her back. There is a positive Darier's sign. The dermatologist takes a skin biopsy, which is stained with toluidine blue. There are an excessive number of the metachromatically-stained cells labeled with the arrows and shown in the inset to the lower left in the photomicrograph below. Which of the following would be the most likely expected symptom in the patient?

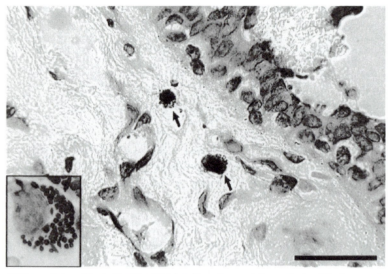

(With permission of the JayDoc Histo Web:http://www.kumc.edu/instruction/medicine/anatomy/ histoweb/.)

a. Inhibition of HCl production by parietal cells
b. Darkening of the skin
c. Osteoporosis
d. Anemia
e. Edema

100. A 46-year-old woman who has been a type I diabetic for 35 years visits your family medicine office. She has foot ulcers on both her right and her left feet. You prescribe Beclaperin gel, a prescription drug for the treatment of diabetic foot ulcers. It contains platelet-derived growth factor (PDGF). Which of the following is the most likely mechanism for the action of PDGF in the improvement of wound healing?

a. Acceleration of chemotaxis of monocytes-macrophages
b. Inhibition of vascular smooth-muscle cell proliferation
c. Inhibition of fibroblast proliferation
d. Inhibition of granulation tissue formation
e. Secretion of type II collagen from fibroblasts

101. A 55-year-old Caucasian man presented with generalized back pain. His physical examination reveals slight right-sided muscular weakness and a pulse of 78/min, regular; blood pressure 140/82 mm Hg. X-ray examination of the spine showed two wedged thoracic vertebrae, T7 and T8; no osteolytic lesions are observed. Peripheral blood: Hb 11 g/dL, WBC 6.0 × 10^9/l (polymorphs 81%, lymphocytes 16%, monocytes 2%, eosinophils 1%), platelets 300 × 10^9/l (300 000/mm³). The blood film was normal. The bone marrow shows an increase in the cells shown in the accompanying light micrograph. Other tests were all normal. The cells in the light micrograph synthesize which of the following?

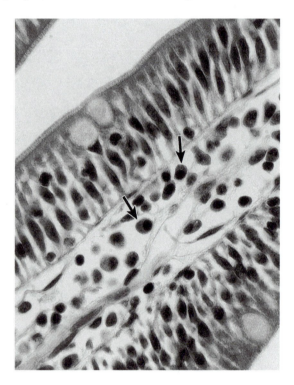

a. Collagen
b. Heparin and histamine
c. Histaminase
d. IgA
e. Myeloperoxidase

102. A 44-year-old African-American woman visits her family physician's office. She has come in for a physical examination at the urging of her husband. She has no current complaints and is taking no medications. She is allergic to erythromycin. She works as a software developer and lives with her 52-year-old husband and 12-year-old daughter. She is a nonsmoker; and drinks an occasional glass of wine when she and her husband go out to dinner. She is involved in no regular exercise. Her mother is 66 and suffers from type II diabetes, hyerlipidemia, and hypertension and had a myocardial infarction last year. The patient's father died of a stroke last year at the age of 72. On examination, the patient's blood pressure is 155/100, pulse 84, weight 215 lb (increased from 180 3 years ago), height 5 ft 7 in. In this patient, during the period of weight gain which of the following responses would be most expected in the cells shown in the photomicrograph?

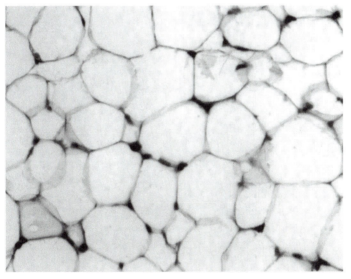

(Micrograph courtesy of Dr. WenFang Wang.)

a. Up-regulation of leptin-receptors
b. Decreased synthesis of leptin
c. Decreased release of leptin into the serum
d. Increased secretion of neuropeptide Y
e. Increased release of norepinephrine from nerve terminals in adipose tissue

103. A 65-year-old African-American man who has a history of both urinary tract infections and urinary stones presents at the urology clinic with hematuria. He has a dietary history high in saturated fats and has been exposed to second-hand smoke both at home (his wife smokes) and at work where many of his coworkers smoke. His work as a machinist exposed him to metal parts. Before working as a machinist he worked as a commercial painter. Cystoscopy identified several bladder tumors and was followed by transuretheral resection and biopsy (TURB). The biopsy shows a transitional cell carcinoma 4.5 cm. in diameter staged as "T3aN1M2." Which of the following would facilitate the processes involved in the "M2" classification?

a. Lysyl oxidase
b. Metalloproteinases
c. Plasminogen
d. Serpins
e. TIMPs

Connective Tissue

Answers

86. The answer is c. (*Alberts, p 1103. Kasper, pp 1481–1484.*) The patient in the scenario suffers from Marfan syndrome, an autosomal dominant disease in which persons develop abnormal elastic tissue. Decreased elasticity of lung tissue causes an increased tendency toward spontaneous pneumothorax, also known as a collapsed lung. The aorta is the most affected organ because of the extensive elastin in the wall, and dissecting aortic aneurysms are common in these patients. Marfan malformations include cardiovascular (valve problems as well as aortic aneurysm), skeletal (abnormal height and severe chest deformities), and ocular systems. The molecular basis of the disease is a mutation in the fibrillin gene. The lens is also often affected in patients with Marfan syndrome. The result is the dislocation of the lens because of loss of elasticity in the suspensory ligament.

87. The answer is b. (*Alberts, pp 1082–1085, 1113–1118.*) The <u>integr</u>ins are transmembrane heterodimers (<u>integr</u>al membrane proteins) that act as membrane receptors for extracellular matrix components. The best examples are the fibronectin receptor and the laminin receptor. The receptor structure includes an intracytosolic portion that binds to the actin cytoskeleton through the attachment proteins talin or α-actinin. The extracellular portion has specificity for extracellular matrix molecules. Proteoglycans (**answer a**) are located on the extracellular surface of the plasma membrane and throughout the extracellular matrix. The cadherins (**answer c**) function as transmembrane glycoproteins involved in the formation of parts of the intercellular junctional complexes. Cadherins are components of the desmosome and zonula adherens. Intermediate filaments and microtubules (**answers d and e**) are found intracellularly and constitute the cytoskeleton.

88. The answer is b. (*Alberts, pp 1094–1096, 1102–1105. Junqueira, pp 91, 115–116.*) Fibronectin is an adhesive glycoprotein that is important for cell attachment and adhesion. It is important for modulation of cell migration in the adult and during development. Neural crest and other cells appear to be guided along fibronectin-coated pathways in the embryo. Fibronectin is found in three forms: a plasma form that is involved in blood clotting; a cell-surface form, which binds to the cell surface transiently; and a matrix form, which is fibrillar in arrangement. Fibronectin contains a cell-binding domain (RGD sequence), a collagen-binding domain, and a heparin-binding domain. Elastin and type III collagen are responsible for elasticity seen in large arteries and the pinna of the ear (**answer a**). Cell-cell interactions involve both transient and more long-term, stable processes. Cell-cell adhesion is mediated by transmembrane proteins called cell adhesion molecules which include the calcium or magnesium-dependent selectins, integrins, and cadherins (**answers c and d**) and the non-calcium-dependent immunoglobulin (Ig) superfamily. The stable adhesion junction, known as the zonula adherens, links the cytoskeleton of adjacent cells through cadherins (transmembrane linker proteins) to actin filaments inside the cell [**answer e** (see feedback for question 199)].

89. The answer is b. *(Junqueira, p 357. Kasper, pp 1547–1550. Kumar, pp 719–723.)* The patient suffers from alpha-1 antitrypsin (AAT) emphysema. AAT protects the lung from neutrophil-derived elastase, which breaks down elastic fibers (**answer d**), which are composed of a core of elastin with a surrounding network of fibrillin. Desmosine and isodesmosine are amino acids unique to elastin and responsible for the covalent binding of elastin fibers to each other. Lysyl oxidase catalyzes the cross-linking of tropoelastin (**answers a**). Microfibrils, composed of fibrillin, facilitate formation of the elastin molecules, but are not directly involved in cross-linking. Elastase (**answer c**) is a serine protease that specifically degrades elastin. Interactions occur between type III collagen and elastic fibers (**answer e**). The collagen may serve to limit the stretch of the elastic components. Elasticity is conferred through the highly hydrophobic nature of elastin. One-third of elastin is composed of the hydrophobic amino acid glycine, which is randomly distributed throughout the elastin molecule. This is in contrast to the even distribution of glycine in collagen. The random distribution of glycine makes elastin hydrophobic. The overall hydrophobicity of elastin molecules allows for their distensibility and facilitates their capacity to slide over one another.

90. The answer is c. *(Alberts, pp 1098–1100. Junqueira, pp 106–110.)* Prolyl and lysyl hydroxylase are the two enzymes that carry out hydroxylation of proline and lysine. The process is both co- and posttranslational and, therefore, occurs during, or more often after, the amino acids are inserted into nascent collagen polypeptide chains in the RER. Those two amino acids are characteristic of collagen. Hydroxyproline, which constitutes 10% of collagen, is often used to determine the collagen content of various tissues. Hydroxylation of proline stabilizes the triple helix through interchain hydrogen bonds, and hydroxylation of lysine is critical for the cross-linking stage of collagen assembly.

91. The answer is c. (*Alberts, pp 1098–1100. Junqueira, pp 106–110.*) Nonhelical registration peptides at the ends of the triple helix prevent tropocollagen assembly in the RER, Golgi apparatus, and secretory vesicles. Collagen is synthesized as pro-α–chains, which are assembled into procollagen molecules (triple helix) in the rough endoplasmic reticulum. Procollagen is subsequently transported in transfer vesicles to the Golgi for packaging into secretory vesicles. Transport of secretory vesicles is an energy- and microtubule-dependent process. Outside of the cell, N-terminal and C-terminal specific procollagen peptidases cleave the nonhelical registration peptides, which results in the formation of tropocollagen. Tropocollagen spontaneously assembles in a staggered array to form collagen fibrils. Lysyl oxidase (**answer a**) is an extracellular enzyme responsible for the formation of covalent cross-links between tropocollagen molecules. Fibrils form collagen fibers under the influence of other extracellular matrix constituents, such as proteoglycans and glycoproteins. Collagenases (**answer d**) specifically cleave tropocollagen in the extracellular matrix.

92. The answer is a. (*Alberts, pp 1099, 1107–1108.*) The primary function of entactin (nidogen) is to cross-link laminin to type IV collagen. The basal lamina is formed by interactions between type IV collagen, laminin, entactin, and the proteoglycan perlecan. Integrins like laminin receptors (**answer b**) bind cells to the basal lamina; fibronectin receptors bind cells to the extracellular matrix (**answer c**). Laminin receptors in the cell membrane also organize the assembly of the basal lamina. Collagen (**answer d**) is cross-linked by covalent intramolecular and intermolecular cross-links that form primarily between the nonhelical segments at the ends of the collagen molecules. Lysyl oxidase is a key enzyme in the cross-linking process; it deaminates lysine and hydroxylysine to form aldehyde groups that react with each other to form the covalent bonds. Actin is cross-linked (answer e) into bundles by actin-binding proteins such as the bundling protein α-actinin and the gel-forming protein (fimbrin). The following table lists the location of the major types of collagen.

Type	Location	Function and Other Information
MAJOR COLLAGEN TYPES		
*I	General C.T., bone, and fibrocartilage	Most abundant type of collagen, 67-nm periodicity, tensile strength
*II	Hyaline and elastic cartilage	Thinner fibrils than type I, tensile strength, electrostatic interactions between type II collagen and proteoglycan aggregates form the molecular basis for the rigidity of hyaline cartilage
*III	Spleen, bone marrow, and lymph nodes	Reticular framework, stains with silver
*IV	Basement membrane	Filtration, support, meshwork scaffolding, interacts with heparan sulfate proteoglycan to produce a polyanionic charge distribution that facilitates selective filtration; synthesized by epithelia; it retains propeptides that are used to form a meshwork; also interacts with fibronectin
V	Placental basement membrane, muscle basal lamina	Linkage function in basement membrane (?)
VII	Basement membrane of skin and amnion	Anchoring fibers
VIII	Endothelium	Angiogenesis, bridging ECM components
IX–XII	Cartilage	Fibril-associated collagens with interrupted triple helices (FACIT) regulate orientation and function of fibrillar collagens

*Most common collagen types and most testable

93. The answer is a. *(Junqueira, pp 107, 111, 367. Alberts, p 1100.)* The patient in the vignette is suffering from Ehlers-Danlos Syndrome (EDS) type IV (also known as EDS of the vascular type). In this disorder there is improperly formed type III collagen, which is responsible for the elasticity of the intestinal and aortic walls. There are errors in the transcription of type III collagen mRNA or in translation of this mRNA. Hyperextensible skin **(answer b)** occurs in Ehlers-Danlos type VI disorder, in which problems with the hydroxylation of the amino acid lysine and subsequent cross-linking result in enhanced elasticity. Type VII Ehlers-Danlos disorder involves a specific deficiency in an amino terminal procollagen peptidase. This results from a genetic mutation that alters the propeptide sequence in such a way that the molecular orientation and cross-linking are adversely affected. The result is hypermobility **(answer c)** of synovial joints. Increased degradation of proteoglycans occurs in osteoarthritis **(answer d)**. Type I collagen is found in dentin **(answer e)**.

94. The answer is c. *(Junqueira, pp 123, 125–127.)* The photomicrograph illustrates the microscopic structure of brown fat. Both types of fat tissue (brown and white) are highly vascularized and function in protection from the cold. Brown fat specifically is involved in heat production, whereas white fat is a true thermal insulator. Brown adipose tissue is multilocular and is found in the human fetus and neonate. Brown fat is involved in nonshivering thermogenesis and generates heat **(answer c)**, probably as a protective device for developing organs in the fetus and neonate. White adipose tissue is specialized for lipid storage and functions as a thermal insulator **(answer b)** and shock absorber. White adipose tissue is unilocular, and the cells have a single, large lipid droplet in the cytoplasm that provides the "signet-ring" appearance often described for fat cells. Brown adipose tissue has a multilocular appearance and is brown because of numerous mitochondria.

In fat, norepinephrine activates the cyclic AMP **(answer d)** cascade through adenylate cyclase. Cyclic AMP activates hormone-sensitive lipase, which removes triglycerides from the stored lipid and hydrolyzes free fatty acids. In white adipocytes, the released fatty acids and glycerol are exported from the cells. In brown adipose tissue, the fatty acids are used within the cell **(answer a)**. However, the electron transport system is uncoupled from oxidative phosphorylation, which results in the production of heat **(answer c)** instead of ATP. Heat is transferred to the blood by the extensive capillary networks found in brown adipose tissue.

Shivering **(answer e)** initiates the mobilization of lipid in white adipose tissue because shivering requires energy.

95. The answer is b. *(Alberts, pp 1113–1118.)* A mutation resulting in loss of integrin function would prevent leukocytes from extravasting from the blood to the lymph nodes (see figure below) and sites of inflammation resulting in increased lymphocytes in the blood (leukocytosis), not leukopenia

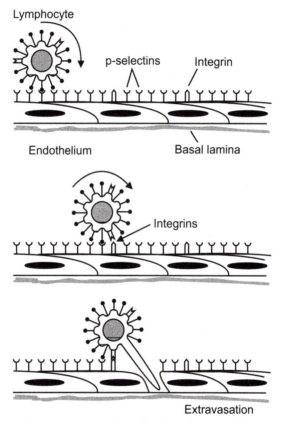

Extravasation

There are several stages in extravasation: *rolling, firm adhesion, and diapedesis.* Cytokines, such as tumor necrosis factor-alpha (TNF-α), are released during inflammation and stimulate the endothelium of veins to express the surface adhesion molecule P-selectin (also E-selectin). E and P-selectins bind reversibly to glycoproteins on leukocytes causing them to *roll* along the endothelial surface. Intercellular adhesion molecules (e.g. ICAM-1) are up-regulated and bind to the leukocyte integrins LFA-1 and CR3. *Adhesion* of leukocytes results in arrest of leukocyte motion, allowing secreted proteases to disrupt endothelial tight junctions and the basement membrane, subsequently resulting in *diapedesis.* L-selectins expressed by leukocytes are also involved in the process.

(answer a). In a rare congenital immunodeficiency disease, known as lymphocyte adhesion disease (LAD), patients suffer from recurrent bacterial infections in which the leukocytes from affected children fail to adhere to endothelial cells and migrate to the site of infection **(answer c)** due to defects in the leukocyte integrin CD18 subunit. In different forms of LAD there may be structural defects in the integrin molecule or a deficiency or absence of CD18. Lymphocyte apoptosis **(answer d)** is not regulated directly by integrins and plasma cells do not normally enter the blood **(answer e)**. The leukocyte adhesion cascade involves several precise ordered steps: rolling, integrin activation and firm adhesion of the leukocytes, all necessary prerequisites to transendothelial migration. Therefore, in LAD, extravasation of leukocytes is not possible.

96. The answer is c. *(Alberts, pp 1098–1102. Junqueira, pp 107.)* Vitamin C deficiency causes scurvy. The woman in the scenario is pregnant, smokes, and has a diet deficient in fresh fruits and vegetables. Scurvy, or vitamin C deficiency, results in an inability to form normal collagen triple helices. In scurvy, the resulting collagen is less stable and is subject to denaturation and proteolytic breakdown **(answer a)**. That results partially from slower secretion of collagen from fibroblasts. The collagen formed is not normally hydroxylated at proline and lysine residues because of the absence of vitamin C, which is a specific cofactor for hydroxylation of proline and lysine **(answer b)**. Bone structure and the dentition may be abnormal and wound and fracture healing delayed **(answer d)**. General tissue instability may occur because collagen synthesis is necessary for maintenance of structural support **(answer e)**. Periodontal bleeding and ulceration are also common symptoms in scurvy.

97. The answer is d. *(Alberts, pp1096–1102.)* The fibrillar collagens establish tensile strength at a number of levels including intra- and intermolecular cross-links. Covalent binding occurs through the OH^- groups of hydroxylysine and hydroxyproline and serves to stabilize the triple helix. The triple helix **(answer b)** itself functions to resist tensile forces. The degree of cross-linking varies from tissue to tissue. For example, it is highly extensive in tendons. The organization of collagen in tissues also varies, depending on function, from the layered appearance in bone to the axial parallel bundles in tendons and the wickered pattern in skin. The interactions with fibril-associated collagens (with interrupted triple helices) regulate orientation and are also important in establishing tissue organization and flexibility **(answer a)**. Electrostatic interactions **(answer c)** do not play a significant role in maintenance of collagen tensile strength. Lysine, along with hydroxylysine, is the substrate for lysyl oxidase that catalyzes the formation of cross-links **(answer e)**.

98. The answer is e. *(Alberts, pp 1081–1088, 1107–1108, Junqueira, pp 67, 91, 115–116.)* Laminin is a glycoprotein and a major component of all basement membranes that is involved in cell adherence to the basal lamina. Laminin in the lamina rara (lucida) of the basal lamina binds to the laminin receptor (integrin) on the epithelial cell **(answer a)**. Cell-cell interactions **(answer b)** are modulated by the cell adhesion molecules [e.g., the Ca^{2+}-dependent cadherins and selectins and the Ca^{2+}-independent CAMs, such as the neural cell adhesion molecule (N-CAM)]. Laminin contains RGD and YIGSR cell-binding sites as well as binding sites for collagen, entactin, and heparan sulfate proteoglycan. Type IV collagen forms the insoluble scaffolding of the basal lamina **(answer c)**. The highly charged glycosaminoglycans are responsible for the filtration characteristics **(answer d)** of the basement membrane (e.g., renal glomerular basement membrane).

99. The answer is e. *(Kasper, pp 228, 1953–1954. Junqueira, pp 97–99, 101–103.)* Mastocytosis is a disease in which there is excessive production of mast cells by the bone marrow. The cells in the biopsy are mast cells that stain metachromatically (change color of the stain from blue to purple). Like basophils, they synthesize and secrete heparin and histamine. The result of mastocytosis is an excessive release of the bioactive products contained in mast cell granules: histamine, heparin, eosinophil chemotactic factor of anaphylaxis (ECF-A), slow-reacting substance of anaphylaxis (SRS-A), and leukotrienes. Mastocytosis induces urticaria pigmentosa (the skin condition from which the patient in the scenario suffers), including edema (caused by the increased vascular permeability induced by histamine and SRS-A). In mastocytosis, there is infiltration of eosinophils (attracted by ECF-A), which causes itching. Excessive production of acid by the parietal cells of the stomach **(answer a)** occurs because of the overstimulation of histamine receptors on these cells. This can result in peptic ulcers and gastritis. Lower GI tract symptoms include increased motility and diarrhea due to the stimulation by mast cell contents. Periportal fibrosis of the liver often occurs in systemic mastocytosis due to the extensive infiltration of mast cells into the liver. Melanocytes **(answer b)** are not affected. Anemia and osteoporosis **(answers c and d)** would occur in either multiple myeloma or plasmacytosis, where there are excessive numbers of plasma cells. The excessive production of plasma cells in the bone marrow disrupts normal hematopoiesis including the production of RBCs, causing anemia. Plasma cells release interleukins (IL-1 and IL-6) and tumor necrosis factor-alpha (TNF-α) that stimulate osteoclastic activity and induce osteoporosis (see clinical case questions in the chapter on bone and cartilage).

The positive Darier's sign is a red wheal and surrounding erythema around the lesions after rubbing due to the release of histamine.

100. The answer is a. (*Alberts, pp 872–874, 1015. Kumar, pp 42, 95, 110, 1198, 1204. Rubin, pp 86–88, 103.*) Platelet-derived growth factor (PDGF) stimulates chemotaxis of monocytes and macrophages as well as fibroblasts to the site of a wound. PDGF also induces proliferation of vascular smooth muscle cells **(answer b)** to facilitate blood vessel repair and fibroblasts **(answer c)** to synthesize type I collagen. PDGF stimulates the formation of granulation tissue **(answer d)** consisting of new connective tissue and small blood vessels that form in the wound site. Type II collagen **(answer e)** is synthesized by chondrocytes in hyaline and elastic cartilage. Wound healing is a complex process initiated by damage to capillaries in the dermis. The clot forms through the interaction of integrins on the surface of blood platelets with fibrinogen and fibronectin. Fibrin is the primary protein that constructs the three-dimensional structure of the clot. A scar is formed as a very dense region of type I collagen fibers. Macrophages remove debris at the wound site and are also involved in the remodeling of the scar. All wound healing processes are slower in diabetics, and the presence of advanced-glycation end products (AGE) and their interaction with the receptor for AGE (RAGE) as well as the endogenous ligand for RAGE (ENRAGE) appear to contribute to inhibited healing in diabetes. AGE are produced by the nonenzymatic glycation and oxidation of proteins/lipids and alter those molecules and therefore the function and structure of tissues and organs such as the kidney (diabetic nephropathy), peripheral nerves (neuropathy), and the retina (diabetic retinopathy).

101. The answer is d. (*Alberts, pp 1367–1368, 1375. Young, pp 11, 16, 78, 200. Goldsby, pp 9, 33, 36–37, 76–78, 88–94.*) The patient in the scenario suffers from multiple myeloma with an increase in the number of plasma cells responsible for producing immunoglobulins (antibodies). The cells delineated by the arrows in the photomicrograph are plasma cells characterized by eccentric nuclei with coarse granules of heterochromatin arranged in a radial pattern about the nuclear envelope. Membrane-bound ribosomes are extremely plentiful, providing the cytoplasm with a characteristic intense basophilia. The ribosomes are involved in antibody production, principally immunoglobulin G (IgG). The juxtanuclear region, which does not stain, represents the Golgi complex, in which the antibodies are processed for secretion. Plasma cells produce all the immunoglobulins— IgG, IgA, IgM, IgD, and IgE—and are derived from B lymphocytes. The differentiation of plasma cells requires antigen-presenting cells (macrophages, dendritic cells, or B cells that phagocytose and present antigen-MHC II complex) and T helper (T_H) cells. The function and origin of the connective tissue cells are summarized in the table below.

CONNECTIVE TISSUE CELLS		
Cell Type	**Origin**	**Function**
Fibroblast	Mesenchyme	Synthesis of fibers (collagen, elastic, reticular) and ground substance (proteoglycans and glycoproteins of connective tissue matrix)
Macrophages (e.g., Kupffer cells, Langerhans cells and microglia)	Monocyte (bone marrow)	Phagocytosis, antigen presentation, produce and respond to cytokines
Lymphocytes T lymphocytes	Bone marrow (thymus-educated)	Cell-mediated immunity (CD_8^+) and helper T cells (CD_4^+)

(*Continued*)

Cell Type	Origin	Function
B lymphocytes	Bone marrow (bone marrow–educated)	Humoral immunity
Plasma cell	B lymphocyte	Immunoglobulin secretion
Neutrophils (PMNs)	Bone marrow	First cells to enter an inflammation site, secrete myeloperoxidase, phagocytose bacteria, and die (forming pus)
Eosinophils	Bone marrow	Source of major basic protein, histaminase (breakdown of histamine), arylsulfatases (degradation of leukotrienes), phagocytosis of antigen-antibody complexes and parasites
Basophils	Bone marrow (different stem cell from mast cell)	Blood source of histamine
Mast cells connective tissue mast cells (CTMC) and mucosal mast cells (MMC)	Bone marrow	CTMC are T-lymphocyte independent, MMC are T-lymphocyte dependent, secrete histamine and slow-reacting substance of anaphylaxis [(SRS-A) increase vascular permeability], heparin (anticoagulant), eosinophil chemoattractant factor of anaphylaxis [(ECF-A), chemoattraction of eosinophils], leukotrienes (smooth muscle contraction)

102. The answer is e. (*Junqueira, p124. Ross & Pawlina, pp 239–241.*) Leptin is a protein hormone produced by adipocytes (shown in the photomicrograph). Leptin binds to receptors in the hypothalamus and has multiple effects including increased release of norepinephrine (NE) from sympathetic nerve terminals that innervate adipose tissue. Adipocyte adrenergic receptors bind NE leading to increased metabolism of fatty acids with dissipation of the energy as heat. As weight increases and adipocytes accumulate triglycerides, the "obese" (ob) gene is up-regulated in adipocytes and leptin synthesis and serum levels of leptin are increased (**answers b and c**). Leptin-receptors in the hypothalamus are up-regulated as leptin levels increase (**answer a**). Leptin inhibits hypothalamic synthesis and secretion of neuropeptide Y, an appetite (orexigenic) peptide (**answer d**).

103. The answer is b. (*Kumar, pp 309–313.*) The patient is diagnosed with transitional cell carcinoma (TCC) that is highly aggressive having penetrated the muscle of the bladder (T3a), with lymph node involvement and metastases (M2). TCC metastasizes primarily to the lymph nodes, lung, bone, liver and brain. The tumor cells normally adhere to the basement membrane. To undergo metastasis they must dissolve the basement membrane and extracellular matrix in order to reach the bloodstream and subsequently migrate to a new site, where they reaggregate and reestablish cell-cell and cell-basal lamina interactions. Metalloproteinases such as the serine, cysteine, and metalloproteinases (MMPs), including type IV collagenase (MMP-2), play a key role in freeing tumor cells to migrate to metastatic sites. Lysyl oxidase (**answer a**) is an extracellular enzyme that is responsible for cross-linking of collagen by deamination of lysine and hydroxylysine residues to form aldehydes. Those aldehydes then interact with each other or with other lysyl side chains to form collagen cross-links. A similar process occurs in the synthesis of elastin. Plasminogen (**answer c**) is an inactive form of plasmin that occurs in plasma and is converted to plasmin by organic solvents. SERPINS (**answer d**) are serine protease inhibitors. Members of that gene family regulate cell division and migration, neurite extension, tumor cell metastasis, and blood coagulation. The SERPINS act as specific inhibitors of cell-surface and extracellular matrix serine proteases that participate in cascade mechanisms in those biological processes. TIMPs (**answer e**), are the tissue inhibitors of the metalloproteases and, like SERPINS, inhibit the degradation of the extracellular matrix.

Specialized Connective Tissues: Bone and Cartilage

Questions

DIRECTIONS: Each item below contains a question or incomplete statement followed by suggested responses. Select the **one best** response to each question.

104. Intramembranous ossification differs from endochondral ossification in which of the following ways?

a. Action of osteoblasts
b. Light microscopic appearance of the adult bone
c. Ultrastructural appearance of the adult bone
d. Presence of woven bone early in the ossification process
e. Microenvironment in which ossification occurs

105. A 7-year-old boy is referred to the endocrine clinic with short stature, rhizomelic shortening of the arms and legs, a disproportionately long trunk, trident hands, midfacial hypoplasia, prominent forehead (frontal bossing), thoracolumbar gibbus, and megalencephaly. Radiological examination by MRI reveals caudal narrowing of the interpedicular spaces of T1 and T2 vertebrae and spinal stenosis at L2–L4. Genetic analysis reveals a gain of function mutation, G1138A, in the fibroblast growth factor receptor-3 (*FGFR3*), band 4p16.3. His parents are requesting the initiation of treatment with growth hormone. The endocrinologist is concerned about harmful growth hormone effects: deposition of abnormally-formed bone and worsening of the patient's kyphoscoliosis. During this child's postnatal development, which of the following is the most likely effect of the FGFR-3 gene mutation?

a. Decreased bone deposition under the periosteum
b. Decreased proliferation of osteoblasts in the primary ossification center
c. Decreased proliferation of osteoblasts in the secondary ossification center
d. Decreased appositional growth of chondroblasts in the primary ossification center
e. Decreased interstitial growth of chondroblasts in the epiphyses

106. The molecular basis for shock absorption within articular cartilage is which of the following?

a. Electrostatic interaction of proteoglycans with type IV collagen
b. Ability of glycosaminoglycans to bind anions
c. Noncovalent binding of glycosaminoglycans to protein cores
d. Sialic acid residues in the glycoproteins
e. Hydration of glycosaminoglycans

107. A 16-year-old girl presents to the pediatric genetic and endocrine clinic with short stature, Tanner stage 2 of pubertal development and lack of menstruation. She is 49 in. tall (normal range for age is 59–68 in. mean 64 in.) and weighs 65 lb (normal range for age is 92–158 lb, mean is 126 lb.). She has a short, broad, webbed neck, short fingers and toes, and *cubitus valgus*. Hormonal profile reveals high levels of the gonadotrophins LH and FSH, and very low levels of estrogen. Ultrasound studies show uterine hypoplasia and poorly-defined gonadal streaks. Genetic analysis shows a 45, X0 pattern. The short stature has been linked to reduced protein expression of the short stature homeobox gene (SHOX). That gene working through specific transcription factors would influence the production of which of the following by the cells delineated by the box in the accompanying photomicrograph.

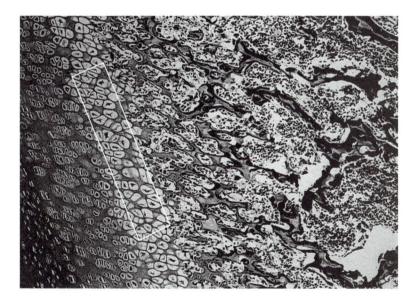

a. Cyclins
b. Acid phosphatase
c. Alkaline phosphatase
d. Type I collagen
e. Osteocalcin

108. A 22-year-old man presents to the orthopedic clinic after a referral from his primary care physician. He has a history of recurrent fractures of the humerus and femur and numerous dental caries and associated abcesses. Three years prior to this referral, he was successfully treated with hyperbaric oxygen and surgery for mandibular and maxillary osteomyelitis. Laboratory results include a serum acid phosphatase of 4 units (0.5–2 is normal range by the Bodanksy method) and a hematocrit of 35 (normal range is 41–50%, mean is 47%). Other blood tests are normal. He complains of joint pain. A spine x-ray shows "sandwich" vertebrae with thickening of the vertebral endplates. X-rays of the long bones show abnormal thickening of the bone. A skull x-ray shows basilar sclerosis. The cell type primarily affected in this patient is shown in the accompanying transmission electron micrograph (A) and labeled as "C" in the light micrograph (B). The activation and stimulation of those cells is involved in which of the following?

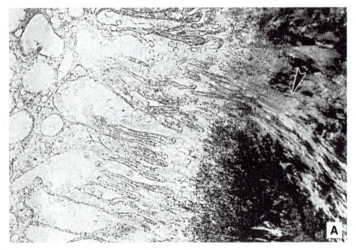

(A. Reproduced, with permission, from Erlandsen SL, Magney JE: Color Atlas of Histology. St. Louis, MO: CV Mosby, 1992.)

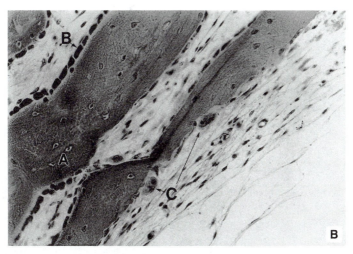

(B. Micrograph courtesy of Dr. John K. Young.)

a. Mechanical grinding of the bone matrix
b. Synthesis of alkaline phosphatase
c. Response to vitamin D through receptors on its cell membrane
d. Regulation by PTH receptors on its cell membrane
e. Proton pump activity similar to a parietal cell

109. LDC is a 45-year-old woman who presents with symmetric polyarticular joint pain, swelling, joint stiffness lasting an hour or more (particularly in the morning), malaise, fatigue, tenderness and pain, and is seropositive for RF. Analysis of synovial fluid reveals synovitis with a white blood cell count of 2500 (normal less than 2000/mm³). Physical examination shows decreased abduction and external rotation of the right and left shoulders. She has some swelling in her right and left knees with full range of motion. Which joint changes will most likely be associated with LDC's disease?

a. Loss of the proteoglycan matrix and fibrillation in the articular cartilage during the early stages
b. Decreased levels of fibrinogen in the synovial fluid
c. Formation of osteophytes at the articular margins and eburnation of large weight-bearing joints in the later stages
d. Decreased number of leukocytes including PMNs in the synovial fluid
e. Heterologous autoantibodies directed against the synovium

110. A 42-year-old woman who has been a type I diabetic for 30 years falls when she trips over her vacuum cleaner hose. She tried to break her fall by placing her hand out to save herself and in the process her wrist is forced backwards. She arrives in the emergency room and an x-ray of her wrist is shown in the accompanying x-ray. The first step in the healing of this injury is?

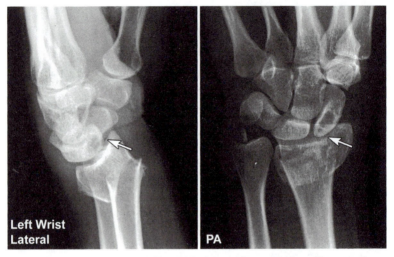

(Image 6120, used with permission from the Radiological Anatomy website, University of Kansas, School of Medicine, http://classes. Kumc.edu/SOM/radanatomy/.)

a. Internal callus
b. External callus
c. Clot
d. Pannus
e. Granulation tissue

111. A 55-year-old woman presents with pain in her right hip and thigh. The pain started approximately 6 months ago and is a deep ache that worsens when she stands or walks. Your examination reveals increased warmth over the right thigh. The only laboratory abnormalities are alkaline phosphatase 656 IU/L (normal 23–110 IU/L), elevated 24-hour urine hydroxyproline, and osteocalcin 13 ng/mL (normal 6 ng/mL). X-ray of hips and pelvis shows osteolytic lesions and regions with excessive osteoblastic activity. Bone scan shows significant uptake in the right proximal femur. Which of the following would you include in your differential diagnosis?

a. Paget's disease
b. Multiple myeloma
c. Osteomalacia
d. Osteoporosis
e. Hypoparathyroidism

112. A 66-year-old man with no previous significant illness presents with back pain. The patient had felt well except for an increase in fatigue over the past few months. He suddenly felt severe low back pain while raising his garage door. Physical examination reveals a well-developed white male in acute pain. His pulse is 88 beats per minute and blood pressure is 150/90 mm Hg. The conjunctivae are pale. There is marked tenderness to percussion over the lumbar spine. The following laboratory data are obtained: hemoglobin 11.0 g/dL (normal 13–16 g/dL), serum calcium 12.3 mg/dL (normal 8.5–11 mg/dL), abnormal serum protein electrophoresis with a monoclonal IgG spike, urine positive for Bence-Jones protein, and abnormal bone marrow smear. X-rays reveal lytic lesions of the skull and pelvis and a compression fracture of lumbar vertebrae. A potential underlying mechanism for the symptoms observed in this case is which of the following?

a. Increased IL-1, IL-6, and TNF-α by plasma cells
b. Increased release of histamine from mast cells
c. Decreased RANK expression on osteoclasts
d. Decreased RANK-L levels
e. Decreased production of M-CSF

113. A 46-year-old woman presents with pain in the left leg that worsens on weight bearing. An x-ray shows demineralization, and a decalcified (EDTA-treated) biopsy shows reduction in bone quantity. The patient had undergone menopause at age 45 without estrogen replacement. She reports long-standing diarrhea. In addition, laboratory tests show low levels of 1, 25-hydroxyvitamin D, calcium, and phosphorus and elevated alkaline phosphatase. A second bone biopsy, which was not decalcified, shows uncalcified osteoid on all the bone surfaces. On the basis of these data, your diagnosis would be which of the following?

a. Osteoporosis
b. Osteomalacia
c. Scurvy
d. Paget's disease
e. Hypoparathyroidism

114. Patients with Cushing's syndrome often show osteoporotic changes. Which of the following is involved in the etiology of osteoporosis induced by Cushing's syndrome?

a. Decreased glucocorticoid levels that result in decreased quality of the bone deposited
b. Excess deposition of osteoid
c. Stimulation of intestinal calcium absorption
d. Decreased PTH levels
e. Bone fragility resulting from excess bone resorption

115. A newborn girl is born with a small mouth, rather widely spaced eyes and low-set ears. Genetic analysis shows a microdeletion on chromosome 22q11.2 leading to a diagnosis of an anomaly which results from failure of the normal development of the third and fourth branchial pouches during embryonic development. Which of the following would be expected to occur in a child with this anomaly?

a. Absence of the parafollicular cells
b. Increased numbers of cells in the deep cortex of the lymph nodes
c. Tetany
d. Excess activity of osteoclasts
e. Increased Ca^{2+} levels in the blood

116. A 56-year-old man with a history of hypertension, type II diabetes, and a 2-year history of end-stage renal disease (ESRD) requiring hemodialysis returns to the internal medicine clinic. The patient is hyperparathyroid (parathyroid hormone, 234 pg/mL; normal 10–55 pg/mL) and hypercalcemic (calcium, 12.2 mg/dL). He also has elevated levels of serum urea nitrogen (52 mg/dL), creatinine (5.2 mg/dL), and hyperphosphatemia (phosphorus, 9.1 mg/dL). Serum levels of 1,25-dihydroxyvitamin D are decreased (10 pg/mL; reference range, 24–65 pg/mL). He has been receiving large doses of calcium supplemented with vitamin D to bind the phosphate. He complains of bone and chest pain, increasing fatigue, and extreme dyspnea. His coronary arteries are examined by electron-beam computed tomography (EBCT) and are found to be calcified. The production of calcified soft tissues is mediated by the structures shown in the accompanying transmission electron micrograph. Which of the following is a possible mechanism of action for those structures?

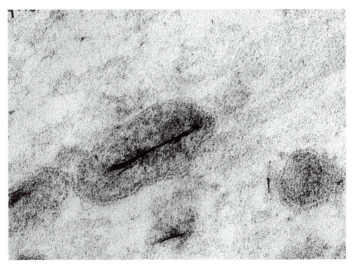

(Micrograph courtesy of Dr. H. Clarke Anderson.)

a. Increased secretion of acid phosphatase
b. Inhibition of alkaline phosphatase
c. Accumulation of calcium and phosphate
d. Increased secretion of osteoprotegerin
e. Increased synthesis of type I collagen

117. The collagenous protein in bone subserves which of the following functions?

a. Growth factor
b. Binding of ionic calcium and physiologic hydroxyapatite
c. Formation of the three-dimensional lattice of the matrix
d. Cell attachment
e. Binding of mineral components to the matrix

118. In the diagram of a joint below, the structure labeled C is which of the following?

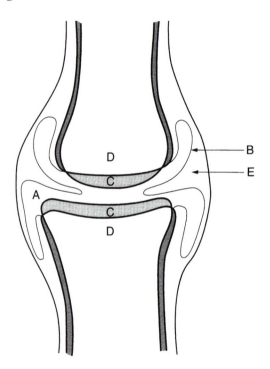

a. Site of macrophage-like cells that phagocytose particles from the synovial fluid
b. Site of cells that synthesize the synovial fluid
c. Initial site of damage in osteoarthritis
d. Initial site of inflammation in rheumatoid arthritis
e. Perichondrium

119. A 58-year-old Caucasian woman is seen in the endocrine clinic. She has been followed for type I diabetes for the past decade. She sustained a Colles' fracture last year when she fell over the hose while watering the garden. She took hormone replacement therapy (HRT) for 3 years at the start of menopause, but was taken off HRT 5 years ago because of her concerns about ovarian cancer. She drinks three glasses of milk a day and eats other dairy products frequently. She drinks socially, a drink, a glass of wine, or a beer twice/week. She does not smoke. She once was a "runner," but now walks 2 miles twice/week when weather permits. She is 5 ft 4 in. and she weighs 122 lb. Her height has decreased by an inch over the past 5 years and her weight has increased by 12 lb. CBC and blood chemistries are normal. Her "T" score on dual-energy absorptiometry (DXA) is -2 for spine and -2.5 for hip. Bisphosphonates are prescribed. Which of the following is the most likely mechanism of action for the bisphosphonates?

a.   Inhibition of osteoblastic activity
b.   Increased RANK-L secretion by osteoblasts
c.   Increased M-CSF secretion by osteoblasts
d.   Apoptosis of osteoclasts
e.   Increased RANK expression by osteoclasts

120. A 12-year-old boy who has grown 3 in. in the past 2 months presents with pain and swelling in his femur just above the knee. Any exercise results in intense pain, and the boy now walks with a limp. X-ray shows a fracture at the distal end of the right femur. Overall, the bone appears immature in the distal femur and there is increased density extending into the metaphysis. There appears to be a soft tissue mass expanding outside the bone. There is also some cortical bone destruction above the lateral condyle. A CT scan shows bone-forming cells in the lung. Once the osteosarcoma cells reach the lungs, enter the lung parenchyma, and clonally expand, they produce bone. In that process, the tumor cells synthesize which of the following?

a.   Type III collagen
b.   Type II collagen
c.   Acid phosphatase
d.   Alkaline phosphatase
e.   Elastin

121. If a laboratory were designing an effective therapy to prevent the spread of metastatic osteosarcoma, which of the following approaches would most likely be successful?

a. Enhancement of fibronectin-integrin interactions
b. Enhancement of laminin-integrin interactions
c. Upregulation of selectins on endothelial cells
d. Upregulation of TIMPs at the primary tumor site
e. Downregulation of angiostatin or endostatin at the primary tumor site

122. A 28-year-old woman visits your family medicine clinic complaining of loss of sense of smell, nosebleeds, problems with swallowing, and hoarseness. She admits to "casual, social use" of cocaine on a regular basis since her sophomore year of college when her "boyfriend turned her on to cocaine at a party." You complete examination of her nose with a speculum and otoscope and determine that she has rhinitis (inflammation). There is also perforation and collapse of the nasal cartilage resulting in a "saddle nose" deformity. You also note erosions in the enamel of her front teeth. The breakdown of the nasal cartilage releases collagen fibers primarily of which type?

a. Type I
b. Type II
c. Type III
d. Type IV
e. Type VII

Specialized Connective Tissues: Bone and Cartilage

Answers

104. The answer is e. *(Junqueira, pp 141–147. Ross and Pawlina, pp 232–235.)* The difference between endochondral and intramembranous ossification is the microenvironment in which bone formation occurs. In both cases, bone development occurs by essentially the same process, the synthesis of collagen and other matrix components by osteoblasts **(answer a)** and the calcification of the matrix through the action of alkaline phosphatase from osteoblasts. Bone development occurs in two different locations, which differ in the presence or absence of cartilage models of the bones. For example, in the flat bones of the skull, bone formation occurs through the differentiation of osteoprogenitor cells from mesoderm and is accompanied by vascularization. This is known as intramembranous ossification. In the other form of ossification (endochondral), chondrocytes establish a cartilage model of the long bone that is subsequently replaced by bone. This method occurs in bones such as the humerus and femur. The cartilage model of each bone is used as a scaffolding for bone formation. Bone formed by the two methods cannot be distinguished with the light or electron microscope **(answers b and c)**. In both endochondral and intramembranous ossification, the first bone formed is woven bone **(answer d)**, also known as primary bone. This bone is replaced by adult, lamellar bone through a remodeling process.

105. The answer is e. *(Sadler, pp 129–131.)* In achondroplasia, the common mutations cause a gain of function of the *FGFR3* gene, resulting in decreased endochondral ossification, inhibited proliferation of chondroblasts in growth plate cartilage, decreased cellular hypertrophy, and decreased cartilage matrix production **(answers b and c)**. Growth in the length of long bones after birth (postnatally) occurs through cell proliferation of chondroblasts (immature chandrocytes) in the secondary ossification centers of the epiphyses. The primary ossification centers "close" soon after birth **(answer d)**. Fetal development of long bones occurs by the process of endochondral ossification in which a cartilage model is replaced by bone. Before birth, growth in length of the long bone occurs primarily through the proliferation of chondroblasts within the diaphysis of the cartilage model (primary ossification center). Growth in the width of the long bone occurs by the addition of osteoblasts from the periosteum and deposition of a periosteal collar **(answer a)**. This is appositional growth without a cartilage intermediate (intramembranous ossification). It is one of the best examples of intramembranous ossification, even though it occurs in the development of a long bone. The action of osteoblasts is to deposit bone matrix and secrete alkaline phosphatase; they do not proliferate in either the primary or the secondary ossification centers.

106. The answer is e. *(Alberts, pp 1093–1094. Junqueira, pp 113–114.)* Hydration of the glycosaminoglycans plays an important role in shock absorption and enhances the resiliency of the cartilage. This role is particularly important in the articular cartilages, which receive pressure during joint movement and are required to resist strong compressive forces. Proteoglycans are the major component of the ground substance of cartilage. They possess a large anionic charge because of the presence of sulfate, hydroxyl, and carboxyl groups within the glycosaminoglycans, which join to form proteoglycan subunits by linking with a core protein **(answer c)**. The proteoglycan subunits (monomers) subsequently form an aggregate by linking noncovalently to hyaluronic acid **(answer c)**. Those aggregates establish the rigidity of hyaline cartilage by reacting electrostatically with type II collagen **(answer a)**, probably through the sulfate groups of the glycosaminoglycans. The negative charge of the glycosaminoglycans facilitates the binding of cations **(answer b)** and the transport of electrolytes and water within the matrix. This is an important aspect of cartilage metabolism because the chondrocytes depend on diffusion to obtain nutrients or to dispose of waste products. Glycoproteins **(answer d)** are not a major constituent of the cartilage matrix.

107. The answer is c. *(Young, pp 184–187.)* The child in the vignette is suffering from Turner's syndrome, gonadal dysgenesis in which the XO karyotype results in multiple medical problems. The short stature has recently been attributed to the short stature homeobox gene SHOX which can affect various stages of endochondral development. The light micrograph illustrates a developing long bone. The zone shown is the region of chondrocyte hypertrophy, and the cells synthesize alkaline phosphatase, which calcifies the cartilage matrix. This secretion results in the eventual death of these cells that depend on diffusion to obtain oxygen and nutrients from the matrix. During development of the long bones of the body, specific zones are established, as a cartilage model of a long bone is converted to mature bone. The zones from the epiphysis toward the center of the shaft (diaphysis) are as follows: resting zone, proliferative zone, hypertrophy zone, and zone of calcified cartilage that is used as the scaffolding for the deposition of bone. The periosteal bud represents the ingrowth of blood vessels (angiogenesis) bringing, bone marrow precursors and osteoprogenitor cells into the diaphysis. Angiogenesis is required for bone formation. Bone is formed by the action of osteoblasts forming type I collagen, noncollagenous proteins (e.g., osteocalcin, osteopontin, and osteonectin), and alkaline phosphatase, which plays an essential role in mineralization of the osteoid. Cyclins are synthesized by cells passing through the cell cycle, cells in the proliferative zone **(answer a)**; acid phosphatase **(answer b)** is synthesized by osteoclasts; and type I collagen and osteocalcin **(answers d and e)** are synthesized by osteoblasts.

108. The answer is e. *(Alberts, pp 1304–1308. Kumar, pp 1281–1283. Guyton, pp 904–910. Greenspan, pp 274, 278–279, 286–287. Junqueira, pp 136, 148. High-Yield Facts, p 20.)* The patient in the vignette is suffering from type II autosomal dominant osteopetrosis (type II ADO), also known as Albers-Schönberg disease with a characteristic radiological image of "sandwich vertebrae." The targets in this disease are the osteoclasts which are indicated in the micrographs. Osteoclast function is altered in osteopetrosis. Osteoclasts function by release of lytic enzymes and protons (derived from carbonic acid) into the calcified matrix beneath the ruffled border and not through a grinding action **(answer a)**. The bone compartment around the ruffled border of the osteoclast is, therefore, analogous to a secondary lysosome in function, albeit extracellular. Osteoclasts use protons derived from carbonic acid, catalyzed by carbonic anydrase, in similar fashion to parietal cells of the stomach. Alkaline phosphatase is synthesized by osteoblasts **(answer b)**; PTH and Vitamin D receptors are found on osteoblasts **(answers c and d)**, *not* osteoclasts.

The electron micrograph illustrates the typical ultrastructure of an osteoclast with its distinctive ruffled border. The light micrograph illustrates the position of the osteoclasts (multinucleate cells) in small depressions in the bone (Howship's lacunae). The arrowhead in the electron micrograph indicates collagen within the degraded bone matrix. The plasmalemma of the osteoclast adjacent to the resorbing bone surface is thrown into folds and villous-like processes with tips that reach and even enter the bone surface (ruffled border). The osteoclast is attached to the bone surface, and the resorption area is sealed off by the presence of contractile proteins in the cytoplasm lateral to the site of the ruffled border. The basolateral membrane of the osteoclast posseses a Na^+,K^+-ATPase pump as do all human cells.

Osteoclasts are of hematopoietic origin and arise from the monocytic lineage. Osteoclasts are responsive to a number of hormones including parathyroid hormone (PTH), calcitonin, and 1, 25(OH) 2-vitamin D3. PTH is the major regulator of osteoclastic activity, increasing the number of osteoclasts as well as ruffled-border activity. The osteoclasts respond to low serum Ca^{2+} by removing calcium from bone. PTH receptors are located on osteoblasts, *not* osteoclasts **(answer d)**, and so PTH affects osteoblasts to release soluble factors (RANK-L and M-CSF) that stimulate osteoclasts. Vitamin D receptors are also present on osteoblasts and absent from the plasma membrane of osteoclasts **(answer c)**. This indirect receptor effect links the osteoblast and osteoclast in the so-called "ARF cycle" [**A**ctivation of osteoclasts → **R**esorption → **F**ormation of new bone]. Calcitonin is only responsible for transient changes in bone resorption. In the presence of high Ca^{2+}, calcitonin is synthesized and released from C (interfollicular, parafollicular) cells of the thyroid, which decreases ruffled-border activity. Calcitonin receptors are located on osteoclasts. Long-term responses to elevated Ca^{2+} are mediated by lowering of PTH levels rather than increased calcitonin production. This is exemplified in patients with an absence of calcitonin secretion (e.g., after thyroidectomy), or with stimulated levels of calcitonin (e.g., in medullary thyroid carcinoma) who exhibit relatively normal bone metabolism. However, calcitonin measurements are an important tool in the diagnosis of medullary thyroid carcinoma, a malignancy of thyroid cells. Calcitonin is also used as a nasal spray for osteoporosis when patients cannot tolerate bisphosphonates. Bisphosphonates are analogues of pyrophosphate and the primary means of treating osteoporosis and Paget's disease. They function by inhibiting osteoclastic activity through apoptosis of osteoclasts.

109. The answer is e. *(Kumar, pp 1304–1309.)* Arthritis involves inflammatory changes in a joint. LDC suffers from rheumatoid arthritis; an autoimmune disease in which a rheumatoid factor (RF) composed of heterologous autoantibodies directed against serum gamma globulin (IgG) appears.

Rheumatoid factor is present in the serum of 85–90% of patients with rheumatoid arthritis. Deposition of rheumatoid factor can be pathogenic and leads to inflammatory destruction of the joint surface. Cell-mediated immunity is also involved in rheumatoid arthritis. Alteration of the synovial membrane results in the formation of a pannus, or inflammatory, hypertrophic synovial villus. The presence of the pannus and release of lysosomal enzymes from the pannus result in degradation of the cartilage. This is followed by hypertrophy and hyperplasia of the articular cartilages, which often leads to bone formation across the joint with welding of the bones together (ankylosis). Because of the inflammation in rheumatoid arthritis, there are elevated numbers of leukocytes **(answer d)**, in particular PMNs, in the synovial fluid. During rheumatoid arthritis, fibrinogen **(answer b)**, another indicator of inflammatory responses, is elevated. Osteoarthritis begins with loss of hydrated glycosaminoglycans, followed by death of chondrocytes, fibrillation, and development of fissures in the articular cartilage matrix **(answer a)**. The severe wear and tear of osteoarthritis increases with age. During the breakdown of the articular cartilages, the width of the underlying bone increases. Osteoarthritis typically includes the formation of reactive bone spurs called osteophytes **(answer c)**, which may break off to form foreign bodies in the joint space (i.e., "joint mice"). In the fingers, osteoarthritis primarily affects distal interphalangeal joints, where it produces painful nodular enlargements called Heberden's nodes. Large weight-bearing joints are also usually involved in osteoarthritis and often exhibit eburnation in the late stages, when the articular cartilages have been worn down, and result in an osseous articular surface.

110. The answer is c. *(Junqueira, pp 145, 147. Kumar, pp 1288–1289.)* The most common type of wrist fracture is a Colles' fracture. The location of the break is between 2 and 3 cm from the wrist joint at the point where the radius narrows from cancellous bone forming the joint to the cortical bone of the shaft of the radius. In the healing of fractures, the first step is clotting of extravasated blood. The clot is organized into a callus by granulation tissue **(answer e)** that consists of fibroblasts, osteogenic cells, and budding capillaries. An internal, bony callus **(answer a)** forms where local bone factors are most active (i.e., in close proximity to the periosteum and endosteum that retain osteogenic potential). An external, cartilaginous **(answer b)** callus forms bone by endochondral ossification following initial chondrogenesis. These steps involve repetition of the cellular events involved in the histogenesis of bone. A bone graft is more important as a method of forming a temporary bridge in a severe defect than a source of osteoprogenitor cells. Other methods useful in stimulating bone repair include electrical forces and bone morphogenetic protein (BMP), a bone growth factor obtained from decalcified bone matrix. BMP stimulates bone formation when implanted at the fracture site. Pannus formation is an inflammatory event within the synovial membrane in patients with rheumatoid arthritis (answer d).

111. The answer is a. (*Favus, pp 321–323. Kumar, pp 1284–1286. Greenspan, pp 326–329. Kasper, pp 2279–2281.*) The correct diagnosis is Paget's disease, also known as osteitis deformans because of its deforming capabilities (e.g., skull or femoral head enlargement). In this disease the serum calcium is normal, but there is an increase in osteoclastic activity (osteolytic lesions and elevated 24-hour urine hydroxyproline) and an increase in osteoblastic activity (elevated osteocalcin and alkaline phosphatase). Patients with Paget's disease exhibit a marked increase in osteoid, and the bone actually enlarges. The osteoid is never normally mineralized in this disease. In this patient, the bone scan shows significant uptake of labeled bisphosphonates, which are incorporated into newly formed osteoid during bone formation. Her proximal femur is enlarged and no longer fits properly into the acetabulum, which results in the hip pain.

There are a number of useful biochemical markers of bone metabolism. Osteoclasts synthesize tartrate-resistant acid phosphatase so that increased osteoclastic activity is reflected in increased serum levels of tartrate-resistant acid phosphatase. Bone resorption fragments of type I collagen and noncollagenous proteins increase as bone matrix is resorbed. Hydroxyproline is a good urinary marker of bone metabolism because hydroxyproline is released and excreted in the urine as collagen is broken down. The presence of pyridinoline cross-links, which are involved in the bundling of type I collagen, is used for measurement of bone resorption. Those cross-links are released only during degradation of mineralized collagen fibrils as occurs in bone resorption. Usually, pyridinoline cross-links are measured by immunoassay over a 24-hour period to detect excess bone resorption and collagen breakdown in disorders such as Paget's disease.

Markers of bone formation include osteocalcin, alkaline phosphatase, and the extension peptides of type I collagen. Osteocalcin is a vitamin K–dependent γ-carboxyglutamic acid protein, that is, synthesized by osteoblasts and secreted into the serum in an unchanged state. Serum concentrations of osteocalcin are, therefore, directly related to osteoblastic activity. It is a more specific marker than alkaline phosphatase, because other organs, such as the liver and kidney, produce that enzyme.

Radiologic methods such as conventional x-ray can be used to detect osteoporosis, but only after patients have lost 30–50% of their bone mass. Dual-beam photon absorptiometry allows a much more accurate diagnosis of loss of bone mass.

112. The answer is a. *(Favus, pp 378–379. Kumar, pp 679–681. Kasper, pp 656–658.)* The patient is suffering from multiple myeloma, which causes increased plasma cell activity and anemia (hemoglobin data and increasing fatigue). Those plasma cells produce elevated levels of interleukin 1 (IL-1), which functions as an osteoclast activation factor, resulting in elevated serum calcium (12.3 mg/dL). Depletion of bone calcium results in lytic lesions of the skull and pelvis as well as compression fractures of the spine. The Bence-Jones protein represents free-immunoglobulin light chains, a diagnostic feature (Bence-Jones proteinuria) in the urine of patients with multiple myeloma. RANK is found on osteoclasts, binds to RANK-L produced by osteoblasts, and stimulates osteoclastic activity ("High-Yield Facts", p 21).

113. The answer is b. *(Favus, pp 330–335. Kumar, pp 453–455. Greenspan, pp 320–322. Junqueira, pp 135, 148. Kasper, pp 2247–2248.)* The patient suffers from osteomalacia, a disease related to malnutrition, specifically vitamin D deficiency. On the basis of the first bone biopsy in which the tissue was decalcified, one could make a diagnosis of osteoporosis. The second, non-decalcified bone biopsy indicates that osteoid is being formed but is not undergoing mineralization. This correlates with the low 25-hydroxyvitamin D levels. Vitamin D replacement and calcium supplementation would be prescribed for this patient.

114. The answer is e. *(Favus, pp 398–401. Kasper, pp 2091, 2226–2231, 2236. Greenspan, pp 310–320. Kumar, pp 1282–1284.)* Osteoporosis is a major problem of normal aging in both sexes but is particularly prevalent in older women. In that disease, the quality of bone is unchanged, but the balance between bone deposition and bone resorption is lost. The disease is prevalent in postmenopausal women because the protective effect of estrogens is no longer present. Osteoporosis may also be induced by other diseases (e.g., hyperthyroidism) or drugs (e.g., alcohol and caffeine). In addition, excess glucocorticoid induces osteoporosis. For example, in Cushing's syndrome, patients produce high levels of corticosteroids that interfere with bone metabolism. A similar pattern may be seen during prolonged steroid therapy. The result is increased bone resorption compared with bone deposition. Intestinal calcium absorption is inhibited and PTH levels may be increased.

115. The answer is c. (*Sadler, pp 172, 176–179. Moore and Persaud, Developing pp 168, 214.*) The child in the vignette is suffering from DiGeorge anomaly, which results in the absence of the thymus and parathyroid glands, which arise from the third and fourth pairs of branchial pouches. The absence of the thymus results in a deficiency in T lymphocyte–dependent areas of the immune system. These areas include the deep cortex of the lymph nodes, periarterial lymphatic sheath (PALS) of the spleen, and interfollicular areas of the Peyer's patches. Parathyroid hormone (PTH) stimulates the development of osteoclasts and the formation of ruffled borders in osteoclasts. The absence of PTH results in: i) a drastic reduction in numbers and activity of osteoclasts, ii) reduced Ca^{2+} levels in the blood, iii) denser bone, iv) spastic contractions of muscle called tetany, and v) excessive excitability of the nervous system. The parafollicular (C) cells arise from the ultimobranchial body that migrates into the thyroid gland and should form normally.

116. The answer is c. (*Kumar p 41. Junqueira, pp 144–145.*) The transmission electron micrograph is a high magnification view of a matrix vesicle that is derived from the cell membrane of osteoblasts, hypertrophied chondrocytes, ameloblasts, and odontoblasts depending on the location. After budding off from the plasmalemma, matrix vesicles accumulate calcium and phosphate in the form of hydroxyapatite crystals and serve as seed crystals for calcification. Exposure of those crystals to the extracellular fluid leads to seeding of the osteoid between the spaces in the collagen fibrils located in the matrix. Matrix vesicular alkaline phosphatase (**answers a and b**) results in local increases in the Ca^{2+}/PO_4^{2-} ratio. Adult lamellar bone contains very few matrix vesicles, suggesting that mineralization in remodeling of adult bone occurs by other mechanisms. The three-dimensional arrangement of collagen with the presence of holes or pores where hydroxyapatite crystals form is involved in the mineralization of adult bone. Osteoprotegerin inhibits osteoclastic activity (**answer d**) and osteoblasts synthesize type I collagen (**answer e**).

117. The answer is c. *(Kumar, pp 1274–1275.)* Type I collagen is responsible for the three-dimensional fiber structure of the matrix. It is synthesized by osteoblasts and accounts for 85–90% of total bone protein. The noncollagenous bone proteins are primarily synthesized by osteoblasts and constitute 10–15% of bone protein. Some plasma proteins are preferentially absorbed by the bone matrix. The noncollagenous proteins include cytokines and growth factors, which are synthesized endogenously and become trapped in the matrix. Also included in the category of noncollagenous proteins are the cell attachment proteins (fibronectin and osteopontin); proteoglycans (e.g., chondroitin 4-sulfate and chondroitin 6-sulfate), which appear to play a role in collagen fibrillogenesis; and the GLA proteins, such as osteocalcin (containing γ-carboxyglutamic acid), which binds Ca^{2+} and mineral components to the matrix.

118. The answer is c. *(Young, pp 189–191. Kumar, pp 1304–1309. Ross and Pawlina, pp 189, 205.)* The structure labeled **C** is the articular cartilage that is the site of wear-and-tear damage, which is the hallmark of osteoarthritis. The joint shown in the diagram is a freely movable joint known as a diarthrosis. Other joints allow limited or no movement (synarthroses) and may be classified by the uniting connective tissue: hyaline cartilage (synchondroses), bone (synostoses), or dense connective tissue (syndesmoses).

The joint cavity (**A**) is lined by an epithelium (**B**), which is surrounded by an external fibrous layer (**E**). The synovial fluid is formed from the synovial capillary ultrafiltrate as well as mucins, hyaluronic acid, and glycoproteins produced by fibroblast-like cells in the synovial epithelium (**B**) that lines the fluid-filled joint cavity (**A**). Macrophage-like cells in the epithelium perform a phagocytic function. The ends of the bone (**D**) are covered by hyaline cartilage that lacks a perichondrium. Synovial fluid, which differs from blood serum in its reduced protein content, acts as a lubricant and becomes more viscous with age. It may be used to diagnose joint disorders such as arthritis. Rheumatoid arthritis is an autoimmune disease in which infiltration of cells from the immune system leads to the destruction of the synovial capsule and the articular cartilages. Inflammation of the synovium leads to the formation of a pannus and eventually to changes in the articular cartilage converting it into a fibrocollagenous structure.

119. The answer is d. *(Favus, pp 58–59, 150–152, 277–282. Kierszenbaum, pp 126–128. Reszka, pp 45–52. High-Yield Facts, p 21.)* The woman in the vignette is diagnosed with osteoporosis. The DXA "T" score of -2 indicates that she is four times more likely to have a spine fracture than a person with a normal bone mineral density (BMD). The -2.5 "T" score indicates she is five times more likely to have a hip fracture than a person with a normal BMD. Bisphosphonate treatment is the most effective current treatment for osteoporosis. Bisphosphonates are analogues of the pyrophosphates and suppress bone resorption by osteoclasts. Inhibition of osteoblastic activity (**answer a**) would inhibit new bone deposition but also inhibit the production of RANK-L (receptor for activation of nuclear factor kappa beta-ligand) and M-CSF (macrophage colony-stimulating factor) by osteoblasts. RANK-L binds to RANK on the osteoclast and stimulates osteoclastic activity. M-CSF stimulates the differentiation of monocytes into osteoclasts. Increased RANK-L (**answer b**) and M-CSF (**answer c**) secretion by osteoblasts and upregulation of RANK (**answer e**) on the surface of osteoclasts will all increase osteoclastic activity. Some of the bisphosphonates are metabolized to a toxic analogue that targets mitochondria and apoptosis of the osteoclasts. Others interfere with cholesterol-dependent pathways in the osteoclast. The interactions of RANK, RANK-L, and osteoprotegerin (OPG) are shown in the figure in "High-Yield Facts" pp 20–21.

120. The answer is d. (*Kumar, pp 1294–1298.*) The patient in the scenario has an osteosarcoma that has metastasized to the lungs. The osteosarcoma cells synthesize bone and function similarly to osteoblasts, from which they are derived. Osteoblasts and osteosarcoma cells synthesize alkaline phosphatase, which is critical in increasing the local calcium: phosphate ratio, thereby inducing the calcification of osteoid (prebone) to form bone. Osteoblasts synthesize type I collagen. Fibroblasts in highly cellular organs such as the spleen synthesize type III collagen (**answer a**), the primary component of reticular fibers. Chondrocytes in hyaline and elastic cartilage synthesize type II collagen (**answer b**). Acid phosphatase (**answer c**) is synthesized by osteoclasts and is essential for the dissolution of bone and its subsequent resorption. Elastin (**answer e**) is synthesized by smooth-muscle cells, endothelial and microvascular cells, chondrocytes, and fibroblasts.

121. The answer is d. (*Kierszenbaum, p 997. Kumar, pp 279–281, 1294–1296. Favus, pp 372–373.*) One possible target for therapy of metastatic tumors, such as osteosarcoma, is to reduce metastases by upregulation of tissue inhibitors of matrix metallo proteinases (TIMPs) at the primary tumor site. TIMPs inhibit the proteolytic activity of the matrix metalloproteinases (MMPs) by inhibiting tumor invasion of the basement membrane or by restraining tumor angiogenesis. TIMPs also appear to modulate tumor growth and apoptosis of tumor cells. Downregulation of the anti-angiogenic peptides, angiostatin and endostain, would enhance tumor growth **(answer e)**. Angiostatin is a cleavage product of plasminogen; endostatin is a cleavage product of type XVIII collagen (see "High-Yield Facts," Page 8 for more information on angiogenesis). Antibodies to fibronectin, integrins, and laminin interfere with metastasis. Enhancement of integrin-integrin receptor interactions would facilitate metastasis **(answers a and b)**. Overexpression of selectins **(answer c)** on endothelial cells could enhance sticking of tumor cells to the endothelium and eventual extravasation.

122. The answer is d. *(Junqueira, pp 103–104.)* Type II collagen is found in the nasal septum. Type I collagen **(answer a)** is ubiquitous, type III collagen forms a reticular network in highly cellular organs **(answer c)**, type IV collagen is found in the basement membrane **(answer d)** and type VII collagen **(answer e)** is found in the basement membrane of skin and forms anchoring fibrils (see table page 184).

Muscle and Cell Motility

Questions

DIRECTIONS: Each item below contains a question or incomplete statement followed by suggested responses. Select the **one best** response to each question.

123. A 5-year-old boy sustains a tear in his gastrocnemius muscle when he is involved in a bicycle accident. Regeneration of the muscle will occur through which of the following?

a. Differentiation of satellite cells
b. Dedifferentiation of myocytes into myoblasts
c. Fusion of damaged myofibers to form new myotubes
d. Hyperplasia of existing myofibers
e. Differentiation of fibroblasts to form myocytes

124. In a given muscle fiber at rest, the length of the I band is 1.0 μm and the A band is 1.5 μm. Contraction of that muscle fiber results in a 10% shortening of the length of the sarcomere. What is the length of the A band after the shortening produced by the muscle contraction?

a. 1.50 μm
b. 1.35 μm
c. 1.00 μm
d. 0.90 μm
e. 0.45 μm

125. A 66-year-old man who lives alone has a severe myocardial infarction and dies during the night. The medical examiner's office is called the following morning and describes the man's body as being in *rigor mortis*. The state of *rigor mortis* is due to:

a. Inhibition of Ca^{++} leakage from the extracellular fluid and sarcoplasmic reticulum
b. Enhanced retrieval of calcium by the sarcoplasmic reticulum
c. Failure to disengage tropomyosin and troponin from the myosin active sites
d. Absence of ATP preventing detachment of the myosin heads from actin
e. Increased lactic acid production

126. The sarcoplasmic reticulum of skeletal muscle functions in which of the following?

a. Cellular Ca^{2+} storage
b. Cellular glycogen storage
c. Glycogen degradation
d. Transport of Ca^{2+} into the terminal cisternae during muscle contraction
e. Ca^{2+} release from the transverse tubules during muscle relaxation

127. Observation of a histologic preparation of muscle reveals cross-striations and peripherally located nuclei. The use of histochemistry shows a strong staining reaction for succinic dehydrogenase. The same tissue prepared for electron microscopy shows many mitochondria in rows between myofibrils and underneath the sarcolemma. Which of the following is the best description of this tissue?

a. White muscle fibers
b. Fibers that contract rapidly but are incapable of sustaining continuous heavy work
c. Red muscle fibers
d. Cardiac muscle
e. Smooth muscle

128. In skeletal muscle contraction, the "powerstroke" is initiated by which of the following?

a. The initial binding of ATP to the myosin heads
b. Release of Pi from the myosin heads
c. Release of ADP and subsequent addition of an ATP molecule
d. Detachment of the myosin head from the actin
e. Phosphorylation of the myosin light chains

129. In muscular dystrophy, the actin-binding protein dystrophin is absent or defective. Dystrophin contains similar actin-binding domains to the spectrins (I and II) and α-actinin and has a similar structure. Which of the following is most likely to occur as a result of this deficiency?

a. Enhanced smooth-muscle contractility
b. Deficiency in skeletal muscle actin synthesis
c. Loss of binding of the I and M bands to the cell membrane
d. Loss of organelle and vesicle transport throughout the muscle cell
e. Loss of integrity of the desmosomal components of the intercalated discs of cardiac muscle

130. DLM is a 32-year-old male homosexual seropositive for HIV. He has HIV-associated periodontitis and intraoral candidiasis. Peripheral neutrophils (PMNs) were isolated from the patient and found to have increased activity as measured by oxidative burst and F-actin assays compared to control patients. Which of the following cellular events would most likely be increased in the peripheral blood PMNs from DLM?

a. Phagocystosis
b. Bidirectional transport of vesicles
c. Fast axoplasmic transport
d. Chromosomal movements
e. Ciliary movement

131. Which of the following is absent in smooth-muscle cells compared to skeletal muscle cells?

a. Troponin
b. Calmodulin
c. Calcium
d. Myosin light-chain kinase
e. Actin and tropomyosin interactions

132. In the transmission electron micrograph of skeletal muscle shown below, which of the following is true of the zone labeled C?

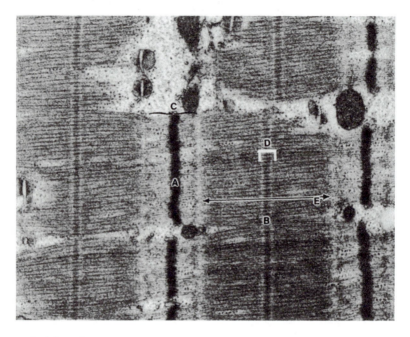

a. It defines the sarcomere
b. Thin filaments are anchored to this structure
c. This structure bisects the H band and is formed predominantly of creatine kinase
d. No overlap of thick and thin filaments occurs in this zone
e. This portion of the A band consists solely of the rodlike portions of myosin

133. The mechanochemical enzyme that can be found on the surfaces of cellular organelles where it mediates movement toward the plus end of microtubules is which of the following?

a. Myosin (myosin II)
b. Minimyosin (myosin I)
c. Dynein
d. Kinesin
e. Filamin

Muscle and Cell Motility

Answers

123. The answer is a. *(Kumar, pp 91, 94, 1327. Alberts, pp 1299–1300.)* Satellite cells in skeletal muscle proliferate and reconstitute the damaged part of the myofibers. They are supportive cells for maintenance of muscle and a source of new myofibers after injury or after increased load. There is no dedifferentiation of myocytes into myoblasts **(answer b)**, or fusion of damaged myofibers to form new myotubes **(answer c)**. Hypertrophy, not hyperplasia **(answer d)**, occurs in existing myofibers in response to increased load. Proliferation of fibroblasts may occur in the damaged area but leads to fibrosis, not repair of skeletal muscle. Fibroblasts do *not* differentiate into myocytes **(answer e)**. The multinucleate organization of skeletal muscle is derived developmentally by fusion and not by amitosis (failure of cytokinesis after DNA synthesis). Mitotic activity is terminated after fusion occurs. In the development of skeletal muscle, myoblasts of mesodermal origin undergo cell proliferation. Myocyte cell division ceases soon after birth. Myoblasts, which are mononucleate cells, fuse with each other end to end to form myotubes. This process requires cell recognition between myoblasts, alignment, and subsequent fusion.

124. The answer is a. *(Alberts, pp 961–965. Junqueira, pp 186–191. High-Yield Facts, p 22.)* During contraction, the sarcomere, the distance between adjacent Z lines, decreases in length, and the length of the A band is almost constant. However, as the degree of overlap of thick and thin filaments is altered, the thin filaments, which form the I band and are anchored to the Z line, are pulled toward the center of the sarcomere. As this occurs, the I band decreases in length and the H band is no longer visible. The filaments themselves do not decrease in length; they slide past one another in the sliding-filament model of muscle contraction. The average length of a sarcomere is 2.5 μm. This distance is measured from one Z line to the next Z line. If the resting length of the A band is 1.5 μm and the length of the I band is 1.0 μm, then the resting length of the sarcomere is determined by adding the length of the I band to the length of the A band. If there is a 20% contraction of the muscle (contraction to 80% of its length), then the sarcomere is reduced in length from 2.5 to 2.0 μm. The size of the A band remains unchanged (i.e., whether the contraction is 10% or 20%), therefore the length of the I band is reduced from 1.0 to 0.5 μm and makes up for the 0.5 μm reduction in length during the muscle contraction. The processes of skeletal muscle contraction and relaxation are shown in the image below and in the "High Yield Facts" section, p. 22.

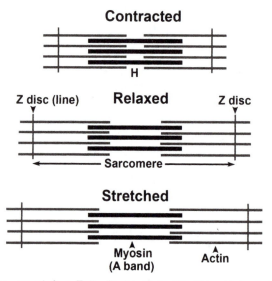

The Sarcomere extends from Z disc (line) to Z disc. The H band is located between the ends of the thin (actin) filaments. The A band is defined by the the width of the thick (myosin) filaments. The I bands are not shown completely on the figure (see High-Yield Facts) because they are found between adjacent A bands.

125. The answer is d. (*Alberts, pp 961–965. Junqueira, p 192.*) There is some small amount of production of ATP after death through anaerobic and phosphagen pathways. However, there is insufficient ATP to induce the detachment of the myosin heads from actin. Ca^{2+} ions continue to leak from the extracellular fluid and the sarcoplasmic reticulum (**answer a**), however, the sarcoplasmic reticulum is no longer able to retrieve the Ca^{2+} ions (**answer b**). Tropomyosin and troponin are disengaged from the myosin active sites (**answer c**). Lactic acid is produced during *rigor mortis* through anaerobic pathways. The high levels of lactic acid cause deterioration of the skeletal muscle and end the state of *rigor mortis* (**answer e**).

126. The answer is a. (*Alberts, pp 961–965. Junqueira, pp 186–191.*) Ca^{2+} is responsible for the coupling of excitation and contraction in skeletal muscle. The sarcoplasmic reticulum (SR) is a modified smooth endoplasmic reticulum. Ca^{2+} is concentrated in the lumen of the SR. Depolarization of the muscle cell membrane during an action potential triggers the opening of ryanidine receptor channels in the membrane of the SR. Ca^{2+} passes through the open ryanidine receptor channels, traveling from the lumen of the SR into the muscle cell cytoplasm. When Ca^{2+} in the muscle cell cytoplasm is high, the Ca^{2+} binds to the troponin complex. The binding of Ca^{2+} to the troponin complex results in a conformational change in the complex, thereby allowing myosin to interact with actin. The interaction of myosin and actin produces force. Ca^{2+} is constantly pumped back into the lumen of the SR by Ca^{2+}-ATPases. As the Ca^{2+} inthe cytoplasm is pumped back into the SR the concentration of Ca^{2+} in the cytoplasm drops, and Ca^{2+} dissociates from the troponin complex. The troponin complex subsequently reverts to the conformational state in which the troponin complex blocks the interaction of myosin with actin **(answer b)**. Glycogen is stored as particles or droplets in the cytoplasm, which contains the enzymes required for the synthesis and breakdown of glycogen **(answer c)**. The transverse tubule system, or T system, is an extension of the plasma membrane of the myofiber (sarcolemma). The T system allows for simultaneous contraction of all myofibrils since it encircles the A-I bands in each sarcomere of every myofibril. In combination with the paired terminal cisternae, the transverse tubules form a triad. Two triads are found in each sarcomere of skeletal muscle—one at each junction of dark (A) and light (I) bands. Depolarization of the T system during contraction is transmitted to the sarcoplasmic reticulum at the triad **(answers d and e)**. It is important to note that cardiac muscle also has a T system, although it is not as elaborate and well organized as that found in skeletal muscle (e.g., diads are present rather than the triads of skeletal muscle and there are fewer T tubules in the atrial vs. ventricular muscle).

127. The answer is c. (*Kumar, pp 1327–1328. Junqueira, p 196.*) The histologic sample contains red fibers. The deductive process is based on the fact that the sample must be skeletal or cardiac muscle due to the presence of cross-striations **(answer e)**. The presence of peripherally placed nuclei eliminates cardiac muscle as a possibility **(answer d)**. Skeletal muscle may be subclassified into three muscle fiber types: red, white, and intermediate fibers. Red muscle fibers have a high content of cytochrome and myoglobin and, beneath the plasmalemma, contain many mitochondria required for the high metabolism of these cells. Mitochondria are also found in a longitudinal array surrounding the myofibrils. The presence of numerous mitochondria provides a strong staining reaction with the use of cytochemical stains such as that for succinic dehydrogenase. Physiologically, red fibers are capable of continuous contraction (high concentrations of myosin ATPase), but are incapable of rapid contraction (**answer b**). The term "red (type I) fibers" is due to the presence of large concentrations of myoglobin, the colored oxygen-binding protein. White (type IIB) muscle fibers (**answer a**) are fast-twitch in function, stain very lightly for succinic dehydrogenase and myosin ATPase, and few mitochondria would be visible at the ultrastructural level. White fibers are capable of rapid contraction but are unable to sustain continuous heavy work. They are larger than red fibers and have more prominent innervation. The white fibers contain relatively little myoglobin. Human skeletal muscle fibers are composed of red, white, and intermediate-type fibers. The intermediate (type IIA) fibers possess characteristics including a size and innervation pattern intermediate between red and white muscle fibers. The intermediate fibers contain a concentration of myoglobin between white and red muscle fibers.

128. The answer is b. (*Alberts, pp 961–965. Junqueira, pp 186–191.*) The "powerstroke" is initiated by the release of Pi from the myosin heads, leading to the tight binding of actin and myosin. The tight binding induces a conformational change in the myosin head. The myosin head subsequently pulls against the actin filament to cause the "powerstroke" of the myosin head walking along the actin filament. This walking process is unidirectional and is based on the polarity of the actin filament (i.e., walking occurs from the minus to the plus end of the actin filament). The cycle of ATP-actin-myosin interactions during contraction begins with the resting state. In the quiescent period, ATP binds to myosin heads (**answer a**); however, hydrolysis occurs slowly and only allows the weak binding of myosin heads to the actin filaments. Tight binding occurs only when Pi is released from myosin heads, leading to the "powerstroke." Recycling occurs through the release of ADP and the subsequent addition of an ATP molecule (**answer c**) and detachment of the myosin head from actin (**answer d**). Rigor results from the lack of ATP because one ATP molecule is required for each myosin molecule present in the muscle. *Rigor mortis* occurs from the absence of ATP. In skeletal muscle, phosphorylation of the light chain is not required for binding to actin (**answer e**).

129. The answer is c. (*Alberts, p 1299. Kasper, pp 2526–2529. Kumar, pp 1336–1338.*) Dystrophin, like α-actinin and spectrin, is an actin-binding protein. It binds actin to the skeletal muscle membrane and therefore binds the I and M bands to the cell membrane. The inability to bind actin to the plasma membrane of skeletal muscle leads to disruption of the contraction process, weakness of muscle, and abnormal running, hopping, and jumping. The Gower maneuver is the method used by persons suffering from muscular dystrophy to stand from a sitting position. Respiratory failure occurs in those persons because of disruption of diaphragmatic function. Dystrophin is found in all muscle types and is part of a complex that regulates interactions of the sarcolemma with the extracellular matrix through associated glycoproteins (dystrophin-glycoprotein complex). Therefore, loss of dystrophin causes destabilization and decreased contractility (**answer a**). Muscular dystrophy refers to a group of progressive hereditary disorders (1/3500 male births) that involve mutations in the dystrophin gene. Dystrophin is similar in structure to spectrins I and II and α-actinin. Dystrophin is absent in Duchenne muscular dystrophy. Becker muscular dystrophy is a less severe dystrophy in which dystrophin is defective. Synthesis of actin (**answer b**) is not reduced in skeletal muscle from these patients; in fact, hypertrophy and pseudohypertrophy (replacement of muscle with connective tissue and fat) occurs. Microtubules perform vesicular and organelle transport functions (**answer d**), and intermediate filaments, not actin, form the intracellular connection in desmosomes (**answer e**).

130. The answer is a. (*Alberts, pp 184, 952, 953, 972.*) DLM's peripheral blood PMNs have increased activity as measured by oxidative burst and F-actin assays. Actin maintains the mechanical strength of the cytoplasm of the cell and is essential for cellular functions that require surface motility. Those functions include phagocytosis, cytokinesis, and cell locomotion. Although movement of vesicles along filaments is regulated by minimyosins (myosin I), movement of vesicles and organelles is predominantly a function of microtubules (**answers b and c**) under the influence of the unidirectional motors kinesin and dynein. The movements of chromosomes (**answer d**) as well as the cilia and flagella (**answer e**) are driven by dynein, and chromosomal movements occur through microtubular kinetics.

131. The answer is a. (*Junqueira, pp 198–202.*) Smooth muscle is the least specialized type of muscle and contains no troponin. The contractile process is similar to the actin-myosin interactions that occur in motility of nonmuscle cells. In the smooth-muscle cell, actin and myosin are attached to intermediate filaments at dense bodies in the sarcolemma and cytoplasm. Dense bodies contain α-actinin and, therefore, resemble the Z-lines of skeletal muscle. Contraction causes cell shortening and a change in shape from elongate to globular. Contraction occurs by a sliding filament action analogous to the mechanism used by thick and thin filaments in striated muscle. The connections to the plasma membrane allow all the smooth-muscle cells in the same region to act as a functional unit. The sarcoplasmic reticulum is not as well developed as that in the striated muscles. There are no T tubules present; however, endocytic vesicles called caveolae are believed to function in a fashion similar to the T tubule system of skeletal muscle.

When intracellular calcium levels increase, the calcium is bound to the Ca^{2+}-binding protein, calmodulin. Ca^{2+}-calmodulin (**answers b and c**) is required and is bound to myosin light-chain kinase (**answer d**) to form a Ca^{2+}-calmodulin-kinase complex. This complex catalyzes the phosphorylation of one of the two myosin light chains on the myosin heads. That phosphorylation allows the binding of actin to myosin. A specific phosphatase dephosphorylates the myosin light chain, which returns the actin and myosin to the inactive, resting state. The actin-tropomyosin interactions (**answer e**) are similar in smooth and skeletal muscle.

Smooth-muscle cells (e.g., vascular smooth-muscle cells) also differ from skeletal muscle cells in that like fibroblasts, they are capable of collagen, elastin, and proteoglycan synthesis.

132. The answer is d. (*High-Yield Facts, p 18. Junqueira, pp 188–191.*) Myofibrils are composed of sarcomeres, which are repeating units that extend from Z disk (**A** on the transmission electron micrograph) to **Z** disk in the TEM. With the use of polarizing microscopy, the **A** (anisotropic) bands (**E** on the TEM) are visible as dark, birefringent structures, and the **I** (isotropic) bands are visible as light-staining bands (**C** on the TEM). The I band consists of thin filaments without overlap of thick filaments. At the center of the myofibril and consisting of thick filaments is the A band, which interdigitates with the I band. Each I band is bisected by the Z disk. The Z disk is composed mostly of the intermediate filament protein desmin and other proteins such as α-actinin, filamin, and amorphin, as well as Z protein. In the center of the A band is a lighter-staining area that consists only of thick (rod-like portions of myosin) filaments and is known as the H band (**D** on the TEM). Lateral connections occur between adjacent thick filaments in the region of the M line (**B** on the TEM), which bisects the H zone and is composed primarily of creatine kinase, an enzyme that catalyzes the formation of ATP.

133. The answer is d. (*Alberts, pp 953, 959, 979, 1037. Junqueira, pp 57–62.*) Kinesin moves vesicles unidirectionally from the minus end to the plus end of the microtubule—for example, from the cell body to the axon terminus in fast axonal transport. Myosin, minimyosin, dynein, dynamin, and kinesin (**answers a, b, c, and e**) are all mechanochemical enzymes or molecular "motors" that hydrolyze ATP and undergo conformational changes that are converted into movement. Cytoplasmic dynein is responsible for movement toward the minus end of the microtubules. Remember **k**inesin **k**icks out and **d**ynein **d**rags them in (see feedback to question 41). Ciliary and flagellar bending is the classic model for microtubule-based motility. The motor is dynein, which causes the relative sliding between microtubules in the axoneme. Structural constraints within the axoneme as a whole convert sliding into ciliary bending.

Dynamin is another ATPase motor that mediates sliding between adjacent cytoplasmic microtubules.

Filamin or other actin cross-linking proteins form a gel network in the cell cortex (the area just beneath the cell membrane). The presence of the actin gel in the cell cortex contributes to the rigidity of the cell and is also involved in changes in cell shape and chromosome movements during mitosis. The sarcomere extends from Z disc (line) to Z disc. The H band is located between the ends of the thin (actin) filaments. The A band is defined by the width of the thick (myosin) filaments. The I bands are not shown completely on the figure because they are found between adjacent A bands.

Nervous System

Questions

DIRECTIONS: Each item below contains a question or incomplete statement followed by suggested responses. Select the **one best** response to each question.

134. A 4-year-old boy is referred to the pediatric neurology clinic. His behavior is described as: difficulty in expressing needs, using gestures instead of words and repeating words in place of normal, responsive language. In the examination room he wanders around repeatedly singing "Baa Baa Black Sheep," then crying and laughing for no apparent reason. His parents say he is nervous, excitable, "will not cuddle or be cuddled" and hyperactive. He has no apparent fear of danger and a constant need to spin objects and jumps while twiddling his fingers. MRI showed a significant reduction in total grey matter volume with localized grey matter reductions within fronto-striatal, parietal, and ventral and superior temporal grey matter. FMRI showed an abnormal activation pattern in cortical as well as limbic/striatal areas. The neurons in the frontal, parietal and temporal cortex originate from which region embryologically?

a. subventricular zone
b. marginal zone
c. intermediate zone
d. mantle zone
e. sulcus limitans

135. The action potential in the neuron results from which of the following?

a. Hyperpolarization
b. The opening of K^+ channels
c. The opening of Na^+ channels
d. Inward flux of K^+
e. Pumping of Na^+ from the neuron

136. An 18-month-old girl flexes the great toe toward the top of her foot and the other toes fan out after the sole of her foot has been firmly stroked by the pediatrician. A year later, the response cannot be evoked by the same stimulus. The change in response is due to which postnatal event?

a. Apoptosis of exuberant neurons in the cortex by microglia
b. Maturation of the cerebellar cortex
c. Myelination of the lumbar spinal nerves by Schwann cells
d. Myelination of the corticospinal tract by oligodendrocytes
e. Formation of new neurons in the cerebral cortex

137. A 2-year-old boy has an acute inflammatory reaction in the region shown in this photomicrograph several weeks after suffering from chicken-pox. Which of the following is the most likely symptom?

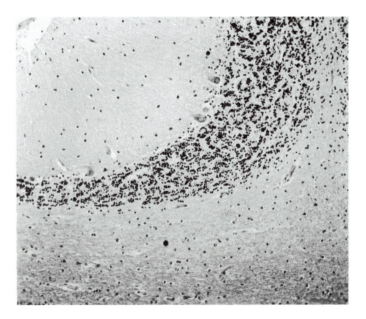

a. Amnesia
b. Ataxia
c. Loss of spinal cord reflex responses
d. Loss of pain sensation
e. Aphasia

138. A febrile 52-year-old male patient receiving glucocorticoid treatment presents with vesicular lesions with intense itching, burning, and sharp pain along the back in a specific dermatomal pattern covering his nipple and extending onto the right side of his back. The vesicular lesions do not cross the midline. A Tzanck test is positive. The cause of this illness is the movement of virus from the structures shown in the photomicrograph toward the surface of the skin. This movement occurs in which direction and by which molecular motor?

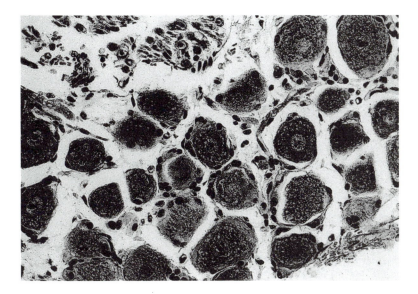

a. Minus end to plus end, dynein
b. Minus end to plus end, kinesin
c. Plus end to minus end, dynein
d. Plus end to minus end, kinesin
e. Minus end to plus end, myosin II

139. A 22-year-old male receives a severe, traumatic compression injury to his radial nerve after a motorcycle crash. He shows an advancing Tinel's sign. Which of the following is true about regeneration of axons after his nerve injury?

a. It occurs in the absence of motor unit potentials
b. It occurs at a rate of 100 mm/day
c. It occurs by a mechanism that is dependent on the proliferation of Schwann cells
d. It occurs in conjunction with degeneration and phagocytosis of endoneurial tubes
e. It occurs in the segment distal to the damage

140. The nodes of Ranvier increase the efficiency of neural transmission by means of which of the following?

a. Decelerating the closing of Na^+-gated channels
b. Enhancing myelination of the internodal segment
c. Sequestration of Na^+ entry into the axon
d. Multiple firings due to local ionic currents around the node
e. Decreasing threshold for the action potential

141. The blood-brain barrier is formed by which of the following?

a. Fenestrations between brain capillary endothelial cells
b. Occluding junctions between brain capillary endothelial cells
c. Astrocytic foot processes surrounding blood vessels entering the brain parenchyma
d. The basement membrane associated with the glia limitans
e. Microglial activity

142. At the neuromuscular junction, action potentials are coupled to neurotransmitter release by which of the following?

a. Ca^{2+}-gated channels
b. Na^+-gated channels
c. K^+-gated channels
d. Cl^--gated channels
e. Gap junctions

143. Following a vehicular accident, a 45-year-old male is transported to the emergency room by ambulance. He presents with motor deficits on his right side and is unable to move his right arm and leg and has slurred speech. The injury has most likely occurred on which side and affects which of the following cells, which predominate in the accompanying photomicrograph?

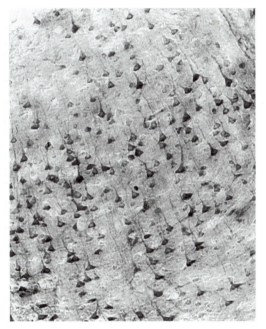

(Micrograph courtesy of Dr. Nancy E. J. Berman.)

a. Right, Purkinje cells
b. Left, Purkinje cells
c. Right, pyramidal cells
d. Left, pyramidal cells
e. Left, basket cells

144. A 36-year-old woman internist completes a 4 week medical mission to rural Bahia, Brazil. Eighteen months after her return she complains of loss of sensation in her hands and feet. Neurologic examination reveals loss of temperature, light touch, pain, and deep pressure on her hands and feet. A hypopigmented macula is present on the dorsum of her hand. A lepromin test is positive and a biopsy reveals inflammation of the structure labeled C in the accompanying photomicrograph. The structure labeled C is which of the following?

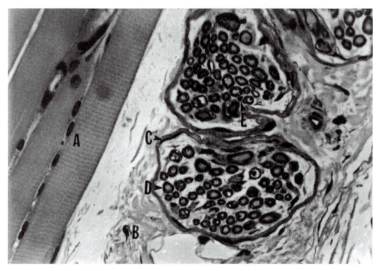

(Micrograph courtesy of Dr. John K. Young.)

a. Perineurium
b. Epineurium
c. Endomysium
d. Perimysium
e. Tunica media

145. The neural crest gives rise to which of the following?

a. Zona glomerulosa of the adrenal gland
b. Pyramidal cells
c. Ventral horn cells
d. Astrocytes
e. Sensory neurons of the cranial ganglia

146. During labor an infant girl went into fetal distress. The child was delivered by a mid-forceps delivery, had seizures soon after births and developed an intracranial hemorrhage with left-sided hemiplegia. She is 6-years-old, has an IQ of about 80, walks with a very severe limp and has a contracted hand on the left side. She barely speaks despite therapy. She is treated with atropine for her sialorhhea. The atropine affects the structure labeled with the arrow to:

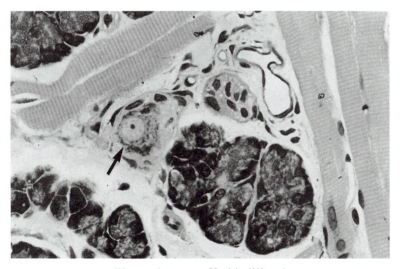

(Micrograph courtesy of Dr. John K. Young.)

a. Block parasympathetic pathways
b. Stimulate parasympathetic pathways
c. Block sympathetic pathways
d. Stimulate sympathetic pathways
e. Bind to acinar cells

147. A 45-year-old man presents at the neurology clinic with memory loss, mood swings, and clinical depression. Laboratory results reveal a CD4 level of 170/mm^3 (normal range is 500–1200) and a CD4 percentage of 12% (normal approximately 40%). His viral load is 12,000 copies/mL. He has previously been treated for pneumocystis pneumonia. The cells in the accompanying photomicrograph, labeled with anti-GFAP, are involved in the progress of this disease. These cells function to do which of the following?

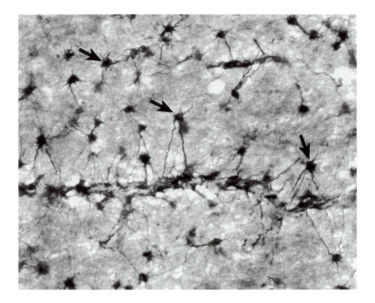

a. Form synaptic contacts with neurons
b. Present antigen
c. Phagocytose dying neurons
d. Form a glial scar following damage
e. Form myelin in the CNS

148. A 47-year-old man is treated with Fluoxetine hydrochloride (Prozac) for clinical depression. This pharmaceutical agent functions through a mechanism that involves the structure labeled "C" in the transmission electron micrograph below. The structure labeled "C" in the accompanying transmission electron micrograph is the site of which of the following?

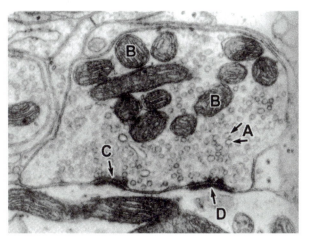

(Micrograph courtesy of Drs. J. F. Hewer and T. S. Reese.)

a. Neurotransmitter reuptake in synaptic vesicles by endocytosis
b. Binding of neurotransmitter to postsynaptic receptors
c. Neurotransmitter-induced alteration of membrane permeability
d. Membrane continuity between adjacent neurons
e. Degradation of neurotransmitter

149. A 35-year-old woman presents with weakness and spasticity in the left lower extremity, visual impairment and throbbing in her left eye, difficulties with balance, fatigue, and malaise. There is an increase in cerebrospinal fluid (CSF) protein, elevated gamma globulin, and moderate pleocytosis. MRI confirms areas of demyelination in the anterior corpus callosum. Imaging identifies plaques which are hyperintense on T_2-weighted and FLAIR images and hypointense on T_1-weighted scans. Which of the following cells are specifically targeted in her condition?

a. Microglia
b. Oligodendrocytes
c. Astrocytes
d. Schwann cells
e. Axons of multipolar neurons

150. A 33-year-old woman is referred to the neurology clinic complaining of weakness of the eye muscles which began 2 months ago. Subsequently she has had diplopia and increasing difficulty in swallowing. Her speech is slurred and she says that she has difficulty clearly enunciating and pronouncing many words. The physical exam reveals bilateral ptosis and an unstable, waddling gait, and some shortness of breath. Laboratory and diagnostic tests reveal a positive edrophonium chloride (tensilon) test and autoantibodies to the acetylcholine receptor. On the accompanying transmission electron micrograph which region is most affected in this disease?

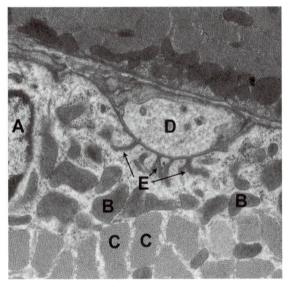

(Micrograph courtesy of Dr. Michael J. Werle.)

a. A
b. B
c. C
d. D
e. E

Nervous System

Answers

134. The answer is a. (*Sadler, pp 296, 300–303. Moore and Persaud, Developing, pp 67–69, 86–87, 442–443.*) Abnormalities in the anatomy and connectivity of cortical regions and the so-called social brain regions (limbic–striatal systems) contribute to the behavioral and brain metabolic differences in autism. In the cerebral cortex, neurons originate from the ventricular and subventricular zones. Before neural tube closure, cell proliferation is the predominant process. After neural tube closure, neurons differentiate. Three layers differentiate from the wall of the neural tube. Mitotic activity occurs in the ventricular zone, closest to the lumen. The mantle (intermediate) zone **(answers c and d)**, is where cell bodies of differentiating motoneurons are located. The most peripheral zone is the marginal zone **(answer b)**, which contains the myelinated axons of the developing motoneurons (adult white matter). In the spinal cord, the layers differentiate into peripheral white matter with a central H-shaped region of gray matter from the marginal and mantle zones, respectively. The sulcus limitans separates the alar (sensory) and basal (motor) plates in the developing brainstem **(answer e)**. The macroglia (astrocytes and oligodendrocytes), arise from the neural epithelium. Microglia (the macrophages of the brain) are bone marrow–derived, arising from monocytes. Cerebral and cerebellar cortex are areas of peripheral gray matter formed through a second wave of cell proliferation. In cerebellar development, the second wave comes from the external granular layer. In the cerebral cortex, layers I to VI form by waves of proliferation and migration from deep to superficial layers with new cells arising from the subventricular zone.

135. The answer is c. (*Alberts, 4/e, pp 638–643. Junqueira, pp 154, 159. Kandel, pp 29–39, 147–148.*) In the resting state, the presence of Na^+/K^+ ATPase builds up high ionic gradients across the axolemma. There are many more Na^+ on the outside of the axon; the inside of the axon is negative relative to the outside (−70 mV resting potential). An action potential is initiated by an exchange of ions across the axonal membrane that will displace the membrane potential toward zero. The first step is the presence of a stimulus that causes Na^+-gated channels to open, Na^+ ions flow through the channels into the neuron. The positive charge of Na$^+$ makes the axon more positive and depolarized. There is a delay in the opening of K$^+$-channels. The opening of K$^+$-channels causes the flow of K$^+$out of the cell, reversing the depolarization. Na$^+$-channels start to close at about this same time. That causes the action potential to return toward -70 mV, repolarizing the membrane. The membrane actually hyperpolarizes (**answer a**) as the potential passes -70 mV. This is due to the fact that the K$^+$-channels remain open longer than required to return to -70 mV. Gradually, the ion concentrations return to resting levels and the membrane returns to -70 mV. K$^+$ channels (**answer b**) serve to bring the membrane potential to the hyperpolarized state. Inward flux of K$^+$ (**answer d**) combined with the closing of Na$^+$-channels (**answer e**), is important in return to the resting membrane potential. The action potential is an all-or-none phenomenon and occurs with constant amplitude and duration for a given axon. Myelination results in a much more rapid conduction of the action potential.

136. The answer is d. (*Young, pp 121, 123–125, 137. Junqueira, pp 170–171. Kandel, pp 20, 147–148.*) The Babinski sign or extensor plantar reflex is an infantile reflex present in children until the age of two years, but abnormal in older children or adults. The Babinski sign is an indication of immaturity of the corticospinal tract which is myelinated after birth (**answers a and e**); the process of myelination is completed by oligodendrocytes in the CNS (**answer c**). Cerebellar cortical development (**answer b**) begins in the second trimester and continues until several years after birth, but is not involved in the Babinski reflex.

A short review of myelination:
Myelination in the CNS and PNS occurs by similar methods, although there are differences in the supportive cells responsible. In the CNS, the oligodendrocytes myelinate axons, whereas Schwann cells myelinate axons in the PNS. In the PNS, formation of myelin is initiated by the invagination of an axon into a Schwann cell. A mesaxon is formed as the outer leaflets of the cell membrane fuse. Subsequently, the mesaxon of the Schwann cell wraps itself around the fiber. In the CNS, oligodendrocytes form myelin around multiple axon segments compared with the 1:1 relationship between Schwann cells and axon segments in the PNS. Myelination occurs in both pre- and postnatal development. CNS myelin is the target for attack by components of the immune system in multiple sclerosis, and PNS

myelin is the target in Guillain-Barré syndrome (GBS), also called acute inflammatory demyelinating polyneuropathy or Landry's ascending paralysis. GBS is an inflammatory disorder of the PNS characterized by rapid onset of weakness and, often, paralysis of the legs, arms, respiratory muscles, and muscles of facial expression.

137. The answer is b. (*Kasper, pp 139–141. Young, p 376. Junqueira, pp 163, 165–166.*) The region shown in the photomicrograph is the cerebellum. An acute childhood infection in the cerebellum (cerebellitis) would result in ataxia: inability to coordinate voluntary muscle movements, unsteady movements, and staggering gait. Ataxia may be classified as axial (trunk) or limb ataxia. In the sitting position, the child's trunk may move side to side and/or back to front and then resume a vertical position in a jerky motion. Nystagmus (jerky eye movements) may also occur. Limb ataxia manifests itself with loss of fine motor control of the hands or legs and appears as though the person is able to coordinate his or her movements. For example, a hand may sway back and forth when reaching for an object. Most often, the cerebellar ataxia that follows a viral infection subsides without treatment over a period of weeks to months. Occasionally, a child will be left with a persistent movement disorder or behavioral problem. Amnesia **(answer a)** would result from a cortical injury; reflexive actions **(answer c)** would occur at the level of the ventral horn cells in the spinal cord; loss of pain sensation is complex and could involve the dorsal root or trigeminal ganglion, the sensory and frontal cortex, limbic system, and thalamus, but not the cerebellar cortex **(answer d)**; and total or partial loss of ability to use or understand language, aphasia **(answer e)**, would be the result of a cortical injury. Damage to the pararhinal–entorhinal–hippocampal–mammillary body–thalamus circuit, the fornix, or the temporal lobe can cause amnesia. There are different types of memory. For example, working memory can be affected by prefrontal lesions or by lesions to specific temporoparietal regions subserving the modality being used. Aphasia can involve several different areas of the cortex including the frontal, parietal, and/or temporal lobes.

Note the three layers forming the cerebellar cortex (molecular layer at left/top, the large Purkinje cell layer, and the granular layer). The mnemonic MPG: Molecular, Purkinje, and Granular may help you remember the layers. White matter is inside of the three layers of gray matter. Basket cells, Purkinje cells, and granule cells compose the cerebellar cortex. Basket cells make profuse inhibitory dendritic contacts with the flask-shaped Purkinje cells. Each Purkinje cell receives about 2×10^5 synapses, mostly onto its dendritic spines which splay out across the molecular layer. Granule cells are small neurons located in the vicinity of the Purkinje cells. Granule cell axons form the parallel fibers that make excitatory synapses onto Purkinje cell dendrites. Each parallel fiber synapses on about 200 Purkinje cells creating an excitation strip across the cerebellum.

138. The answer is b. (*Young, p 133. Junqueira, p 158. Kierszenbaum, pp 28–29. Kasper, pp 1042–1044. Moore and Dalley, pp 85–87.*) Kinesin is a motor protein that uses energy from ATP hydrolysis to move vesicles ($- \rightarrow +$) from the cell body in the dorsal root ganglion (shown in the photomicrograph) in an anterograde direction toward the axon terminal **(answer d)**. The patient in question has shingles caused by the herpes virus known as the varicella-zoster virus (VZV). Shingles begins as erythematous maculopapular eruptions and rapidly evolves to vesicles; it often presents with fever. The patient had chickenpox as a child. Chickenpox is also caused by VZV. The virus is stored in the dorsal root ganglion, primarily in the satellite cells surrounding the perikarya (cell bodies). Kinesin walks along the microtubule toward the plus end of the microtubule. The dyneins **(answers a and c)** are minus-end directed microtubule motors that move organelles, including vesicles, in a retrograde direction toward the cell body (in this case toward the cell bodies of the dorsal root ganglia). The dyneins involved in axonal transport are the cytoplasmic dyneins as compared to the axonemal dyneins seen in cilia and flagella. Myosin II **(answer e)** is an actin-based motor protein that generates the force of muscle contraction. The Tzanck test is a method of testing for the virus; it can detect the presence of the herpesvirus in the cells scraped from a lesion. It cannot detect the difference between herpes simplex virus (HSV) and VZV. PCR of the DNA is required for absolute detection.

The patient's shingles involve dermatomal segment T4, which surrounds the nipple. The nipples are normally found in the middle of T4, although T5 may also innervate this region. A dermatome is the area of skin supplied by nerves originating from a single spinal nerve root.

139. The answer is c. (*Junqueira, pp 179–180. Ross and Pawlina, p 351. Kierszenbaum, pp 30, 216. Alberts, pp 979–981. Kandel, pp 99–103, 1108–1109.*) Regeneration depends on the proliferation of Schwann cells, which guide sprouting axons from the proximal segment toward the target organ. The injury causes Wallerian degeneration distal to the level of injury and proximal axonal degeneration to at least the next node of Ranvier. In more severe traumatic injuries, the proximal degeneration may extend beyond the next node of Ranvier. Electrodiagnostic studies demonstrate denervation changes in the affected muscles, and in cases of reinnervation, motor unit potentials (MUPs) are present (**answer a**). Axonal regeneration occurs at the rate of 1 mm/day (**answer b**) or 1 in./month and can be monitored with an advancing Tinel's sign. The Tinel's sign is observed when tapping over nerve trunk that has been damaged or is regenerating following trauma causes a sensation of tingling and pins in its distribution up to the site of regeneration. A nerve trunk will regenerate about 1 mm/day (see transport rates discussed in the next paragraph). If this sign is absent, there is a poor prognosis. The endoneurial tubes remain intact (**answer d**), and, therefore, recovery is complete, with axons reinnervating their original motor and sensory targets.

The process of response to injury is referred to as Wallerian degeneration. Axonal regeneration occurs in neurons if the perikarya survive following damage. The segment distal (**answer e**) to the wound, including the myelin, is phagocytosed and removed by macrophages. The proximal segment is capable of regeneration because it remains in continuity with the perikaryon. Chromatolysis is the first step in the regeneration process, in which there is breakdown of the Nissl substance (RER, ribosomes), swelling of the perikaryon, and migration of the nucleus peripherally. Degeneration of perikarya and neuronal processes occurs when there is extensive neuronal damage. Transneuronal degeneration occurs only when there are synapses with a single damaged neuron. In the presence of inputs from multiple neurons, transneuronal degeneration does not occur.

Axonal transport occurs by several different mechanisms. Slow axonal transport/dendritic transport (1–5 mm/day) involves the movement of cytoskeletal elements such as actin, tubulin, and neurofilaments from the perikaryon down the axon. Rapid anterograde (away from the perikaryon) transport and retrograde (toward the perikaryon) transport (200–300 mm/day) transports membrane-bound organelles, for example, newly formed secretory vesicles and mitochondria anterogradely. Receptors, recycled membranes, and worn-out organelles are transported retrogradely.

140. The answer is c. *(Kierszenbaum, pp 216–217. Junqueira, pp 154, 171, 174. Kandel, pp 21–22, 148, 160.)* The nodes of Ranvier increase the efficiency of nodal conduction because of restriction (sequestration) of energy–dependent Na$^+$ influx to the node. The nodes of Ranvier represent the space between adjacent units of myelination. This area is bare in the CNS, whereas in the PNS the axons in the nodes are partially covered by the cytoplasmic tongues of adjacent Schwann cells. Most of the Na$^+$-gated channels are located in the bare areas. Therefore, spread of depolarization from the nodal region along the axon occurs until it reaches the next node. This is often described as a series of jumps from node to node, or saltatory conduction.

141. The answer is b. *(Kierszenbaum, pp 216–217. Junqueira, p 168. Kandel, pp 1288–1295.)* The barrier function of the blood-brain barrier is formed by occluding junctions (zonulae occludens) between endothelial cells that comprise the lining of brain capillaries. Adding to the impermeability are the nonfenestrated nature of the capillary endothelium and the paucity or absence of pinocytotic vesicles that represent the physiological pores seen in other endothelia. Astrocytes form foot processes around the brain capillaries that induce and maintain the blood-brain barrier. Surrounding the CNS is a basement membrane with a lining of astrocyte foot processes; this forms the glia limitans. Oligodendrocytes function in myelination of CNS axons. Microglia function as brain macrophages and are involved in antigen presentation and phagocytosis.

142. The answer is a. *(Alberts, pp 645–648. Junqueira, pp 194–195. Kierszenbaum, pp 183–184. Kandel, pp 43, 175–177, 183, 210–211.)* Ca^{2+} entry through specific channels results in fusion of acetylcholine-containing synaptic vesicles with the presynaptic membrane and ultimately the release of neurotransmitter. Neuromuscular (myoneural), junctions represent the site at which end feet (boutons terminaux) approximate the surface of skeletal muscle cells. The arrangement is similar to the synapse; a neuromuscular junction can be considered the best-studied synapse. Na$^+$, K$^+$, and Cl$^-$ voltage–gated channels **(answers b, c, and d)** are involved in transmission of nerve impulses, but do not couple action potentials (an electrical signal) to neurotransmitter release (a chemical alteration). Ca^{2+} influx into the end feet may have a direct effect on phosphorylation of synapsin I, a vesicular membrane protein, which in its nonphosphorylated state blocks vesicle fusion with the presynaptic membrane. Gap junctions are not involved **(answer e)**.

143. The answer is d. *(Junqueira, pp 154, 156–157, 163–165.)* The left hemisphere regulates language and speech and the right hemisphere controls nonverbal, spatial skills such as the ability to draw or play music. If the right side of the brain is damaged, movement in the left arm and leg, vision to the left, or hearing in the left ear, may be affected. An injury to the left side of the brain affects speech and movement on the right side of the body. Pyramidal neurons are labeled with the arrows in the photomicrograph. Axons are evident in the histologic section arising from the axon hillock. Neither the axon nor the axon hillock contains Nissl substance (rough ER), which is dispersed throughout the soma and dendrites. Dendrites generally are wider than axons, are of nonuniform diameter, and taper to a point. Motor neurons, such as those illustrated in the photomicrograph, usually display large amounts of euchromatin, distinct nucleoli, and Nissl (if stained appropriately) characteristic of high synthetic activity.

144. The answer is a. *(Junqueira, pp 172–173, 175. Kasper, pp 966–969.)* The woman in the scenario has contracted leprosy with infection of the peripheral nerves by *Mycobacterium leprae*. Perineurial inflammation of cutaneous nerves leads to distal anesthesia and paralysis, which are major clinical features of the early stages of leprosy. Those neuropathic changes are eventually responsible for the deformities that elicit most of the social stigma associated with leprosy. The neuropathy of leprosy primarily affects the facial, ulnar radial and peroneal nerves with ascending degeneration of the nerves. In the later stages, endoneurial inflammation, infection of Schwann cells, demyelination, and reduced conduction velocity occurs. In the high-magnification light micrograph, several cross-sections through small peripheral nerves are visible. C indicates the perineurium, a layer of two to three fibroblast-like cells with contractile properties that surround individual fascicles. Cells of the perineurium are joined by tight junctions and form a barrier to macromolecules. B indicates the dense, irregular connective tissue part of the epineurium surrounding the entire nerve. There are numerous nerve fibers surrounded by myelin sheaths **(D)** produced by Schwann cells (nucleus visible at **E**). Other nuclei visible within the fascicle include those of fibroblasts, which secrete the reticular connective tissue elements forming the endoneurium surrounding the individual neuronal fibers, and nuclei of capillary endothelial cells. Neuronal perikarya are not present in peripheral nerves. Label **A** indicates skeletal muscle, identifiable by its striations and peripherally located nuclei.

145. The answer is e. *(Sadler, pp 286, 290–291, 311, 313, 315. Junqueira, p 155. Kandel, pp 880, 883, 1027, 1046–1048. Moore and Persaud, Developing, pp 90, 202, 303–304, 428–435, 486–487, 494, 522.)* The neural crest forms most of the peripheral nervous system, in contrast to the neural tube, which is the embryonic source of the central nervous system. The sensory neurons of the cranial and spinal sensory ganglia (e.g., dorsal root ganglia), sympathetic chain ganglia, postganglionic sympathetic and parasympathetic fibers of the autonomic nervous system, cells of the pia and arachnoid, Schwann cells, and satellite cells of the dorsal root ganglia are neural elements derived from the neural crest. Nonneuronal structures formed from the neural crest include melanocytes of the skin, odontoblasts in teeth, derivatives of the branchial arch cartilages (e.g., pinnae of ear), and the adrenal medulla, but not the adrenal cortex, e.g., zona granulosa **(answer a)**. The adrenal medulla represents postganglionic sympathetic fibers that respond to inputs from preganglionic sympathetic fibers in splanchnic nerves. Ventral horn and pyramidal cells **(answers b and c)** as well as astrocytes **(answer d)** are derived from the neuroepithelium of the neural tube.

146. The answer is b. *(Junqueira, p 179. Ross and Pawlina, p 336. Kasper, p 140. Kumar, p 1356.)* The structure in the photomicrograph delineated by the arrow is a single intramural parasympathetic ganglion cell distinctly characterized by its large, euchromatic nucleus and prominent nucleolus. Several small satellite cells surround the ganglion cell. Parasympathetic stimulation of the salivary glands produces a profuse, watery secretion. Atropine blocks parasympathetic responses. The child in the scenario is suffering from cerebral palsy (CP). Sialorrhea is excessive drooling and is a common symptom in children with CP. Children with CP are at increased risk of aspiration, skin maceration, and infection. Sialorrhea also impedes social integration. Parasympathetic ganglia are located in close proximity to or in the wall of the organs they innervate. Other structures within the field include serous acini from an exocrine gland, a small peripheral nerve, a venule, and several skeletal muscle fibers.

147. The answer is d. *(Junqueira, pp 45, 47, 153–154, 160–163.)* The cells labeled with GFAP are activated astrocytes. Astrocytes are the most abundant cell type in the human brain. Astrocytes are activated following CNS damage and form the glial scar. These glial cells interact with neurons, blood vessels and the *pia mater* by their stellate processes. Regulation of the microenvironment including the concentrations of ions, metabolites and neurotransmitters (e.g., glutamate) is an important function of astrocytes. Astrocytes are also the source of the most common glioma, astrocytoma. The barrier function of the blood-brain-barrier is established by tight junctions (*zonula occludentes*) between endothelial cells in the blood vessels of the brain. However, astrocytes establish and maintain the blood-brain barrier and thus control the entry of compounds into the brain parenchyma. During development the astrocytes are critical to normal migration of developing neurons. The patient in the vignette suffers from NeuroAIDS. In that disease, astrocytes are believed to be infected with the AIDS virus. Astrocytes can be infected with HIV-1, however, there appears to be only limited replication. Infection can lead to changes in gene expression (of the cell) and some of the released products can have deleterious effects on neurons. Astrocytes integrate neuronal inputs, exhibit calcium excitability, and communicate bidirectionally with neighboring neurons and synapses, but do not synapse with neurons **(answer a)**. Microglia present antigen and phagocytose dying neurons **(answers b and c)**. Oligodendrocytes myelinate axons in the CNS **(answer e)**.

148. The answer is a. (*Kasper, pp 2554–2556. Junqueira, pp 158–161, 166–169. Kandel, pp 265–269.*) Clinical depression is associated with reduced levels of the monoamines, such as 5-hydroxytryptamine (serotonin, 5-HT) in the CNS. The selective serotonin reuptake inhibitors (SSRIs), such as Fluoxetine hydrochloride (Prozac), bind to the 5-HT reuptake transporter in the presynaptic membrane, blocking reuptake, and subsequent degradation of serotonin in the synaptic cleft **(answer e)**. Therefore, serotonin levels increase in the synaptic cleft as a result of SSRI-treatment. The structure labeled "D" is the postsynaptic membrane. The electron micrograph of the synapse shows the presynaptic membrane (C), postsynaptic membrane (D), mitochondria (B), and synaptic vesicles (A). Recycling of synaptic vesicle membrane occurs at the presynaptic membrane in conjunction with neurotransmitter release by exocytosis. Neurotransmitter release is induced by membrane depolarization, leading to transient opening of calcium channels followed by calcium influx. There is no cytoplasmic continuity between adjacent neurons **(answer d)**. Transmission from neuron to neuron occurs by chemical transmission in the form of neurotransmitter release. The neurotransmitter (from the synaptic vesicles) crosses the synaptic cleft (between the pre- and postsynaptic membranes) and interacts with receptors on the postsynaptic membrane (**answer b**), which results in changes in the permeability of this membrane (**answer c**). Numerous mitochondria and synaptic vesicles are typically found on the presynaptic side of the synapse. The postsynaptic surface typically is denser than the presynaptic membrane.

149. The answer is b. (*Kasper, pp 2461–2463. Kumar, pp 1382–1384. Kierszenbaum, pp 210–212. Junqueira, p 163.*) The patient is suffering from multiple sclerosis (MS), a demyelinating disease in which both CD4$^+$ and CD8$^+$-T cells as well as autoantibodies are targeted to oligodendrocytes. MS is twice as prevalent in women as in men and demyelination is most commonly found in the anterior corpus callosum. Alterations in the CSF shows pleocytosis (increase in the number of mononuclear cells above normal levels), increase in protein, elevated gamma globulin (antibodies to oligodendrocytes as represented by oligoclonal bands on gel electrophoresis). Microglia (**answer a**) are the phagocytes of the CNS, astrocytes (**answer c**) induce and maintain the blood-brain barrier and form the glial scar following injury, and Schwann cells (**answer d**) are responsible for myelination in the PNS. On autopsy, plaques are found that contain lymphocytes and monocytes in infiltrates around small veins in what is known as perivascular cuffing. Axons (**answer e**) are generally preserved. The main identifying feature on histopathological examination is the paucity of oligodendrocytes. Astrocytic proliferation and gliosis may increase with the duration of MS.

150. The answer is e. (*Junqueira, pp 154, 194. Ross and Pawlina, pp 291–292, 311–313. Kasper, pp 2518–2521. Kumar, pp 212, 1344.*) The junctional folds are the site of acetylcholine (ACh) receptors which are reduced in number in myasthenia gravis. The normal neuromuscular junction releases acetylcholine (ACh) from the motor nerve terminal in discrete packages (quanta). The ACh quanta diffuse across the synaptic cleft and bind to receptors on the folded muscle end-plate membrane. Stimulation of the motor nerve releases many ACh quanta that depolarize the muscle end-plate region and then the muscle membrane causing muscle contraction. In myasthenia gravis, the postsynaptic muscle membrane is smooth and lacks the normal folded shape. The concentration of ACh receptors on the muscle end-plate membrane is reduced, and antibodies are attached to the membrane. ACh is released normally, but its effect on the postsynaptic membrane is reduced. The postjunctional membrane is less sensitive to applied ACh, and the probability that any nerve impulse will cause a muscle action potential is reduced. The edrophonium chloride (tensilon) test uses a rapid acting and degrading acetylcholine esterase inhibitor. It causes neuromuscular transmission to be increased in the patient. The physician injects the tensilon and then looks for rapid relief of the symptoms, particularly the eyelids and the diplopia. Other structures labeled in the electron micrograph are: A = nucleus, B = mitochondria, C = myofilaments, and D = nerve terminal.

Cardiovascular System, Blood, and Bone Marrow

Questions

DIRECTIONS: Each item below contains a question or incomplete statement followed by suggested responses. Select the **one best** response to each question.

151. Vasa vasorum provide a function analogous to that of which of the following?

a. Valves
b. Basal lamina
c. Coronary arteries
d. Endothelial diaphragms
e. Arterioles

152. The cell labeled A is best described as which of the following?

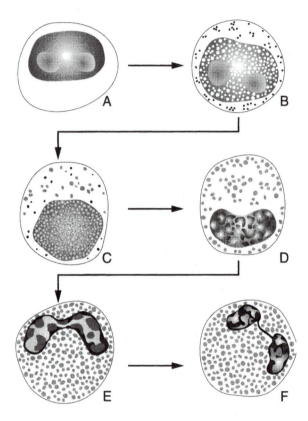

a. Myeloblast
b. Proerythroblast
c. Metamyelocyte
d. Myelocyte
e. Promyelocyte

153. A newborn girl presents with a mutation in the erythropoietin receptor gene which leads to primary familial erythrocytosis (familial polycythemia). During the 5th to 9th months of fetal development, the primary effect was on red blood cell production in which of the following?

a. Liver
b. Yolk sac
c. Spleen
d. Thymus
e. Bone marrow

154. A 64-year-old man presents with splenomegaly, lymphadenopathy, persistent fever, night sweats, and weight loss. Bone marrow aspiration and biopsy are scheduled. Which of the following would be the best place to sample bone marrow?

a. Iliac crest
b. Sternum
c. Scapula
d. Humerus
e. Tibia

155. Organs such as the brain and thymus have a more effective blood-barrier because their blood capillaries are of which of the following types?

a. Continuous type with few vesicles
b. Fenestrated type with diaphragms
c. Fenestrated type without diaphragms
d. Discontinuous type with diaphragms
e. Discontinuous type without diaphragms

156. A 62-year-old African-American man presents with exercise-induced angina. His serum cholesterol is 277 mg/dL (normal <200), LDL is 157 (normal <100), HDL is 43 (normal >35), and triglycerides 170 (normal <150). His BMI is 34 and his coronary risk ratio is 6.84 (normal <5). On cardiac catheterization there is occlusion of the left anterior descending and the origin of the right coronary artery. The disease process is initiated by which of the following?

a. Proliferation of smooth muscle cells
b. Formation of an intimal plaque
c. Attraction of platelets to collagen microfibrils
d. Adventitial proliferation
e. Injury to the endothelium

157. A 66-year-old man patient who was diagnosed with type II diabetes 10 years ago presents with an aching pain in the muscles of his lower extremity. He says the pain is relieved by rest and worsened by resumed physical activity. His lower limbs appear cold, pale, and discolored, and he has a sore on the skin of his left calf. He has a weak tibial pulse on both sides and poor skin filling from capillaries. In this patient, which of the following functions would be primarily affected in the blood vessel from the lower extremity shown in the accompanying transmission electron micrograph?

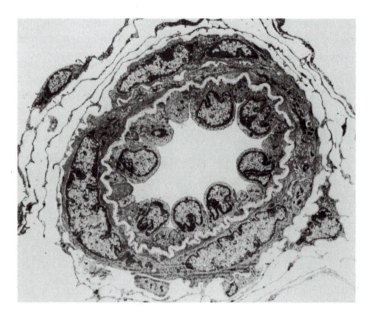

a. Adaptation to systolic pressure
b. Distribution of blood within an organ
c. Blood flow from the aorta to specific organs
d. Return of lymphocytes to the blood
e. Return of venous blood to the heart

158. A 35-year-old woman's physician orders laboratory blood tests. Her fresh blood is drawn and centrifuged in the presence of heparin as an anti-coagulant to obtain a hematocrit. The resulting fractions are which of the following?

a. Serum, packed erythrocytes, and leukocytes
b. Leukocytes, erythrocytes, and serum proteins
c. Plasma, buffy coat, and packed erythrocytes
d. Fibrinogen, platelets, buffy coat, and erythrocytes
e. Albumin, plasma lipoproteins, and erythrocytes

159. As a hematologist in the clinic, you diagnose a 34-year-old woman with idiopathic thrombocytopenic purpura (ITP). Which of the following symptoms/characteristics would you expect in this patient?

a. Decreased clotting time
b. Normal blood count
c. Abnormal bruising
d. Hypercoagulation
e. Light menstrual periods

160. A 47-year-old man presents to his family physician complaining of unusual thirst, increased frequency of urination, dizziness, blurred vision, and numbness in his left foot. His BMI is 32. He reports that his lifestyle is sedentary with very rare exercise. His diet consists largely of what he describes as "fast and junk food." A finger stick reading indicates a blood glucose level of 190 mg/dL and two fasting blood sugars are 156 and 166 mg/dL. Over time, which of the following describes the changes that may occur in the structure labeled "A" in the accompanying light micrograph?

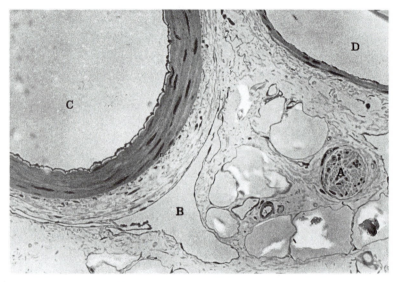

(Micrograph courtesy of Dr. John K. Young.)

a. Loss of beta cells
b. Arteriosclerosis
c. Progressive decrease in nerve conduction velocity
d. Altered smooth muscle glucose transporter function
e. Altered lymphatic flow

161. Erythrocytes may have abnormal shapes and sizes in certain diseases. In iron deficiency you would expect to see which of the following?

a. Microcytic, hypochromatic anemia with smaller mature erythrocytes
b. Macrocytic, hyperchromatic anemia with fewer, larger mature erythrocytes
c. Poikilocytosis and more fragile erythrocytes
d. Spherocytosis
e. No change in erythrocyte size or shape, but a substantial drop in the hematocrit

162. A 43-year-old woman who has suffered from diabetes for 30 years comes into the clinic. Her hematocrit is 21 and she has a reduced RBC count. Her serum creatinine is 3.0 (normal 2.0 or below). She has a negative pregnancy test and is a nonsmoker. Which of the following would best explain her condition?

a. Decreased hepatic production of erythropoietin leading to decreased numbers of circulating reticulocytes in the bloodstream
b. Increased erythropoietin production by the liver resulting in increased numbers of reticulocytes
c. Decreased renal erythropoietin production leading to reduced red blood cell production
d. Decreased estrogen levels stimulating hepatic production of erythropoietin
e. Decreased estrogen levels directly inhibiting red blood cell production by the bone marrow

163. Which of the following is a metabolic function of the cells labeled with arrows in the accompanying light micrograph?

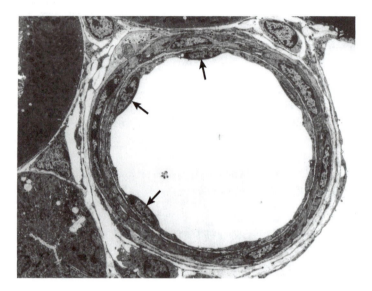

a. Receptors for endothelin
b. Release of serotonin
c. Production of type III collagen
d. Synthesis of plasminogen activator
e. Production of thromboxane

164. You are working in a research laboratory studying cardiovascular function. The studies in that laboratory use a "knockout" mouse in which the gene for atrial natriuretic peptide (ANP) is deleted. Which of the following would you most likely find elevated?

a. ANP levels in the bloodstream
b. Excretion of urine
c. Excretion of sodium
d. Peripheral vasoconstriction
e. Capillary permeability

165. A 43-year-old anatomy professor is working in her garden, pruning rose bushes without gloves. She has a thorn enter the skin of her forefinger. The area later becomes infected and she removes the thorn, but there is still pus remaining at the wound site. Which of the following cells functions in the formation of pus?

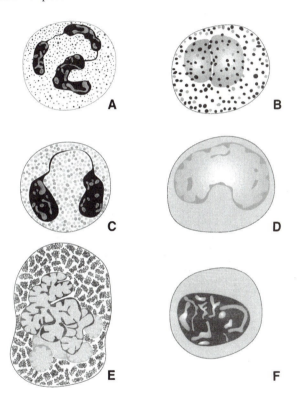

a. A
b. B
c. C
d. D
e. E
f. F

166. A 27-year-old man returns from a climbing trip to Ouray, Colorado. He spent 2 weeks camping with his fellow climbing friends. He is dehydrated and complains that he has been vomiting and has had "foul-smelling" diarrhea since his return from camping. He says that he has noticed several large worms in the vomitus and had a visible worm in his loose stool last week. A stool sample is positive for ova and parasites. How do the structures labeled in the accompanying electron micrograph assist in defending against this condition?

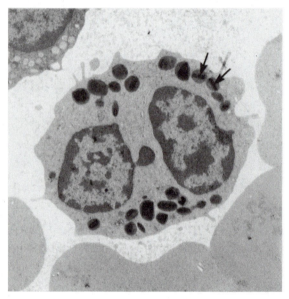

(Electron micrograph courtesy of Dr. Amy Klion)

a. Phagocytose parasites
b. Release IL-1 which activates antigen presenting cells (APCs) and CD4⁺ lymphocytes
c. Release IL-2 which stimulates the proliferation and activation of B-cells and T-cells.
d. Produce IL-5 which stimulates the production and maturation of eosinophils during inflammation
e. Contain a toxin for parasites

Cardiovascular System, Blood, and Bone Marrow

Answers

151. The answer is c. *(Junqueira, pp 206–207, 211. Kumar, p 512.)* Vasa vasorum (VV) are vessels within a vessel and are found primarily in the adventitia of large arteries and veins. They provide nutrition and oxygenated blood to the thick media and adventitia of these vessels, which are unable to obtain nutrition by diffusion from the lumen. Coronary arteries fulfill a similar function for the myocardium.

152. The answer is a. *(Junqueira, pp 245–247. Ross, pp 268, 270–271.)* The first stage in granulopoiesis is the myeloblast (A), a large cell with prominent light-staining nucleoli with only a little cytoplasm, generally without granules. The lineage shown in the figure illustrates eosinophilic development in the bone marrow. Basophils may be bilobed or segmented, but with larger and more irregular granules that obscure the nucleus in Wright-stained blood smears. The promyelocyte (**B**) is the next cell in the lineage. It is larger than the myeloblast, nucleoli are less visible, and primary granules are present in the cytoplasm. Granule specificity is attained in the myelocyte with flattening of the nucleus. The eosinophilic myelocyte (**C**) differentiates into the eosinophilic metamyelocyte (**D**) when invagination of the nucleus begins. Further invagination leads to the formation of an eosinophilic band (**E**) and ultimately a mature eosinophil (**F**). An eosinophil has a bilobed nucleus and plays an important role in allergic and parasitic infections. The granules stain with eosinophilic dyes and contain major basic protein, histaminase, peroxidase, and some hydrolytic enzymes. Eosinophils have an affinity for antigen-antibody complexes and, although phagocytic, are not as active against bacteria as neutrophils. The histaminase secreted by eosinophils counteracts the release of histamine from basophils and mast cells, essential in hypersensitivity reactions. B lymphocytes differentiate into antibody-producing plasma cells; T lymphocytes are responsible for cell-mediated responses including graft rejection; and neutrophils are responsible for phagocytosis of bacteria.

153. The answer is e. *(Ross, p 254. Junqueira, p 238. Kumar, p 620.)* The bone marrow begins to function in the second month and becomes the predominant hematopoietic site during months 5 to 9 of gestation, The first site of blood cell development (hematopoiesis) is extraembryonic, in the yolk sac **(answer b)**, which produces hematocytoblasts and primitive erythroblasts from the third week through the second month of gestation. Hepatic erythropoiesis **(answer a)** begins during the sixth week, reaches its maximum in the third month, and then ceases about the seventh month. Whereas, the spleen **(answer c)** is involved specifically in the production of red blood cells (erythropoiesis) from months 2 to 5 of gestation with some activity continuing postnatally. The spleen continues to produce monocytes and lymphocytes throughout life. From the second month of gestation, the lymph nodes produce lymphocytes, and the thymus **(answer d)** is responsible for the education of T cells. Those T lymphocytes are seeded to T-dependent areas, such as the deep cortex of the lymph node and periarteriolar lymphoid sheath (PALS) of the spleen.

154. The answer is a. *(Kumar, p 620. Ross, p 254. Junqueira, p 238.)* The iliac crest is the best location for bone marrow sampling. The sternum is not as safe a place for bone marrow aspiration and biopsy because of possible damage to thoracic structures **(answer b)**. The patient in the vignette suffers from chronic lymphocytic leukemia CLL more common in adults over 60 years old. Hematopoiesis occurs in the flat bones **(answer c)** and other bones in the adult human. Although most bones in the body are involved in hematopoiesis during growth, the marrow of the sternum, ribs, vertebrae, iliac crest, skull, and proximal femora are the primary sites of blood cell development by the time that skeletal maturity is achieved. It also occurs in the long bones **(answers d, and e)** during development, but many of those areas become dominated by yellow marrow that contains many fat cells (adipose tissue). The inactive yellow marrow can be reactivated on exposure to the proper stimulus (e.g., severe blood loss).

155. The answer is a. *(Young, pp 139, 203. Junqueira, pp 168, 212–213, 266–267. Ross, pp 423–424. Kierszenbaum, pp 327–330.)* The capillary endothelia in the brain and thymus are continuous, as is the basal lamina. The blood-thymus barrier provides the appropriate microenvironment for education of T cells without exposure to self. The capillary is further surrounded by perivascular connective tissue and epithelial cells and their basement membrane. In the blood-brain barrier, there is also a continuous endothelium with a basal lamina and an absence of fenestrations. Surrounding the basal lamina in the brain are the foot processes of astrocytes, which form the glia limitans; however, it is important to note that the barrier function of the blood-brain barrier is formed specifically by endothelial cell occluding junctions with many sealing strands. Other capillary endothelia (**answers b → e**) in the body are fenestrated (transcellular openings) or discontinuous (sinusoids). The fenestrae are transcellular openings that occur in many of the visceral capillaries. In hematopoietic organs, there are large gaps in the endothelium, and the capillaries are classified as discontinuous. Diaphragms (thinner cell membrane) are present in some fenestrated capillaries and produce an intermediate level of molecular transit. Diaphragms contain proteoglycans with particularly high concentrations of heparan sulfate. This results in numerous anionic sites that repel anionic proteins. The diaphragms facilitate the passage of water and small molecules dissolved in fluid. Physiologically, the large pores (50 to 70 nm) of endothelia are represented by pinocytotic vesicles. Intercellular junctions, particularly the tight junctions, function as the small endothelial pores (approximately 10 nm in diameter) observed in physiologic studies. Plasmalemmal vesicles and channels are neutrally charged and rich in galactose and N-acetylglucosamine. Vesicular and channel pathways are required for transport of anionic proteins such as insulin, transferrin, albumin, and low-density lipoprotein (LDL).

156. The answer is e. *(Junqueira, pp 206–209. Moore and Dalley, p 160. Kierszenbaum, pp 335–336.)* The site at which coronary arteries become occluded are: first, at the left anterior descending (thus affecting both ventricles anteriorly); second, at the origin of the right coronary artery affecting both the right atrium and ventricle and disrupting cardiac rhythm; and third, the circumflex branch (affecting both left atria and ventricle). Atherosclerosis is initiated by damage to the endothelial cells, which exposes the subjacent connective tissue (subendothelium). The loss of the antithrombogenic endothelium results in aggregation of platelets. Atherosclerosis is one form of arteriosclerosis (hardening of the arteries) that involves deposition of fatty material primarily in the walls of the conducting arteries. The intima and media become infiltrated with lipid. Intimal thickening occurs through the addition of collagen and elastin with an abnormal pattern of elastin cross-linking. Platelets release mitogenic substances that stimulate proliferation of smooth muscle cells. The thickening of the intima is also called an atheromatous plaque and worsens with repeated damage to the endothelium. It is most dangerous in small vessels, particularly the coronary arteries, where occlusion can result in a myocardial infarction. Atherosclerotic plaques also lead to thrombi and aneurysms.

157. The answer is b. (*Young, pp 147, 149. Junqueira, pp 208, 211, 215. Ross, p 371.*) The blood vessel in the electron micrograph is an arteriole (small artery) involved in intraorgan blood flow. There is only one layer of smooth muscle, but a distinct internal elastic membrane is present.

There is no visible internal elastic membrane in a venule. A capillary lacks smooth muscle and is composed only of a single layer of endothelial cells.

The aorta and large arteries (**answer a**) contain extensive elastic fibers that permit rapid arterial wall stretch in response to the force of ventricular contraction during systole (120 to 160 mm Hg) followed by sudden relaxation (60 to 90 mm Hg) during diastole. Blood is ejected from the left ventricle into the large arteries only during systole; however, blood flow is uniform because of the elasticity of the large, conducting arteries.

The muscular (distributing) arteries regulate blood flow to organs (**answer c**). Muscular (medium) arteries contain more smooth muscle than the arteriole (**answer b**) in the figure and distribute blood to organs. Contraction of muscular arteries is regulated by local factors as well as sympathetic innervation. The degree of contraction regulates blood flow between organs. When the tunica media of the muscular artery is contracted, less blood flow occurs to the organ. In a more relaxed state, there is increased blood flow to the same organ.

The thoracic duct (**answer d**) returns lymphocytes from the lymphoid compartment to the circulation. The thoracic duct shows complete disorganization in the wall with no distinct media or adventitia. The large veins (**answer e**), such as the vena cava, that return blood to the heart contain smooth muscle bundles in the adventitia and are also the only vessel in which one sees both cross sections and longitudinal sections of smooth muscle in the same vessel.

158. The answer is c. (*Junqueira, p 223. Ross, p 248.*) After blood is removed from the body, a clot forms that contains platelets, erythrocytes, leukocytes, and a clear, yellow fluid known as serum. Hematocrit is the volume of erythrocytes per unit volume of blood (e.g., 40 to 50% in adult human males). When centrifuged with anticoagulants, blood separates into three layers. The uppermost layer is the plasma; the buffy coat is a thin white layer consisting of leukocytes found beneath the plasma; and the packed erythrocyte layer at the bottom of the tube.

159. The answer is c. (*Junqueira, p 250. Kierszenbaum, p 156. Kasper, pp 674–676.*) Idiopathic thrombocytopenic purpura (ITP) is primarily a disease of increased peripheral platelet destruction and/or reduction in platelet production by the bone marrow. The main symptom is bleeding, which can include bruising ("ecchymosis") and tiny red dots on the skin or mucous membranes ("petechiae"). In some instances bleeding from the nose, periodontal ligament ("gums"), urinary or gastrointestinal tracts may occur. Cerebral hemorrhage occurs rarely in ITP. Red and white cell counts are normal, but platelet counts range from 10,000 to 30,000/mL^3 (**answer b**) with 150,000 mL^3 as normal and higher than 100,000 mL^3 is safe.

The reduction in platelets increases clotting time (**answer a**), decreases coagulation (**answer d**), and would result in heavier menstrual bleeding (**answer e**). ITP appears to be an autoimmune disease since most patients have autoantibodies to specific platelet membrane glycoproteins. ITP patients often show diminished platelet production by the bone marrow. Acute ITP often follows an acute infection or in response to pharmaceutical administration. It can also occur during pregnancy and in chronic diseases such as hepatitis C, HIV, and lupus.

160. The answer is c. (*Ross and Pawlina, p 395. Junqueira, pp 208, 211–212, 214.*) The photomicrograph shows several types of blood or lymphatic vessels. Frequently, peripheral nerves are found in association with blood vessels (neurovascular bundle). In this section, a small peripheral nerve is labeled **A**. It is characterized by an outer covering of perineurium. The dark nuclei visible within the cross section belong mostly to Schwann cells. Neuronal cell bodies (perikarya) are not found within peripheral nerves. The structure labeled **B** is a small lymphatic vessel. Small lymphatic vessels are characterized by a wall consisting only of an exceedingly thin, single layer of endothelium. The lumen is usually larger than that of comparable venules. As observed in the photomicrograph, valves are also present in lymphatic vessels. A small muscular artery (**C**) and comparable vein (**D**) are also present in the field. The patient is diabetic with neuropathy.

161. The answer is a. *(Junqueira, pp 224–226. Kasper, pp 330–335. Kumar, pp 622–628.)* Iron deficiency leads to anemia with the presence of smaller, pale-staining erythrocytes (microcytic, hypochromatic). Hyperchromatic, macrocytic anemia results from vitamin B_{12} deficiency **(answers b and e).** The presence of spherical rather than biconcave erythrocytes is known as spherocytosis **(answer d).** The RBC membrane undergoes deformation due to the inability of ankyrin to bind spectrin. The shape change results in trapping in the splenic sinusoids and excessive destruction of red blood cells in that organ. Poikilocytosis is the generic term for abnormally shaped erythrocytes **(answer c).** Hereditary elliptocytosis and hereditary poikilocytosis are inherited diseases in which there is RBC membrane fragility and abnormal shape due to spectrin mutations. Mutations in Band 3 (anion exchanger 1) result in RBCs that are hyperchromatic with poikilocytosis.

162. The answer is c. *(Kasper, pp 329–330, 1658. Junqueira, pp 240, 242, 373.)* Normal hematocrit for a woman is 37 to 47%. The most likely cause of the anemia is renal failure leading to decreased production of the kidney-derived red blood cell growth factor, erythropoietin **(answers a and b).** In the initial stages of renal failure the kidneys will increase their production of erythropoietin, but as renal damage continues, the cells that produce this factor are destroyed. Therefore, there are initially increased levels of reticulocytes (immature red blood cells) in the bloodstream, but this is later reversed, as in the anemia of renal disease, low production of reticulocytes is a hallmark of the disease. Although the patient may have decreased estrogen levels, estrogen decreases hematocrit **(answers d and e).** Also, women who are pregnant (third trimester) can have slightly decreased hematocrits [37 ± 6 (third trimester women) vs. 40 ± 6 (adult women) and 42 ± 6 (postmenopausal women)]. However, this patient had a negative pregnancy test. Administration of recombinant erythropoietin (EPO) is the preferred treatment for anemia caused by advanced renal disease. Generally, EPO is administered if the hematocrit is less than 30%. Erythropoietin is synthesized by the peritubular (interstitial) cells of the kidney cortex, stimulates the differentiation of cells from the erythrocyte colony–forming units (E-CFUs), and the differentiation and release of reticulocytes from the bone marrow. Colony-forming units (CFUs) are distinct cell lineages derived from pluripotential stem cells in the bone marrow.

163. The answer is d. (*Kumar, pp 65–68, 513–514. Kierszenbaum, pp 334–335. Junqueira, pp 75, 206. Kasper, p 337.*) Endothelial cells synthesize a number of antithrombogenic factors including plasminogen activator and prostacyclin. Prostacyclin functions through cyclic AMP to inhibit thromboxane production by platelets (**answer e**). Endothelial cells synthesize the basal lamina including type IV collagen. Fibroblasts synthesize type III collagen (**answer c**). Serotonin is released from platelets and enteroendocrine cells (**answer b**). Other endothelial cell functions include: secretion of endothelin [the most potent vasoconstrictor (**answer a**)], plasminogen inhibitor (a coagulant), and nitric oxide [NO, also known as endothelium-derived relaxing factor (EDRF)]. Angiotensin-converting enzyme (ACE) on the endothelial cell surface converts angiotensin I to angiotensin II (a potent vasoconstrictor), but also serves as an inactivation enzyme (bradykininase) for bradykinin, a vasodilator. Von Willebrand factor (factor VIII) is found in Weibel-Palade granules localized in the endothelial cells of vessels larger than capillaries. A deficiency of factor VIII leads to decreased platelet aggregation and hemophilia.

164. The answer is d. (*Kierszenbaum, p 323. Kumar, p 8. Junqueira, pp 198, 201, 217. Kasper, pp 213, 2131.*) Atrial natriuretic peptide (ANP) is an important diuretic and natriuretic molecule that is released from the atria in response to atrial stretch and/or endothelin-1 stimulation. In the absence of ANP, peripheral vasoconstriction increases due to the absence of the ANP-induced relaxation of vascular smooth muscle and the increase in aldosterone levels. Aldosterone increases Na^+ permeability of the luminal membrane in the distal renal tubule and the activity of Na^+ pumps. The increased salt causes water retention, expanded blood volume, and elevated blood pressure. ANP would not be expressed in ANP knockout mice (**answer a**). Excretion of urine [diuresis (**answer b**)] and sodium [natriuresis (**answer c**)], and capillary permeability (**answer e**) all decrease in the absence of ANP. The main targets of ANP are the kidneys and vascular smooth muscle. ANP decreases blood pressure due to a direct relaxation of vascular smooth muscle. In addition, it increases salt and water excretion, enhances capillary permeability, and inhibits the release or action of several hormones, in addition to aldosterone, such as angiotensin II, endothelin, renin, and vasopressin. The natriuretic effect results from a direct inhibition of sodium absorption in the renal collecting duct, increased glomerular filtration rate (GFR), and inhibited aldosterone production and secretion. ANP counteracts the renin-angiotensin-aldosterone system. Increased ANP levels are detected in congestive heart failure, chronic renal failure, and in severe essential hypertension.

165. The answer is a. *(Young, pp 47–57. Junqueira, pp 226–235.)*
Neutrophil. The neutrophil **(A)** contains neutrophilic granules. Neutrophils are involved in the acute phase of inflammation and are responsible for the phagocytosis of invading bacteria. Neutrophils contain lysozyme and alkaline phosphatase within their granules. They die soon after phagocytosing bacteria and are added to the pus, which consists of dead neutrophils, serum, and tissue fluids.

Basophil. The basophil **(B)** is about the same size as the neutrophil **(A)** and contains granules of variable size that may obscure the nucleus. The nucleus of the basophil is irregularly lobed with condensed chromatin. Basophils are involved in the attraction of eosinophils to the site of infection. This occurs in parasitic and nonparasitic infections and involves chemoattraction by histamine and eosinophil-chemoattractant factor of anaphylaxis (ECF-A). Basophils are similar in structure and function to the connective tissue mast cell. Basophils are also phagocytic granulocytes, but are involved in inflammation through the release of histamine and heparin. Immunoglobulin E (IgE) produced by plasma cells becomes bound to the cell surface of mast cells and basophils on first exposure. At the time of secondary exposure, the antigen binds to the IgE and stimulates the degranulation of mast cell and basophil granules releasing histamine and heparin. Basophils and mast cells are involved in anaphylactic and immediate **hypersensitivity reactions.**

Eosinophil. The eosinophil **(C)** is bilobed with more regular granules than the basophil **(B)**. Eosinophils have less phagocytic ability than neutrophils and may kill parasites by either phagocytosis or exocytotic release of granules. Eosinophils contain major basic protein, histaminase, acid phosphatase, and other lysosomal enzymes. Eosinophils are essential for the destruction of parasites such as trichinae and schistosomes.

Monocyte. The monocyte **(D)** contains an eccentric nucleus, which is often kidney-shaped. The chromatin generally has a ropelike appearance and, therefore, is less condensed than the chromatin of a lymphocyte (**F**). The monocyte has some phagocytic activity in the blood, but its major role is as a source of macrophages throughout the body including Langerhans cells (skin), microglia (brain), and Kupffer cells (liver).

Megakaryocyte. The megakaryocyte (**E**) is a large cell with a multi-lobular appearance and is the source of platelets. Megakaryocytes fragment to form the platelets, which are key elements of the blood.

Lymphocyte. The lymphocyte (**F**) is considered an agranular cell with an ovoid nucleus and scanty cytoplasm. The shape and the arrangement of chromatin vary, depending on the classification of the lymphocyte: small, medium, or large. Small and medium are involved in chronic inflammation, whereas, large lymphocytes are the source of T and B cells. Lymphocytes are either T or B cells based on their education in the thymus or bone marrow. Plasma cells differentiate from B lymphocytes that undergo mitosis and form a plasma cell and a memory cell after exposure to appropriate antigen. An antigen-presenting cell and a specific subtype of T lymphocyte called a helper T cell are required for B cell differentiation into antibody-producing plasma cells.

166. The answer is e. (*Junqueira, pp 229, 231. Ross and Pawlina, pp 257–258. Kasper, pp 349, 351, 356.*) The patient returning from a camping trip most likely has contracted a parasite. The cell in the transmission electron micrograph is an eosinophil. Eosinophil granules contain a number of important substances including histaminase, eosinophil peroxidase, eosinophil cationic protein, and major basic protein (MBP). MBP forms the core of the eosinophilic granules and is a toxin for parasites. MBP binds to and disrupts the membrane of the parasite. The binding is mediated by the Fc receptor. MBP also causes basophils to release histamine. Eosinophils phagocytose parasites, but MBP is not directly involved (**answer a**). IL-1 and IL-2 carry out the functions of activating APCs and stimulating proliferation of B- and T-cells, respectively. However, the eosinophil does not release IL-1 and IL-2 (**answers b and c**). IL-5 stimulates production and maturation of eosinophils, but is not released by eosinophils (**answer d**).

Lymphoid System and Cellular Immunology

Questions

DIRECTIONS: Each item below contains a question or incomplete statement followed by suggested responses. Select the **one best** response to each question.

167. Clonal selection functions to do which of the following?

a. Create the optimal immune response to one specific antigen
b. Stimulate immunoglobulin class switching
c. Stimulate the production of self-reacting lymphocytes
d. Form specific colony-forming units for erythropoiesis and granulopoiesis in the bone marrow
e. Choose the appropriate homing receptors for lymphocytes

168. Tacrolimus (FK506) is prescribed for a patient who received an allogeneic liver transplant. The mechanism of action of tacrolimus is blockage of signal transduction pathways in which of the following cells?

a. T lymphocytes
b. Plasma cells
c. Monocytes
d. Eosinophils
e. Mast cells

169. The shortage of human organs for transplant has focused attention on xenotransplantation as a potential solution for obtaining donor organs. Rejection of a pig pancreas transplanted into a human would occur primarily through which of the following mechanisms?

a. Preformed antibodies recognize carbohydrates on endothelial cells in the graft.
b. T_C lymphocytes recognize dendritic cells in the graft
c. T_H lymphocytes recognize macrophages in the graft
d. Plasma cell response to antigens in the β cells of the islets
e. Hyperacute response of T cells to the pancreatic acinar cells

170. This organ, shown at low magnification (A) and high magnification (B) is which of the following?

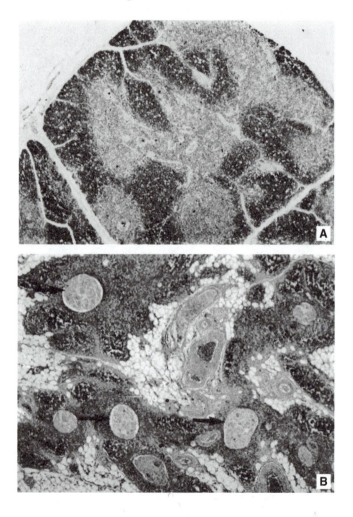

a. A site of antibody production
b. The site of filtration of the lymph and blood
c. Derived embryologically from the 3rd branchial arch
d. The site of production of CD4⁺ and CD8⁺ cells
e. A major site of red blood cell degradation and bilirubin recycling

171. Gene rearrangement of cytotoxic T cells occurs primarily in which of the following?

a. Bone marrow
b. Spleen
c. Germinal centers
d. Thymus
e. Mesenteric lymph nodes

172. Gene products of class II major histocompatibility complex (MHC) present antigenic peptides primarily to which of the following?

a. Helper T cells
b. Cytotoxic T cells
c. Antigen-presenting cells
d. B cells
e. Plasma cells

173. Expression of antigen associated with class I MHC molecules is recognized primarily by which of the following?

a. B cells
b. CD4$^+$ T lymphocytes
c. CD8$^+$ T lymphocytes
d. Plasma cells
e. Macrophages

174. Interleukin 2 is produced by which of the following?

a. Plasma cells
b. Natural killer cells
c. CD4$^+$ T lymphocytes
d. CD8$^+$ T lymphocytes
e. Macrophages

175. Martin Causubon weighed 3.5 kg at birth and appeared to be perfectly normal. Through his first 2 years of life, Martin had persistent otitis media, dry cough, and on one occasion bilateral pneumonia. At 5 months, Martin had oral *Candida spp.* and a red rash in the diaper area. He was not gaining weight; Martin was admitted to the hospital with tachypnea. His tonsils were observed to be very small, he had hepatomegaly, and cultures of his nasal fluid grew *Pseudomonas aeruginosa*. He also had coarse, harsh breath sounds from both lungs. Blood work showed a white blood count = 4800 cells μL^{-1} (normal 5000–10,000 cells μL^{-1}), absolute lymphocyte count = 760 cells μl^{-1} (normal 3000 lymphocytes μL^{-1}). None of his lymphocytes reacted with anti-CD3; 99% of his lymphocytes bound antibody against the B-cell molecule CD20 and 1% were natural killer cells reacting with anti-CD16. His serum contained IgG at a concetration of 30 mg dL^{-1}, IgA at 27 mg dL^{-1}, IgM at 42 mg dL^{-1} (IgG levels are normally 400 mg dL^{-1}; the IgA and IgM levels were at the low end of the normal range for Martin's age). His blood mononuclear cells were completely unresponsive to phytohemagglutinin (PHA), concanavalin A (ConA), and pokeweed mitogen (PWM), as well as to specific antigens to which he had been previously exposed by immunization or infection—tetanus and diphtheria toxoids, and *Candida* antigen. His B lymphocytes did not react with an antibody to the γ chain of the interleukin-2 receptor (IL-2Rγ).

The accompanying images are low magnification (A) and high magnification (B) photomicrographs. In Martin's case what would you expect to find immediately surrounding the region labeled with the arrow?

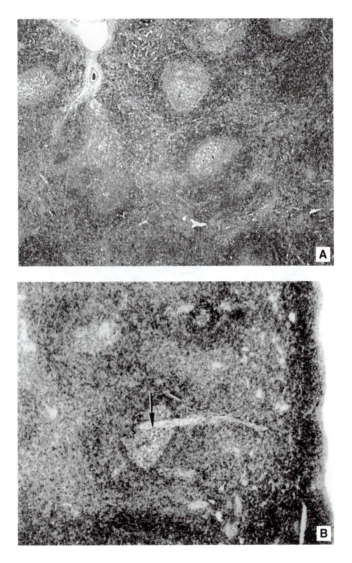

a. Absence of T cells
b. Proliferation of T cells
c. Proliferation of B cells
d. Absence of B cells
e. Absence of antigen-presenting cells (APCs)

176. A 6-year-old boy is brought to the pediatrics clinic. His mother reports that after her son eats peanut butter he complains of a tingling feeling on the lips and in his mouth. After eating an ice cream cone at a local dairy he developed an itchy rash with some swelling on his face. He also had some difficulty in swallowing or breathing. This was followed by complaints of "tummy pain" and cramping with diarrhea. During the patient's reaction, the cells in the accompanying micrograph, treated with fluorescein-labeled antihuman immunoglobulin, would most likely be developing in which organ where and would be producing which of the following?

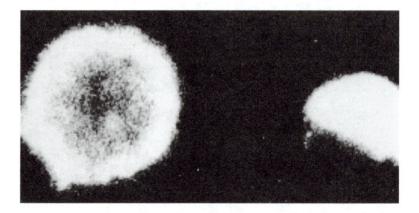

a. Deep cortex of the lymph node, IgE
b. Germinal center of the lymph node, IgE
c. Germinal centers in the lymph node, IgA
d. Skin-associated lymphoid tissue, IgG
e. Perioarteriolar lymphoid sheath of the spleen, IgE

177. Where does immunoglobulin switching from IgM to IgG primarily occur?

a. Bone marrow
b. Peripheral blood
c. Germinal centers
d. Thymus
e. Splenic red pulp

178. A 32-year-old woman has a positive tuberculin skin test, helper T cells assist in which of the following ways?

a. Autocrine-mediated inhibition of proliferation of helper T cells
b. The downregulation of IL-2 receptors on helper T cells
c. Secretion of interleukins that promote T cell proliferation
d. Secretion of IL-1
e. Inactivation of macrophages by release of γ-interferon

179. A 27-year-old school teacher "catches" the flu from her students. Which of the following would occur during the influenza infection?

a. Phagocytosis of virus by CD4⁺ T cells
b. Presentation of antigen by CD4⁺ T cells
c. Killing of virus-infected cells by CD4⁺ T cells
d. Formation of memory T and B cells
e. Killing of virus-infected cells by neutrophils

180. The mechanism for lymphocyte circulation from the lymphoid compartment in the region marked with the asterisk to the blood involves which of the following?

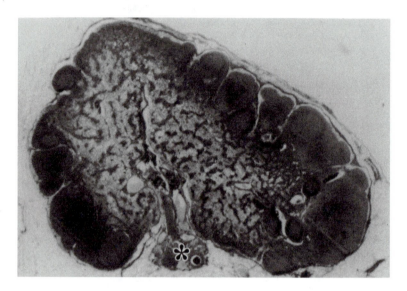

a. Homing receptors on lymphocytes that recognize vascular addressins on high endothelial venule cells
b. Lymphocyte binding to endothelial integrins followed by passage through endothelial cells lining the high endothelial postcapillary venules
c. Lymphocyte passage through the zonulae occludentes by diapedesis after dissolution of the junctions by proteolytic enzyme release
d. Lymphocyte passage from the efferent lymphatic vessel to the thoracic duct and subsequently the venous system
e. Passage of lymphocytes through the discontinuous sinusoidal wall into the blood

181. Macrophages are directly involved in immune responses in which of the following ways?
a. Production of IL-2
b. Presentation of antigen
c. Specific killing of tumor cells
d. Production of antibodies
e. Inactivation of helper T cells

182. A police officer in New York receives a vaccine for anthrax. The immunological basis for the vaccine is based on which of the following facts?

a. The primary response has a longer lag period
b. The secondary response has a shorter duration
c. The primary response is primarily an IgM response
d. The primary response lacks specificity
e. The primary response generates memory B and T cells

Lymphoid System and Cellular Immunology

Answers

167. The answer is a. (*Alberts, pp 1368–1369. Kindt, pp 7, 16–18. Abbas, pp 7, 72, 269.*) Clonal selection is the immune system's way of fine-tuning the immune response. Clonal selection is the means by which the immune system makes antigen receptor sites (T cells) or antibodies (B cells) more and more specific to create the optimal response to one specific antigen.

In clonal selection a clone of lymphocytes is committed to respond to a particular antigen. The antigenic determinants, which consist of specific amino acids or monosaccharides, actually induce many clones and a wide variety of humoral and cell-mediated responses. This occurs during the development and maturation of the immune system and is responsible for the specificity of lymphocyte cell surface receptors for antigens. Immunoglobulin class switching (**answer b**) occurs during the maturation of B cells after antigen stimulation. Homing receptor differentiation (**answer e**) is an important part of naïve T- and B-cell maturation in the thymus and bone marrow, respectively. Regulatory T cells (T_{reg}) actively suppress activation of the immune system and inhibit pathological self-reactivity and autoimmune disease (**answer c**). Clonal selection does not lead to formation of CFUs (**answer d**).

168. The answer is a. (*Abbas, pp 184–190. Kindt, pp 426–434.*) Transplant (acute graft) rejection is mediated by the action of T cells. Helper T (T_H) cells recognize peptides associated with MHC antigens from the donor tissue and become activated. Activated T_H cells release interleukin 2 (IL-2) and interferon-γ (IFN-γ), which activate cytotoxic T (T_c) cells, B cells, and macrophages. Although all of these cells may be involved in the rejection process, T_C cells are the primary agents of transplant rejection in an acute graft rejection response. This has been confirmed by animal studies: animals deficient in T cells are incapable of rejecting grafts. Tacrolimus (FK506) blocks signal transduction pathways leading to IL-2 production and therefore preventing T cell activation.

169. The answer is a. *(Abbas, pp 188, 191. Kindt, pp 434–435.)* Because of the shortage of human organs for transplant, xenotransplantation is considered as the main potential solution for obtaining donor organs. Xenotransplantation induces hyperacute graft rejection since human preformed antibodies recognize [alpha]Gal(1–3)[beta]Gal terminal carbohydrates present on animal endothelial cells in the graft. Interestingly, Old World monkeys and humans do not express that xenoantigen on their endothelial cells.

170. The answer is d. *(Abbas, pp 81–82. Kindt, pp 40–41, 245–248. Alberts, pp 1406–1409.)* The organ in the photomicrograph is the thymus, which produces $CD4^+$ (helper) and $CD8^+$ (cytotoxic) T cells. It functions in the generation of self/nonself discrimination because self-reactive T cells are deleted and self-MHC-restricted cells are expanded during their education within the thymus. T cell receptors for antigen develop develop during the education of T cells in the thymus. Those T cells also develop homing receptors for subsequent seeding to T-dependent areas of lymph nodes, spleen, and other lymphoid tissues throughout the body. The thymus can be identified at low magnification (A) from the lobulation with cortex and medulla in each lobule and the absence of germinal centers. At high magnification (B) the presence of Hassall's (thymic) corpuscles is an identifying characteristic. Hassall's corpuscles contain degenerating epithelial cells in concentric arrays that increase with age and instruct thymic dendritic cells to induce development of regulatory T cells (T_{reg}). The thymus is derived from the third and fourth branchial pouches, *not* the third branchial arch **(answer c).** Production of memory B cells as well as effector and memory T cells occurs in the secondary lymphoid organs. Production of antibodies is the responsibility of plasma cells, which arise from B lymphocytes and are found in germinal centers in lymph nodes throughout the body as well as in the spleen and tonsils **(answer a).** The lymph nodes filter the lymph and blood, **(answer b).** The spleen is the site of erythrocyte degradation and bilirubin recycling **(answer e).**

171. The answer is d. *(Alberts, pp 1393–1394, 1401–1402, 1419. Kindt, pp 223–225, 231–235, Abbas, pp 63–66, 70–73.)* T cell gene rearrangement occurs during the education of T cells in the thymus in fetal and early neonatal development. The T cell receptor (TCR) is composed of α and β chains. Each chain contains a variable amino-terminal portion and a constant carboxyl-terminal portion. These chains are encoded for by V, D, J, and C gene segments, which undergo rearrangement during development in the thymus. There are three types of T cells: cytotoxic T cells, T regulatory (T_r)cells, and helper T cells. Helper T cells possess the specific cell membrane marker CD4, whereas the regulatory and cytotoxic subgroups have CD8 on their cell surface. T cells require close contact with other cells to perform their cell-mediated function. This is quite different from B cells, where antibodies are secreted into the bloodstream. B cell gene rearrangement occurs in the bone marrow during B cell education by a similar process. It must be remembered that T cell receptors are antibody-like heterodimers. Gene rearrangement in B and T cell education involves similar V(D)J recombinations.

172. The answer is a. (*Abbas, pp 47–52, 58–59. Alberts, pp 1396–1397, 1412–1420. Junqueira, pp 258–261.*) Fragments of antigen associated with class II MHC glycoproteins are recognized by helper T cells. Activation of helper T cells is required as an early step in the immune response. For B and T_c cells to respond to most antigens, helper T cells are required. However, in the case of some bacterial polysaccharides, B cells respond to the antigens in the absence of helper T cells. The primary cell type for expression of class II MHC is the macrophage or dendritic cell (antigen-presenting cells, APCs), but thymic epithelial cells and B cells can also present antigen under appropriate conditions.

173. The answer is c. (*Abbas, pp 91–92. Alberts, pp 1394–1406.*) Cytotoxic T cells possess the CD8 cell surface marker. CD8$^+$ T cells recognize foreign antigen in association with class I MHC molecules. Cytotoxic T cells are effective in killing virus-infected cells because those cells express fragments of viral proteins combined with MHC I molecules on their surfaces. In contrast, helper T cells (CD4$^+$) recognize antigen in association with class II MHC molecules. MHC Class I is present on the surface of most cells, whereas antigen-presenting cells (including B lymphocytes) and thymic epithelial cells possess MHC Class II.

174. The answer is c. (*Abbas, pp 93–94. Kindt, pp 68, 307–312. Junqueira, pp 260–262.*) Interleukin-2 (IL-2) is produced by helper T cells (cell surface marker CD4). IL-2 stimulates proliferation of T and B cells. IL-2 is a cytokine, that affects the proliferation and differentiation of other cells. Antigen-presenting cells make interleukin (IL)-1 with helper T cells as the primary target. Helper T cells are greatly diminished during the immunodeficiency that follows AIDS infection. Natural killer (NK) cells comprise about 10–15% of circulating lymphocytes. They produce products that kill tumor cells.

Interleukin-1 (IL-1) plays a critical role in inflammation and in the immune response mediating pathogenetic events. IL-1 is mainly secreted by monocytes and macrophages and binds to T cells that have been activated by exposure to antigenic or mitogenic stimuli. Binding of IL-1 induces activated T cells to produce IL-2. There are two forms of IL-1: keratinocytes secrete IL-1α and monocytes/macrophages secrete IL-1β. IL-1 binds to receptors on activated T cells to induce production and release of IL-2. IL-1 has a wide variety of other effects including induction of chemokine expression [e.g., monocyte chemoattractant protein-1, (MCP-1)], upregulation of vascular adhesion molecules (e.g., selectins) by capillary endothelium, and upregulation of matrix metalloproteases (MMPs) that degrade the extracellular matrix and degrade IL-1. IL-1 is also required for IFN-γ production. See the diagram that illustrates the role of IL-1 and IL-2 in communication between immune cells.

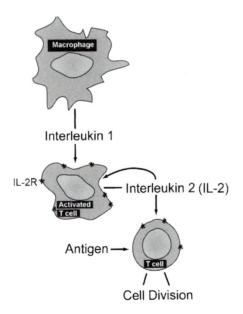

175. The answer is a. *(Young, pp 203, 207–221. Junqueira, pp 258, 268, 271, 272, 274. Kindt, pp 29–30, 494–498. Abbas, pp 211–213.)* Martin Causubon suffers from severe combined immunodeficiency (SCID) and has no T cells. The CD3 antibody recognizes a group of five proteins that are associated with the α and β chains of the T cell receptor (TCR). Recognition of antigen-MHC by the TcR-CD3 complex does not require any other molecules. Other "accessory molecules" on T cells (T_H or T_c) and their partner ligands on APCs or target cells provide a "second signal" to stimulate T cells. The region shown is a T-dependent region of the spleen. The photomicrograph shows an area of white pulp with a central artery. The sheath surrounding the central artery is known as the periarterial lymphoid sheath (PALS) and is analogous to the deep cortex (paracortex) of the lymph node or the interfollicular zone of Peyer's patches, the other T-dependent regions within lymphoid tissue.

The histologic structure of the spleen includes the presence of a connective tissue capsule with extensions into the parenchyma, forming trabeculae. The parenchyma consists of red pulp, which represents areas of red blood cells, many of which are undergoing degradation and phagocytosis by macrophages lining the sinusoids of the red pulp, and white pulp, which represents lymphocytes involved in the filtration of the blood. The germinal centers within the white pulp are the B-dependent regions of the spleen.

(The Case of Martin Causubon is provided courtesy of the Jeffrey Modell Foundation and "The Primary Immunodeficiency Resource Center:" http://www.info4pi.org/patienttopatient/index.cfm?section=patienttopatient&c)

176. The answer is b. *(Abbas, pp 68–69, 133–136. Kindt, pp 372–375. Kasper, pp 1912, 1916, 1947–1948. Junqueira, pp 97–101. Alberts, pp 1208–1211.)* The patient in the scenario suffers from peanut allergy. Allergic reactions involve IgE produced by plasma cells (shown in the fluorescein-labeled micrograph) in the germinal centers of the lymph nodes or spleen **(answers c and d).** Allergens, like peanut antigen, are originally recognized by T cell receptors on T_H2 cells. The T_H2 cell produces IL-4 which stimulates B cells to differentiate into plasma cells (like those in the photomicrograph), which synthesize and secrete IgE. IgE binds specifically to the high affinity receptor, Fc epsilon RI, on mast cells and basophils. The presence of IgE primes the mast cell; it is then capable of an allergic response by secreting histamine and heparin when the child is again exposed to the allergen (peanut antigen). Histamine alters vascular permeability leading to edema and in severe cases to anaphylaxis. Differentiation of IgE-plasma cells is regulated by the low affinity IgE receptor,

Fc epsilon RII, also known as CD23. Immunoglobulin-producing cells are found in the germinal centers of the white pulp of the spleen and other secondary lymphoid organs (i.e., germinal centers in the cortex of the spleen and in the tonsils and lymphoid follicles in the MALT and SALT). B-lymphocytes can be identified by the presence of immunoglobulin on their surface membranes and differentiate into antibody-secreting plasma cells under the appropriate conditions. T lymphocytes, on the other hand, do not have readily detectable cell membrane immunoglobulin. The thymus is the site of T cell education and the deep cortex of the lymph node and the periarteriolar lymphoid sheath (PALS) are T-dependent regions (**answers a and e**).

177. The answer is c. (*Alberts, pp 1375–1384. Kindt, pp 128–130. Abbas, pp 134, 136, 156.*) Immunoglobulin switching normally occurs in the germinal centers during the maturation of B cells. Synthesis of B cell antibody begins as IgM inserted into the cell membrane and then switches to membrane-bound IgM and IgD. After antigen stimulation, a switch to surface IgM, IgA, IgG, or IgE occurs, and those antibodies are secreted. Most antibody production occurs in the germinal centers of the lymph nodes, tonsils, and spleen. It occurs to a lesser extent in the bone marrow (**answer a**), but the bone marrow functions in the education of B cells as well as representing the major site of hematopoiesis in the adult. The thymus is responsible for the education of T cells (**answer d**). The splenic red pulp is the site of red blood cell breakdown (**answer e**).

Recognition of antigen by B cells is accomplished by the expression of IgM molecules on the cell surface. Some investigators use the term pre-B cell, or virgin B cell, to distinguish those B cells that have not yet synthesized IgM from those that have synthesized and inserted IgM into their cell membranes. IgD, which is produced later by maturing B cells, also serves as an antigen receptor. Immunoglobulin switching does not occur in peripheral blood (**answer b**).

178. The answer is c. (*Alberts, pp 1410–1418. Kindt, p 393. Junqueira, pp 260–262.*) In a tuberculin skin test, T cell proliferation is increased by secretion of interleukins. An extract of tuberculin (an antigen of lipoprotein composition obtained from the tubercle bacillus) is injected into the skin of a person who has had tuberculosis or has been immunized against tuberculosis. Memory helper T cells react to the tuberculin and secrete IL-2, which upregulates IL-2 receptors. IL-2 binding to IL-2 receptors on the same cell is an example of autocrine regulation in which a cell secretes a ligand for a receptor on its own surface. The result of this upregulation and ligand-receptor binding is an increase in T cell proliferation. T cell–derived cytokines such as tumor necrosis factor-alpha and -beta (TNF-α and β) induce leukocyte recruitment. Production of gamma-(γ)-interferon (γ-IFN) by helper T cells attracts and activates macrophages (monocytes comprise most of the cellular infiltrate). γ-IFN also converts other cells (such as endothelial cells) to antigen-presenting cells by induction of class II MHC expression, which further augments the response. The result of the activity of helper T cells is a dramatic increase in the number of lymphocytes and macrophages at the test site, which produces swelling. IL-1 is synthesized by antigen-presenting cells and macrophages with helper T cells as the targets.

179. The answer is d. (*Alberts, pp 1396–1400. Abbas, pp 58–59, 91–92, 148. Kindt, pp 448–454.*) There are some viruses in which antibody-mediated immunity is critical to prevention/recovery, whereas with others cell-mediated immunity is the key. Therefore, both memory T and memory B cells will be formed. B cells will divide to form a plasma cell and a memory B cell. Activated T cells enlarge to form large lymphocytes and subsequently undergo cell proliferation to form T cells and memory T cells. In these responses, macrophages phagocytose virus **(answer a)**. Cells that become infected with virus can be killed by CD8$^+$ cytotoxic T cells **(answers c and e)**, which can react to the antigen in the presence of MHC class I molecules. T and B cell areas of the spleen and lymph nodes will be involved in the filtration of blood and lymph, respectively. B cell differentiation requires the presence of CD4$^+$ helper T cells and an antigen-presenting cell (APC). The APC will phagocytose the virus and present it to helper T cells in the presence of MHC class II molecules **(answer b)**. The B cell also presents antigen during viral infections.

180. The answer is d. (*Alberts, pp 1372–1374. Junqueira, p 274. Ross and Pawlina, pp 410, 412.*) Passage of lymphocytes from the lymphoid compartment of the lymph node to the bloodstream involves passage from the efferent lymphatic vessel to the thoracic duct and eventually into the venous system (at the juncture of the left brachiocephalic and subclavian veins). The region of the lymph node marked with the asterisk in the photomicrograph is the hilus of the lymph node. Passage from the blood to the lymphoid compartment involves specific homing receptors on lymphocytes, which are complementary to addressins on the postcapillary high endothelial venules (HEVs) and explains the specificity of lymphocyte homing. The cells that line the HEVs permit the selective passage of lymphocytes by diapedesis through the intercellular junctions. Lymphocytes have specific homing receptors on their cell surfaces that provide entry for mucosal (versus lymph node) seeding. High endothelial venules (HEVs) provide a mechanism for lymphocytes to leave the bloodstream and enter specific areas of the lymph nodes. HEVs are also found in Peyer's patches and during inflammation of tissues (e.g., the synovium in rheumatoid arthritis). Under normal conditions, HEVs are found in the T-dependent areas, that is, the deep cortex (paracortex) of the lymph nodes and the interfollicular regions of the Peyer's patches. T cells home to T-dependent areas of the lymph nodes, spleen, and Peyer's patches. The circulation and recirculation of lymphocytes is a constant process that allows lymphocytes to continuously monitor the presence of antigen. The circulation process also allows augmentation of the immune response to infection. Plasma cells do *not* enter the bloodstream under normal conditions, but secrete antibodies into the circulation from the medulla of the lymph nodes or the marginal zone of the spleen. Lymphocytes and other cells (e.g., monocytes and neutrophils) that leave the blood never pass through the endothelial cells.

In the histologic section of a lymph node, there is a distinctive cortex and medulla with a connective tissue capsule. The organ possesses the classic bean shape with a hilus (marked by an asterisk in the figure). Afferent lymphatics enter the lymph node on the convex side, and lymph percolates through the subcapsular, cortical, and medullary sinuses. The medullary sinuses converge on the hilus, where the efferent lymphatic vessel drains the node. The hilus also contains an artery and a vein.

181. The answer is b. (*Alberts, pp 1366, 1394. Junqueira, pp 93–97. Kindt, pp 65–68, 263–264.*) Macrophages are a group of monocyte-derived phagocytic cells that present antigen and synthesize IL-1. Macrophages arise from the bone marrow (monocytes) and include the Kupffer cells of the liver, Langerhans cells of the skin, and microglia of the central nervous system. Antigen presentation is the process by which macrophages, dendritic cells, and B cells phagocytose antigen and partially degrade the antigen in the endosomal system. Certain portions of the antigen are returned to the cell surface in combination with type II MHC as a complex. IL-1 activates the helper T cell. Although macrophages may be required for the differentiation of plasma cells from B cells, they are *not* directly involved in antibody production. Also note, B cells can present antigen in addition to the more traditional APCs.

182. The answer is e. (*Kindt, pp 289–290, 481–484. Alberts, pp 1370–1371. Abbas, pp 144, 146.*) The goal of all vaccines is to promote a primary immune reaction so that when the organism is again exposed to the antigen, a much stronger secondary immune response will be elicited. Any subsequent immune response to an antigen is called a secondary response. A secondary immune response is more rapid, of longer duration, and more intense than the primary immune response (**answers a, b, and d**). The secondary response is more specific to the invading antigen because of the generation of memory cells produced during the primary response. The design of an immunizing vaccine hinges on the specificity and cross-reactivity of antigen and receptor. Vaccines are more effective and long-lived when live attenuated virus is used to develop the vaccine. Vaccines developed to inactivated virus are not as effective. Live attenuated virus undergoes limited replication in the host cells resulting in a strong, site-specific response to the antigen. Anthrax vaccine is made to inactivated virus and requires boosters at yearly intervals. The primary immune response involves primarily IgM while the secondary response predominantly involves IgG antibodies (**answer c**). Humoral immunity and cell-mediated immunity involve retention of immunologic memory through memory B and T cells, respectively. A secondary immune response may involve memory T cells, helper cells, macrophages, and memory B cells. The proliferation of either T or B cells during the first exposure to antigen results in the production of memory cells. Specificity is retained. For example, the introduction of a different (new) antigen induces a primary rather than a secondary response. However, exposure to an antigen again, will produce a secondary immune response.

Respiratory System

Questions

DIRECTIONS: Each item below contains a question or incomplete statement followed by suggested responses. Select the **one best** response to each question.

183. A 52-year-old man, who has smoked two packs of cigarettes per day for the past 38 years, presents with diminished breath sounds detected by auscultation accompanied by faint high-pitched rhonchi at the end of each expiration and a hyperresonant percussion note. He is afebrile. In addition, he shows discomfort during breathing and is using extra effort to involve accessory muscles to lift the sternum. The diminished lung sounds in this patient are primarily due to which cellular events?

a. Monocytic infiltration leading to collagenase destruction of bronchiolar connective tissue support
b. Neutrophilic infiltration leading to destruction of bronchiolar and septal elastic fibers
c. Monocytic infiltration leading to breakdown of the bronchiolar smooth muscle
d. Neutrophilic infiltration leading to excess production of antiprotease activity in the lung parenchyma
e. Monocytic infiltration leading to excess production of antiprotease activity in the lung parenchyma

184. Which of the following is the smallest active functional unit (including conduction and air exchange) of the lung?

a. An alveolus
b. A respiratory bronchiolar unit
c. A bronchopulmonary segment
d. Segmental bronchi
e. An intrapulmonary bronchus

185. The lung cells known as "congestive heart failure cells" are which of the following?

a. Type I pneumocytes
b. Type II pneumocytes
c. Macrophages
d. Erythrocytes
e. Fibroblasts

186. A newborn child is diagnosed with Cystic fibrosis (CF). Abnormalities of CF include which of the following?

a. A decreased concentration of chloride in the sweat
b. Increased chloride secretion into the airways
c. Decreased water resorption from the lumen of the airways
d. Decreased active sodium absorption
e. Accumulation of mucus in airways

187. A 35-week gestation, 5 lb 5 oz female infant was born to a 30-year-old G2P2 woman. The infant had rapid and labored breathing that was viewed as transient tachypnea of the newborn. The infant's 1- and 5-min APGAR scores were 8 and 9, respectively. She initially breastfed, but now has respiratory distress, with a normal pulse and no heart murmurs. She is transported to the neonatal intensive care unit with worsening tachypnea. In that infant, the cells labeled with the arrow fail to do which of the following?

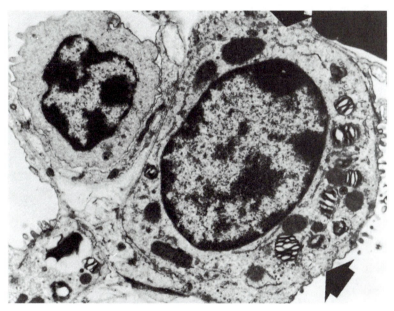

(Electron micrograph courtesy of Dr. Kuen-Shan Hung.)

a. Form during gestation
b. Proliferate sufficiently during gestation
c. Differentiate sufficiently during gestation
d. Produce sufficient amniotic fluid
e. Form its basal lamina resulting in an incomplete blood-air barrier

188. A teenage girl presents in the emergency room with paroxysms of dyspnea, cough, and wheezing. Her parents indicate that she has had these "attacks" during the past winter, and that they have worsened and become more frequent during the spring allergy season. Which of the following cell types and their location is correctly matched to a function it may perform in this patient's disease?

a. Cilia in alveoli, enhanced mucociliary transport
b. Plasma cells in BALT, bronchoconstriction
c. Eosinophils in BALT, bronchodilation
d. Goblet cells in bronchioles, hyposecretion
e. Mast cells in BALT, edema

189. Signal transduction in the epithelium lining the region with the arrow differs from that in rod cells stimulated by light in which of the following ways?

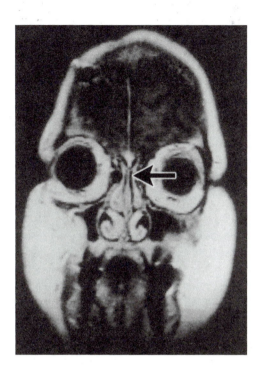

a. Sodium influx into receptor cells
b. Involvement of specific G proteins
c. Stimulation of a cyclic nucleotide
d. Stimulation leading to depolarization
e. Bypass of the protein kinase system

190. Which of the following is part of the minimal blood-air barrier in the lungs?

a. Fused basal laminae of epithelial and endothelial cells
b. Alveolar pores of Kohn
c. Alveolar macrophages
d. Type II pneumocytes
e. Smooth-muscle cells of the pulmonary arteries and veins

191. Major defense mechanisms of the respiratory system include which of the following?

a. Phagocytic activity of type II pneumocytes to ingest microorganisms
b. Cell specific killing by type I pneumocytes
c. Alveolar mucociliary action for clearance of microorganisms
d. IgA activation of complement in the alveolar fluid
e. IgM and IgG activation of complement in the alveolar fluid

192. A 56-year-old man presents to his family medicine physician. He is a 41 year pack/day smoker. He reports that he has had a "typical smoker's cough" for years; however, the morning cough has turned into a chronic productive cough with hemoptysis. He has dyspnea, chest pain, cachexia, increasing dysphonia. He has been treated for 4 respiratory infections in the past 18 months. Examination of the sputum reveals the presence of malignant cells confirmed by fine needle aspiration. Imaging reveals a tumor that is 3 cm in greatest dimension, surrounded by lung parenchyma. Bronchoscopic evaluation reveals a cavitary lesion of a proximal bronchus. Surgical resection is completed and the pathologist classifies the tumor as a T1, N2, MO nonsmall cell lung cancer (NSCLC), specifically a squamous cell carcinoma. Tumor vascularity assessed by bronchial arteriography (BAG) and immunocytochemistry indicates a highly vascular tumor with many microvessels. Vascularity of the tumor is inhibited by upregulation of which of the following?

a. Vascular endothelial growth factor (VEGF)
b. Platelet-derived growth factor (PDGF)
c. Extracellular matrix synthesis
d. Endostatin
e. Periendothelial cell recruitment and proliferation

Respiratory System

Answers

183. The answer is b. *(Junqueira, p 357. Kumar, pp 717–721. Kasper, pp 1547–1550.)* The patient suffers from emphysema, in which neutrophils enter the lung parenchyma and secrete elevated levels of elastase, leading to the destruction of the bronchiolar and alveolar septal elastic tissue support. The destruction of the elasticity in emphysema leads to diminished breath sounds. This is coupled with faint high-pitched rhonchi at the end of expiration and a hyperresonant percussion note. The rhonchi are adventitious (not normally present) sounds that may be high pitched, generally because of bronchospasm, or low pitched, generally because of the presence of airway secretions. Emphysema is a disease characterized by parenchymal tissue destruction and, therefore, is not associated with adventitious breath sounds. However, because most emphysema is due to cigarette smoking, there is almost always some degree of chronic bronchitis, and therefore, rhonchi can be auscultated.

There are genetic and environmental causes of emphysema. The environmental causes include smoking and air pollution, whereas deficiency in α1-antitrypsin (antiprotease) activity is the genetic cause of the disease. The balance between normal elastase-elastin production and protease-antiprotease activity is altered in emphysema. Persons with a deficiency in α1-antitrypsin activity lack sufficient antiprotease activity to counteract neutrophil-derived elastase. When there is an increase in the entry and activation of neutrophils in the alveolar space, more elastase is released, and elastic structures are destroyed. In smoking there is an increase in the number of neutrophils and macrophages in alveoli and increased elastase activity from neutrophils and macrophages. Those changes are coupled with a decrease in antielastase activity because of oxidants in cigarette smoke and antioxidants released from the increased numbers of neutrophils. The increased protease activity causes breakdown of the alveolar walls and dissolution of elastin in the bronchiolar walls. The loss of tethering of the bronchioles to the lung parenchyma leads to their collapse. The bronchioles, unlike the trachea and bronchi, do *not* contain hyaline cartilage. A relatively thick layer of smooth muscle is found in the bronchioles, but the bronchioles are tethered to the lung parenchyma by elastic tissue, which plays a key role in the stretch and recoil of the lungs during inhalation and exhalation.

184. The answer is b. (*Ross and Pawlina, pp 623–625. Moore and Dalley, pp 104, 106, 108.*) The smallest functional unit of the lung is the respiratory bronchiolar unit, which contains a respiratory bronchiole and the alveoli associated with it. This unit allows for air conduction and gas exchange. The alveolus (**answer a**) is only associated with gas exchange, and the bronchi form part of the conduction system. The bronchopulmonary segment (**answer c**) is a functional unit of lung structure, but it is not the smallest unit. Bronchopulmonary segments are particularly important in surgical resections of the lung because they represent functional units with connective tissue boundaries and individualized vasculature, including pulmonary and bronchial arteries, pulmonary lymphatics, and pulmonary nerves, all of which follow the air-conducting system of the bronchial tree and its branches. Segmental bronchi and intrapulmonary bronchi are part of the conduction system (**answers d and e**).

185. The answer is c. (*Kumar, p 698. Junqueira, p 357.*) The alveolar macrophage (containing hemosiderin) has been called the "congestive heart failure cell." The presence of large numbers of these cells, containing hemosiderin granules, is an indicator of edematous lung changes. During congestive heart failure, edema results in leakage of erythrocytes into the alveoli. Transferrin and hemoglobin are also present in the edematous fluid released from the capillaries. These two products are phagocytosed by alveolar macrophages, which convert those products to hemosiderin.

186. The answer is e. (*Kumar, pp 490–492. Kasper, pp 1543–1546.*) Accumulation of mucus in the airways is a common finding in children with cystic fibrosis (CF). CF is a frequent occurrence in Caucasian children (1 in 200 births). It is a genetic disease in which the defect often occurs in the CFTR protein that functions as a chloride channel. In the sweat glands, a decrease in sodium transport results in increased chloride levels in the sweat [(the original detection test for CF) **answer a**]. In the airways, decreased chloride secretion (**answer b**) occurs in conjunction with active sodium absorption (**answer d**), resulting in loss of water from the lumen as water follows sodium (**answer c**). The result is increased viscosity of mucous secretions and obstruction of the airways and other organs. The pancreas and salivary gland secretions are affected in a similar way, although those abnormalities do *not* occur in all cases. In the case of the lungs, the loss of the mucociliary escalator action results in susceptibility to opportunistic lung infections.

187. The answer is c. *(Junqueira, pp 349–357. Kumar, pp 481–483. Moore and Persaud, Developing, pp 107, 247–248, 251–252.)* Differentiation of type II pneumocytes (shown in the electron micrograph) occurs late in gestation and is, therefore, incomplete at birth in premature infants. Those newborn "premies" have a deficiency of surfactant because of the immaturity of the type II pneumocytes. The deficiency of surfactant inhibits normal expansion of the alveoli and results in idiopathic respiratory distress syndrome [(RDS); hyaline membrane disease]. The lecithin/sphingomyelin ratio is a test that can be performed on a sample of amniotic fluid obtained by amniocentesis. It is used to determine whether the type II pneumocytes are mature and are synthesizing and secreting surfactant. Maternally administered glucocorticoids may be used to induce surfactant production prior to birth, and exogenous surfactant may be given intratracheally to premature infants to reduce the severity of RDS.

The surfactant is produced by type II pneumocytes in the lung and is stored in the form of lamellar bodies (the whorls seen in the electron micrograph). Surfactant consists of an aqueous layer, or hypophase, that contains proteins and mucopolysaccharides. That layer is covered by a functional layer of phospholipid that consists predominantly of dipalmitoyl phosphatidylcholine (lecithin). The release of lamellar bodies by exocytosis is followed by their general unraveling to form tubulomyelin figures. The tubulomyelin consists of a crisscross lipid bilayer that covers the type II pneumocytes. Surfactant-associated proteins (SAP) stabilize surfactant, activate surfactant recycling, enhance surfactant-induced reduction of surface tension, and possess antiviral and antibacterial activities. Turnover occurs by both endocytosis (type I and II pneumocytes) and phagocytosis (macrophages); 90% of surfactant is recycled.

The blood-air barrier is formed by the type I pneumocyte, the capillary endothelial cell, and their fused basal laminae.

G2P2 refers to two pregnancies and two children.

188. The answer is e. *(Kumar, pp 723–727. Kasper, pp 1508–1511. Junqueira, p 349.)* The teenage patient is suffering from an asthmatic attack, probably allergen-induced. Mast cells are a key player in this airway disease. Mast cells in the bronchioles are stimulated to release histamine and heparin that induce the contraction of smooth bronchiolar muscle [bronchoconstriction, (**answers b and c**)] and edema in the wall. If the bronchoconstriction is chronic, the long-term result is thickening of the bronchiolar musculature. There are no cilia in the alveoli (**answer a**) alveolar macrophages (dust cells) ingest particulate matter that enters the alveoli. Hypersecretion of viscous mucus from goblet cells in the bronchi (not bronchioles) can obstruct the airway (**answer d**). Eosinophils, neutrophils, lymphocytes and macrophages signal to each other through a complex cytokine network using a variety of mediators: bradykinin, leukotrienes, and prostaglandins, which enhance bronchoconstriction, vascular congestion, and edema. The airway epithelium responds to those mediators. Eosinophils (**answer c**) release proteins that destroy the airway epithelium (releasing Creola bodies). T lymphocytes are also present in more severe "attacks" and, along with B lymphocytes, may play a role in the initiation of allergic asthma. T lymphocytes also release cytokines that activate cell-mediated immunity pathways.

189. The answer is d. (*Alberts, pp 866–867, 1268.*) The region shown on the MRI is the olfactory area lined by the olfactory epithelium. The response of rod cells to light causes hyperpolarization, whereas olfactory stimuli result in depolarization. The olfactory epithelium and rod cells are two examples of signal transduction that bypass a protein kinase system. In the case of the olfactory epithelium, an odorant molecule binds to an odor-specific transmembrane receptor found on the modified cilia at the apical surface. The binding activates an odorant-specific G protein, G_{olf} , which binds GTP. (For summary of 6 proteins, see table page 106). The resulting dissociation of the α-subunit stimulates adenylate cyclase to produce cyclic AMP (cAMP). cAMP directly stimulates the opening of the cation channels on the membrane of the bipolar olfactory receptor cells, leading to Na^+ influx. The resulting membrane depolarization is transmitted from the modified cilia to the olfactory vesicle through the neuron to the basal axon. Axonal processes traverse the lamina propria as the olfactory nerve and pass through the cribriform plate of the ethmoid to terminate in the olfactory bulb. In the case of the rod, the cyclic nucleotide involved is cGMP.

190. The answer is a. (*Junqueira, pp 349–353, 357.*) Oxygen moving from the alveolar air to the capillary blood and carbon dioxide diffusing in the opposite direction pass through a three-component blood-air barrier. This barrier consists of type I pneumocytes, endothelial cells, and their fused basal laminae. Pulmonary capillaries are sometimes in direct contact with the alveolar wall, whereas in other locations, the alveolar wall and capillaries are separated by cells and extracellular fibers. The areas of direct contact are the location of gas exchange, whereas the other areas represent sites of fluid exchange between the interstitium and air spaces. Macrophages are present for the phagocytosis of debris and surfactant. The pores of Kohn are connections from one alveolus to another, and macrophages travel through these passageways. The pores normally equalize air pressure between alveoli and can, in the disease state, provide collateral circulation of air in the event that a bronchiole is blocked. However, they also provide a passageway for the spread of bacteria.

191. The answer is e. (*Kumar, pp 718–719.*) IgM and IgG are serum antibodies present in the alveolar fluid that activate complement by the classic pathway. In that pathway, fixation of C1 to antibody combined with antigen leads to activation of C3b, which binds to bacterial cell walls and enhances opsonization. Neutrophils and macrophages have C3b receptors that facilitate the opsonization. IgG also functions as an opsonin. The type II pneumocytes resorb as well as secrete surfactant and surfactant-associated proteins that have some antiviral and antibacterial function, but they do not ingest microorganisms **(answer a)**. CD8$^+$ T cells carry out cell-specific killing **(answer b)**. Mucociliary action is a critical component of the immune function of the respiratory system, but clearance occurs in the bronchioles → bronchi → trachea as part of the mucociliary apparatus. Microorganisms are entrapped in mucus and then cilia propel them toward the oropharynx. Microorganisms phagocytosed in the alveoli need to be transported to the bronchioles in order to ride on the mucociliary escalator **(answer c)**. IgA functions to prevent attachment of microorganisms to the epithelium, particularly in the upper respiratory tract **(answer d)**.

Overall defense mechanisms of the respiratory system include nasal clearance of material, which occurs through sneezing, whereas other material may be swept into the nasopharynx and subsequently swallowed. The mucociliary action within the trachea and bronchi is often called the mucociliary, or tracheobronchial, escalator. At the distal end of the system, the alveolar macrophages phagocytose foreign material and secrete and respond to an array of cytokines. Neutrophils are attracted by chemokines and factors derived from macrophages and other cells and phagocytose bacteria.

In the bronchi, there is extensive associated lymphoid tissue (BALT), which is analogous to the mucosa-associated lymphoid tissue (MALT) of the gut and the skin-associated lymphoid tissue (SALT). There are B and T cell areas throughout the BALT. The B cells are precursors of plasma cells and synthesize immunoglobulins such as IgA associated with the bronchial secretion. Helper T cells recognize foreign antigen in association with class II major histocompatibility complex (MHC) molecules. Cytotoxic T cells recognize fragments of antigen (specifically viral fragments) on the surface of viral-infected cells in association with class I MHC. Antigen-presenting cells (i.e., alveolar macrophages) also function in a similar fashion to those found elsewhere in the body; they present antigen to helper T cells in conjunction with class II MHC.

192. The answer is d. *(Kumar, p 109. Lobov, pp 11205-11210).* Angiostatin and endostatin are cleavage products of plasminogen and type XVIII collagen respectively and function as anti-angiogenic peptides. Vascular endothelial growth factor (VEGF, **answer a**) stimulates the recruitment and growth of endothelial cells through the VEGF-R located on endothelial cell precursors as well as endothelial cells. Platelet-derived growth factor (PDGF) recruits smooth muscle cells **(answer b)** and transforming growth factor-beta (TGF-β) stimulates and stabilizes extracellular matrix production. Recruitment and proliferation of periendothelial cells **(answer e)**, smooth muscle cells, pericytes, and fibroblasts are required for development and maturation of new blood vessels. The angiopoietins (Ang) 1 and 2 bind their receptor, Tie2, a receptor tyrosine kinase which regulates endothelial cell proliferative status. Ang 1 binds Tie2 leading to periendothelial cell recruitment and therefore vascular maturation.

Ang 2 is found in organs of the female reproductive tract and blocks Ang 1 effects when VEGF is absent. The result is regression of the blood vessel. Ang 2 in the presence of VEGF leads to loosening of the surrounding cells permitting multiplication of endothelial cells and angiogenesis.

Integumentary System

Questions

DIRECTIONS: Each item below contains a question or incomplete statement followed by suggested responses. Select the **one best** response to each question.

193. A 43-year-old woman presents with a cyst on her labia majora with foul-smelling drainage. She says the drainage occurs spontaneously and recently the cyst has enlarged and has become painful. The cyst is associated with the structure in the photomicrograph delineated by the arrow. The mechanism of secretion normally used by this structure is which of the following?

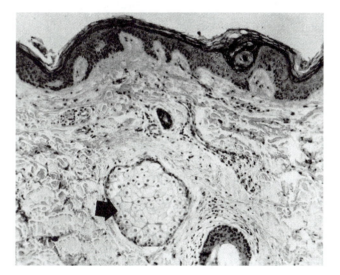

a. Holocrine
b. Merocrine
c. Apocrine
d. Endocrine
e. Autocrine

194. Merkel cells are modified epidermal cells that function primarily in which of the following?

a. Phagocytosis
b. Expression of Fc, Ia, and C3 receptors
c. Detection of texture and shape during active touch
d. Detection of transient vibratory stimuli
e. Two-point discrimination

195. The layer at the tip of the pointer is which of the following?

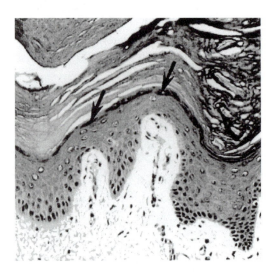

a. Proliferative zone of the vaginal epithelium
b. Proliferative zone of the epidermis
c. Source of the granules that form part of the water impermeability barrier of the skin
d. Layer of the epidermis that shows prominent desmosomes and is the target of autoantibodies in pemphigus
e. Source of new cells following a dermal wound

196. SWL is a 37-year-old woman with a suspected Schwanoma. The radiology report reads as follows: "a soft tissue mass to the right of L1 at the level of the L1-L2 neural foramen. The mass cannot be differentiated from the L1 nerve root and extends into the neural foramen such that it has a 'dumbbell' configuration with components lateral to the neural foramen, a waist in the foramen itself, and a component within the spinal canal to the right of the thecal sac." The neurologist, Dr. Jane Motumbo, applies the base of a vibrating 128 CPS tuning fork to the skin overlying SWL's right and left thighs and asks her to describe the sensation. She asks SWL to close her eyes and then to tell her whether the tuning fork is vibrating or not. Vibration sense is impaired on the right side. Tests for pain and temperature indicate impairment on the left side. Using the tuning fork, Dr. Motumbo is primarily testing the function of which of the following sensory receptors?

a. Ruffini endings
b. Pacinian corpuscle
c. Meissner corpuscle
d. Merkel corpuscle
e. Free nerve endings

197. A woman presents with blisters on her back and buttocks (Figure A). She has autoantibodies to one of the cadherins that is distributed as shown in Figure B. The cause of this disease is disruption of which of the following?

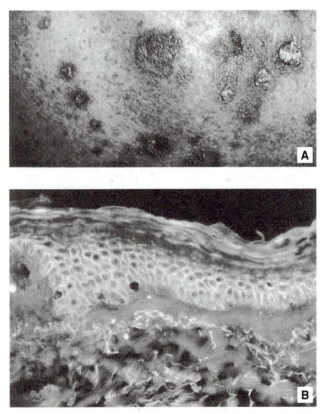

(Micrograph courtesy of Dr. Kristin M. Leiferman and the University of Utah, Department of Dermatology site:http://uuhsc.utah.edu/derm/.)

a. Macula adherens
b. Hemidesmosome
c. Gap junction
d. Zonula occludens
e. Connections between the lamina densa and lamina rarae in the basal lamina

198. A first-year woman medical student presents with patches of raised red skin covered by a flaky white buildup on her knees and elbows. The patches enlarge and become itchy and burning immediately before and during major exams during the first year of medical school. A biopsy from her skin is shown below. Which of the following is the underlying cause of this disorder?

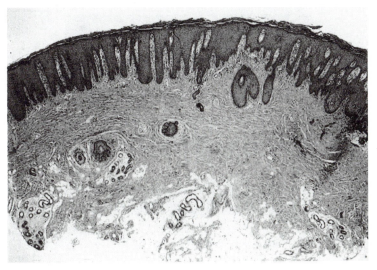

(Micrograph courtesy of Dr. Wolfram Sterry.)

a. Hyperplasia of dermal cells
b. A longer keratinocyte cell cycle
c. Production of cytokines by infiltrating inflammatory cells
d. Microabscesses of the dermis
e. Abnormal microcirculation in the epidermis

199. A 52-year-old woman patient presents with severe blistering over her buttocks. Analysis of sera with immunofluorescence demonstrates autoantibodies localized as shown in the accompanying photomicrograph. A biopsy indicates extensive inflammatory infiltrates with numerous eosinophils present. You are asked to look at the biopsy. The underlying cell biological mechanism most likely involves an abnormality in which of the following structures?

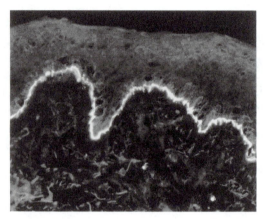

(Micrograph courtesy of Dr. Kristin M. Leiferman and the University of Utah, Department of Dermatology site: http://uuhsc.utah.edu/derm/.)

a. Macula adherens
b. Hemidesmosomes
c. Gap junctions
d. Zonula occludens
e. Zonula adherens

200. A boy is born with blonde hair, blue eyes and very fair complexion, dramatically lighter features than both of his parents. A PKU test is positive. The boy's lighter skin and hair is most likely due to which of the following?

a. Fewer melanocytes differentiating from the neural crest
b. Reduced proliferation of melanocytes in the basal layer of the epidermis
c. Elevated levels of tyrosinase in melanocytes
d. Deficiency in tyrosine in keratinocytes throughout the epidermis
e. Competitive inhibition of phenylalanine for tyrosinase in melanocytes

Integumentary System

Answers

193. The answer is a. *(Young, pp 95, 164, 168. Junqueira, pp 79–80, 370–372.)* The cyst in the vignette is an epidermoid or sebaceous cyst and the gland shown in the photomicrograph is a sebaceous gland, located in the dermis and associated with a hair follicle. Secretion from sebaceous glands is classified as holocrine (i.e., shedding of the disintegrated cell along with sebum into the hair follicle). Blockage of sebaceous gland ducts, presumably from injury, infection or irritation, results in cyst formation. Sebaceous cysts are prone to infection and can have foul-smelling drainage with inflammation and pain. The lesion usually consists of an enlarged sebaceous gland with numerous lobules grouped around a centrally located sebaceous duct, which has become obstructed causing the cyst. The photomicrograph represents a microscopic section obtained from thin skin. The presence of sebaceous glands/hair follicles identifies the section as thin skin. Sebaceous glands and hair follicles are not found in thick skin. Another difference between thick and thin skin is the virtual absence of the stratum lucidum in thin skin. There are two types of sweat glands: merocrine and apocrine. The merocrine glands release their secretion through exocytosis with conservation of membrane **(answer b)**. In anal, areolar, and axillary regions, sweat glands are apocrine **(answer c)**; the apical part of the cell is released with the secretion. Endocrine secretion occurs into the blood **(answer d)**; autocrine secretion is self-stimulation **(answer e)**. For example, activated T cells stimulate their own proliferation by secreting IL-2 and synthesizing IL-2 receptors that bind the IL-2.

194. The answer is e. *(Junqueira, pp 95, 97, 260, 360, 366, 368.)* The Merkel cell is a neuroendocrine cell. It is a modified keratinocyte found in areas in which fine tactile sensation is critical, such as the fingertips. A Merkel cell is associated with an unmyelinated nerve ending, forming a Merkel corpuscle (disk), essential for two-point discrimination: the ability to discriminate two closely placed points as separate. Two point discrimination is dependent on the size of receptive fields and the density of Merkel corpuscles. Langerhans cells function in phagocytosis **(answer a)**, antigen presentation (APCs), cytokine production, and expression of Fc, Ia, and C3 receptors **(answer b)**. They phagocytose epidermal antigens and present them in association with class II MHC molecules to a helper T cell. Meissner's corpuscles detect texture and shape during active touch and are found in the thick skin of the digits **(answer c)**. Transient vibratory stimuli are detected by Pacinian corpuscles **(answer d)**.

195. The answer is c. (*Junqueira, pp 360–366. Kumar, pp 1256–1257.*) The cells labeled with the arrows contain numerous Keratohyalin granules and are located in the stratum granulosum. Those cells also produce lamellar granules, which form a bidirectional lipid bilayer barrier to penetration of substances. The skin or integument is composed of an epithelial layer (epidermis) and underlying connective tissue (dermis). The epidermis consists of four to five strata (from the basement membrane to the skin surface): stratum basale, stratum spinosum, stratum granulosum, stratum lucidum, and stratum corneum. The basal layer contains most of the mitotic cells **(answers a and b)** and is attached to the basement membrane with hemidesmosomes. The stratum spinosum contains cells, with numerous cytoplasmic tonofilaments and intercellular desmosomes **(answer d)**. The stratum basale + stratum spinosum = stratum Malpighii). Those layers are hyperproliferative in psoriasis. Normally, gradual replacement occurs in the epidermis; new cells are produced in the stratum basale, and migration toward the surface occurs as they gradually differentiate. The stratum lucidum is a translucent layer typical of thick skin. The stratum corneum contains as many as 20 layers of flattened cells.

In deep wounds, new epithelial cells are obtained from the epithelium of the hair follicles and sweat glands located in the dermis **(answer e)**.

196. The answer is b. (*Guyton, pp 540–542. Junqueira, pp 367–368. Ross and Pawlina, pp 452–455, 472–473.*) The Pacinian corpuscle is the primary sensory receptor for vibratory sensation. The Ruffini endings are the simplest encapsulated receptor and are associated with collagen fibers **(answer a)**. Mechanical stress results in displacement of the collagen fibers and stimulation of the receptor. The Meissner and Merkel's corpuscles respond to texture and 2-point discrimination, respectively **(answers c and d)**. Free nerve endings detect light pressure and touch **(answer e)**. In the vignette, the Schwannoma (a nerve sheath tumor arising from Schwann cells) results in impairment of proprioception (position sense) and vibratory sense ipsilaterally while pain and temperature are impaired contralaterally.

It is compressing the spinal cord from its lateral or anterolateral aspect causing impairment of pain and temperature sensation on the contralateral side to the Schwannoma, with weakness, spasticity and loss of proprioception and vibratory sense on the ipsilateral side to the tumor. Damage to the anterolateral system (ALS; spinothalamic tract) of the spinal cord causes impairment or loss of pain and temperature sensation *contralateral* to the lesion, and damage to the corticospinal tract in the spinal cord (lateral corticospinal tract; LCST) results in upper motor neuron syndrome *ipsilateral* to the lesion. This is classical Brown-Sequard syndrome.

197. The answer is a. (*Alberts, p 1072. Kasper, pp 303, 311–313. Kumar, pp 1260–1262.*) In pemphigus, autoantibodies to desmogleins (a member of the cadherin protein family) result in disruption of the macula adherens or desmosomes. The desmogleins are the transmembrane linker proteins of the desmosome. Specific desmogleins are the target of the autoantibodies in different forms of the disease. Cadherins are Ca^{2+}-dependent transmembrane-linker molecules essential for cell-cell contact, so their disturbance in pemphigus leads to severe blistering of the skin because of disrupted cell-cell interactions early in the differentiation of the keratinocyte (epidermal cell) and excessive fluid loss. Hemidesmosomes **(answer b)** contain different proteins than desmosomes and are not affected in pemphigus. Therefore, the basal layer of the epidermis remains attached to the basal lamina in pemphigus. In contrast, in bullous pemphigoid (BP), antigens develop that are specific for the hemidesmosomes. In that disease the entire epithelium separates from the basal lamina. For more details on junctional complexes, see the table in feedback for question 199.

198. The answer is c. (*Kierszenbaum, pp 301, 303. Kasper, pp 291–292. Kumar, pp 1256–1257.*) Psoriasis is a chronic disease that affects both the epidermis and dermis of the skin. There is hyperplasia of the epidermis and abnormal microcirculation in the dermis as venules predominate in the capillaries resulting in increased extravasation of inflammatory cells. Thus, the underlying cause is the infiltration of inflammatory cells into the dermis with further migration of neutrophils into the epidermis. Those inflammatory cells release cytokines that induce an inflammatory response. There is hyperplasia of the epidermis **(answer a)** as keratinocytes traverse the cell cycle in a shorter period of time **(answer b)**. Microabcesses form in the epidermis **(answer d)** and epithelia are avascular **(answer e)**.

199. The answer is b. (*Kierszenbaum, pp 301, 303. Kasper, pp 303, 311–313. Kumar, pp 1260–1262.*) The patient is suffering from bullous pemphigoid in which BP antigens are produced to proteins specific to the hemidesmosomes. The immunofluorescence image shows specific labeling of the epidermal-dermal interface. Therefore, the entire epidermis separates from the basal lamina in contrast to pemphigus in which the desmosomes disaggregate due to antibodies to the desmogleins causing a disruption of the macula adherens [desmosomes **(answer a)**] in the stratum spinosum. The gap junction **(answer c)** is a communicating junction; the zonula occludens **(answer d)** prevents material from flowing between cells; and the zonula adherens **(answer e)** is a belt-like component of the junctional complex that links to the actin cytoskeleton. Below is a helpful "memory grid" to remind you of the components of the junctional complexes and their attachments to the cell. You can move down or across, but not diagonally.

Memory Grid			
	Cadherins	**Integrins**	
Actin	**Adhesion Belts**	**Focal Adhesions**	**No Plaque**
Intermediate Filaments	**Desmosomes**	**Hemidesmosomes**	**Plaque**
	Cell to Cell	**Cell to Matrix**	
No fair going diagonally!			

(Table courtesy of Dr. Ronal R. MacGregor.)

200. The answer is e. *(Kumar, pp 487–488. Kasper, pp 371, 376, 2332–2334.)* In patients with phenylketonuria (PKU), there is a diffuse pigmentary dilution due to elevated levels of L-phenylalanine resulting from a deficiency in the enzyme L-phenylalanine hydroxylase that converts L-phenylalanine to L-tyrosine. The high levels of phenylalanine provide competitive inhibition for tyrosinase **(answers c and d).** The characteristic blonde hair of PKU can undergo darkening when the patient is on a low phenylalanine diet. The number of melanocytes that differentiate from the neural crest would be normal **(answer a).** Melanocytes do not proliferate **(answer b).**

Gastrointestinal Tract and Glands

Questions

DIRECTIONS: Each item below contains a question or incomplete statement followed by suggested responses. Select the **one best** response to each question.

201. A 50-year-old woman presents to the family medicine clinic. She admits to drinking a six-pack of beer each day with a little more intake on weekends. Lab tests show elevated ALT/SGPT and AST/SGOT. Her sclerae appear jaundiced and her serum bilirubin is 2.5 mg/dL (normal 0.3–1.9 mg/dL). A biopsy of her liver shows eosinophilic intracytoplasmic inclusions (Mallory bodies) derived from intermediate filament proteins. What is the most likely source of Mallory bodies?

a. Hepatic stellate cells
b. Kupffer cells
c. Vimentin
d. Keratin
e. Desmin

202. The resting parietal cell does not secrete acid for which of the following reasons?

a. The Na^+,K^+-ATPase is inserted into the apical membrane
b. The chloride channel of the apical plasma membrane is closed
c. The H^+,K^+-ATPase is sequestered in tubulovesicles
d. Carbonic anhydrase is not produced
e. Histamine receptors are uncoupled from their second messengers

203. Enteroendocrine cells differ from goblet cells in which of the following ways?

a. The direction of release of secretion
b. The use of exocytosis for release of secretory product from the cell
c. Their presence in the small and large intestine
d. Their origin from a crypt stem cell
e. Secretion by a regulated pathway

204. In regard to the enteroendocrine cells and the cells composing the enteric nervous system of the gut, which of the following applies to both types of cells?

a. They are derived from neural crest
b. They secrete similar peptides
c. They are essential for the intrinsic rhythmicity of the gut
d. They are turned over rapidly
e. They are found only in the small intestine

205. A 17-year-old with counterfeit identification has a piercing done at a local tattoo/piercing establishment. She chooses to have a stainless steel barbell inserted in the piercing through the anterior 2/3 of her tongue. There is damage to the structures shown in the associated photomicrograph. Primary afferents from those structures travel through which of the following cranial nerves?

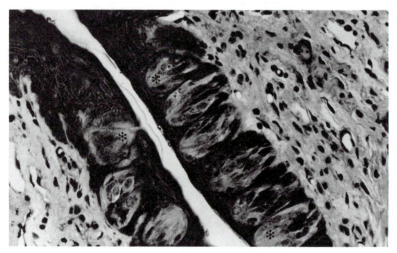

(Micrograph courtesy of Dr. John K. Young.)

a. V
b. VII
c. IX
d. X
e. XII

206. Hirschsprung's disease and Chagas' disease result in disturbance of intestinal motility. The site of this disruption is most likely which of the layers on the accompanying micrograph?

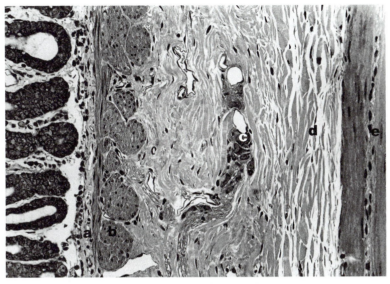

(Micrograph courtesy of Dr. John K. Young.)

a. Layer a
b. Layer b
c. Layer c
d. Layer d
e. Layer e

207. A 48-year-old woman presents to the allergy and rheumatology clinic with itching eyes, dryness of the mouth, difficulty swallowing, loss of sense of taste, hoarseness, fatigue, and swollen parotid glands. She reports increasing joint pain over the past 2 years. She complains of frequent mouth sores. Laboratory tests show a positive antinuclear antibody (ANA) and rheumatoid factor levels of 70U/mL (normal levels less than 60U/mL) by the nephelometric method. A parotid gland biopsy shows inflammatory infiltrates in the interlobular connective tissue with damage to acinar cells and striated ducts. In this case, resorption of which of the following will be most altered by destruction of the striated ducts?

a. Na^+
b. K^+
c. HCO_3^-
d. Cl^-
e. Ca^{2+}

208. Which of the following is the primary regulator of salivary secretion?

a. Antidiuretic hormone
b. Autonomic nervous system
c. Aldosterone
d. Cholecystokinin
e. Secretin

209. A young child presents with hepatomegaly and renomegaly, failure to thrive, stunted growth, and hypoglycemia. A deficiency in glucose 6-phosphatase is identified and the diagnosis is von Gierke disease. In the liver, the structures labeled with the arrows in the accompanying transmission electron micrograph accumulate during this disease. What are the labeled structures?

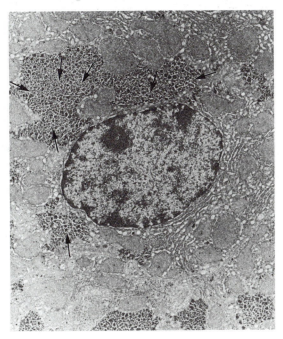

a. Chylomicra
b. Glycogen
c. Mitochondria
d. Peptide-containing secretory granules
e. Ribosomes

210. The branching structures shown in the photomicrograph below (a scanning electron micrograph taken from the region between two hepatocytes) are involved in which of the following?

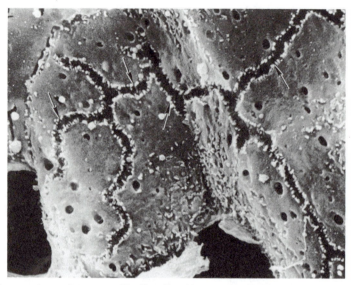

(Electron micrograph courtesy of Dr. Kuen-Shan Hung and Karen Grantham, KUMC Electron Microscopy Center.)

a. Communication between the hepatocytes
b. Preventing flow between adjacent hepatocytes
c. Bile flow
d. Blood flow
e. Spot welds between hepatocytes

211. The following question refers to the photomicrograph below of a plastic-embedded, thin section. The structure labeled A is which of the following?

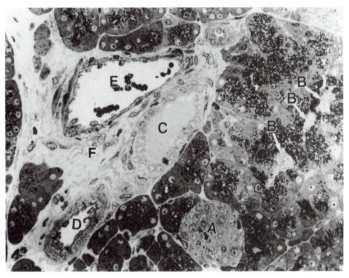

(Micrograph courtesy of Eileen Roach.)

a. A parasympathetic ganglion
b. A cluster of hepatocytes
c. A serous acinus
d. An intralobular duct
e. An islet of Langerhans

212. A pathologist views the following tissues (A and B) in a biopsy. She determines that the tissues are normal. The presence of both of these tissues indicates that the sample was taken from the region of the junction between which of the following?

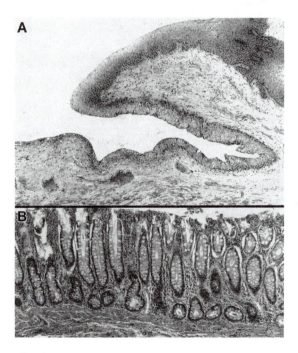

a. Anal canal and rectum
b. Esophagus and stomach
c. Skin of the face and mucous epithelium of the lip
d. Stomach and duodenum
e. Vagina and cervix

213. A 52-year-old woman with a provisional diagnosis of celiac disease presents with bouts of diarrhea and extreme fatigue. Verification was sought through performance of esophagogastroduodenoscopy to obtain small bowel biopsies. Biopsies of the region shown in the accompanying light micrograph disclose hyperplasia of the structures labeled with the asterisks. The labeled structures produce which of the following?

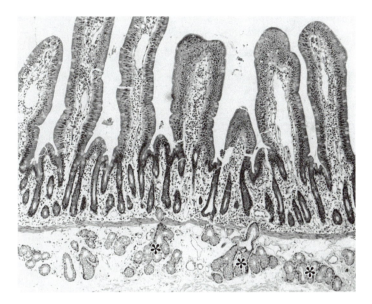

a. Acid
b. Mucus and HCO_3^-
c. Pepsinogen
d. Lysozyme
e. Enterokinase

214. Inflammation in the organ shown in the photomicrograph may result in referred pain to which of the following areas?

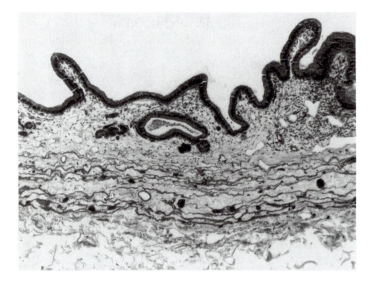

a. Top of the right shoulder
b. Neck
c. Spine between the scapulae
d. Groin
e. Umbilical region

215. The cells labeled with the asterisks in the center of the transmission electron micrograph below function in which of the following processes?

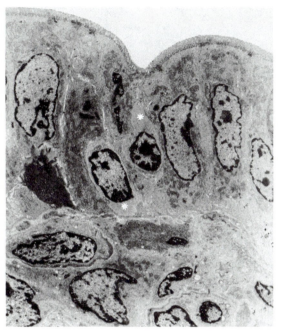

(Reproduced with permission, from McKenzie, Klein, Am. J. Anat. 164: 175–186, 1982.)

a. Immune defense mechanisms
b. Mucus secretion
c. Heparin and histamine secretion and release
d. Endocrine secretion
e. Regulation of the flora of the small bowel

216. In hemolytic jaundice, the structure labeled with the arrow in the accompanying photomicrograph will contain which of the following?

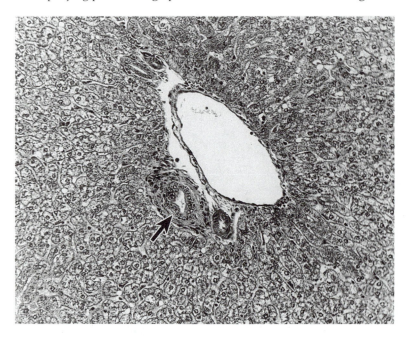

a. Elevated urobilinogen levels
b. Elevated bilirubin levels
c. Decreased urobilinogen levels
d. Decreased bilirubin levels
e. Elevated numbers of lymphocytes undergoing diapedesis

217. A 4-day-old boy weighing 7 lb, 6 oz is brought to the emergency room by his parents. The examining emergency room physician notes that his skin and sclerae are icteric. A blood test indicates elevated unconjugated bilirubin in the serum. The elevated bilirubin levels in this patient are most likely the result of which of the following?

a. Deficiency of enzymes regulating bilirubin solubility
b. Hepatocellular proliferation
c. Decreased destruction of red blood cells
d. Dilation of the common bile duct
e. Increased hepatocyte uptake of bilirubin

218. A 42-year-old woman (5 ft, 3 in., 170 lb) complains of sudden onset of severe pain in the right upper abdomen "under the ribs" accompanied by sweating, nausea, and a feeling of imminent collapse. The pain lasts for about 2 hours and then persists as a dull ache. When seen several hours later, she has normal bowel sounds, is tender throughout the abdomen, especially in the right upper quadrant, and is faintly icteric. She has noticed her urine is darker than usual but has not passed stool recently. She recalls occasional episodes of "indigestion" referred to the right upper abdomen and radiating to the shoulder. This has occurred especially after eating fried foods or after eating a meal following a long period of fasting. She has no fever but is anxious and tachycardic. The test results available are a blood count and blood chemistry including liver enzymes, alkaline phosphatase, and bilirubin. She has a WBC of 10,000. Her cellular hepatic enzymes are: AST/SGOT = 52 (normal 3–33) and ALT//SGPT = 70 (normal 4–44), alkaline phosphatase = 300 (normal 17–91), bilirubin = 6.3 (normal 0.2–1.0). Which of the following is the most probable diagnosis ?

a. Hepatitis A
b. Hepatitis B
c. Carcinoma of the head of the pancreas
d. Gallstone obstructing common bile duct
e. Biliary cirrhosis

219. A 14-month-old girl is brought to the pediatric dentistry clinic because her erupted deciduous teeth are opalescent with fractures and chips in the surface. X-rays reveal bulb-shaped crowns and thin roots. Structure D on the diagram is abnormally large in her teeth. The structure labeled "B" on the diagram is prepared for histology and shows disoriented, irregular, widely-spaced tubules with wide vascular channels. Which of the following applies to the layer labeled "B?"

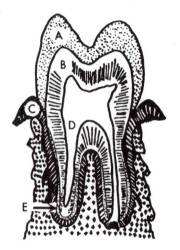

a. It has a composition similar to that of bone and is produced by cells similar in appearance to osteocytes
b. It is formed on a noncollagenous matrix that is resorbed on mineralization by the same cells that secreted it
c. It contains abundant nerves, blood vessels, and loose connective tissue
d. It consists of mineralized collagen secreted by cells derived from neural crest
e. It is the site of inflammation in diabetic patients and is sensitive to deficiency in vitamin C

220. A 39-year-old woman presents with dyspnea, fatigue, pallor, tachycardia, anosmia, and diarrhea. Laboratory results are: hematocrit 32% (normal 36.1–44.3%), MCV 102 femtoliters (fL) [(normal 78–98 fL)], 0.3 % reticulocytes (normal 0.5–2.0%), 95 pg/mL vitamin B12 (normal 200–900 pg/mL), and an abnormal stage I of the Schilling test. Autoantibodies are detected to a cell type that is found in a region shown in the accompanying diagram. In which region would those cells be found?

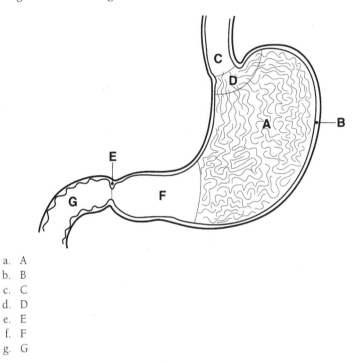

a. A
b. B
c. C
d. D
e. E
f. F
g. G

221. A 43-year-old man who recently returned from a trip to rural Peru presents with severe watery diarrhea, vomiting, and dehydration. He also has marked leg cramps and has lost 8 lb since his return from the trip. Fecal culture is positive for V. cholerae. How does this bacterium exert its effect?

a. Activation of enterokinase on the brush border of epithelial cells
b. Activation of cholecystokinin effects on pancreatic secretion
c. Closure of chloride channels in the enterocyte cell membrane
d. Inhibition of cyclic AMP in the enterocytes
e. ADP-ribosylation of G_s of the GTP-binding protein in enterocytes

222. A 35-year-old man visits his family medicine physician complaining of bloating, a sense of urgency, cramping abdominal pain, meteorism, diarrhea with excessive flatulence several hours after ingestion of milk or dairy products. He says that he has always enjoyed milk and dairy products without any problems, but now eating them causes him abdominal distress. In this disorder, the area shown by the arrows would have a decrease in which of the following?

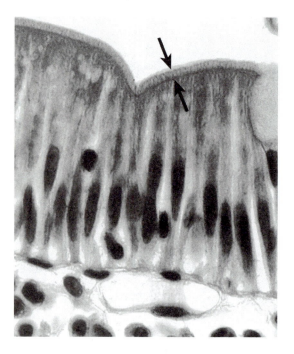

a. Specific disaccharidase activity
b. Glucose/galactose transporter activity
c. Passive diffusion of monosaccharides
d. Uptake of triglycerides by endocytosis
e. Active transport of glycerol

Gastrointestinal Tract and Glands

Answers

201. The answer is d. (*Ross and Pawlina, p 63. Kumar, pp 34, 423.*) Mallory bodies are derived from keratin intermediate filaments within hepatocytes. Hepatic stellate cells **(answer a)** secrete the collagen that replaces normal liver parenchyma in cirrhosis. Kupffer cells **(answer b)** are the macrophages of the liver. Vimentin **(answer c)** is the intermediate filament protein found in cells of mesenchymal origin; the liver and hepatocytes are epithelial in origin. Desmin **(answer e)** is the intermediate filament protein associated with muscle. ALT/SGPT and AST/SGOT are hepatic aminotransferases. When found in the blood they are indicative of liver damage.

202. The answer is c. (*Johnson, pp 1123–1124. Junqueira, pp 293–294, 296–297. Ross and Pawlina, pp 528–530.*) In the resting parietal cell, the proton pump (H⁺,K⁺-ATPase) is found in the tubulovesicle membranes that are located intracellularly **(answer a)**. The sequestration of the proton pump in intracellular tubulovesicles in the resting state prohibits secretion. On activation of the parietal cell through Ca^{2+} and diacylglycerol second messengers, the tubulovesicle membranes fuse with the plasma membrane by exocytosis. Histamine **(answer e)**, along with gastrin and acetylcholine, activate the parietal cell. Na⁺,K⁺-ATPase located in the basal membrane, and the chloride channel **(answer b)** of the apical plasma membrane maintain the appropriate ionic gradients to facilitate acid secretion. Carbonic anhydrase, a cytoplasmic enzyme, catalyzes the formation of carbonic acid (H_2CO_3) from carbon dioxide, which is the source of protons in the parietal cell and other cell types, such as the osteoclast, that also depend on a proton pump **(answer d)**. After dissipation of the stimulus (i.e., gastrin, acetylcholine, or histamine) or exposure to an H_2 blocker, the parietal cell returns to the resting state. This involves the recycling (endocytosis) of membrane to reform the tubulovesicular arrangement within the cytoplasm.

203. The answer is a. (*Junqueira, pp 83, 299–303.*) Goblet cells secrete mucus from their apical surface (domain), whereas enteroendocrine cells release peptides from their basal surface (domain). The goblet cells are unicellular mucus-secreting glands analogous to the enteroendocrine cells that are unicellular endocrine glands. Enteroendocrine cells secrete into the bloodstream (endocrine function) or into the local area to affect nearby cells (paracrine function). The enteroendocrine cells may be identified by their staining response to silver or chromium stains, hence the older terms argentaffin and enterochromaffin, respectively. Examination of such preparations indicates that the enteroendocrine cells are rare compared with other mucosal cell types, including the mucous cells. Enteroendocrine and goblet cells and release granules by a regulated exocytotic secretion **(answer b)**. Both cells are formed by stem cells in crypt base of both the small and large intestinal glands [(of Lieberkühn) **answers c and d**].

204. The answer is b. (*Kierszenbaum, pp 404–405, 430. Junqueira, pp 300, 311. Ross and Pawlina, pp 521, 530, 534.*) The enteroendocrine cells and the enteric (intrinsic) nervous system secrete similar peptides and are found throughout the gastrointestinal tract **(answer e)**. Enteroendocrine cells are derived from the same stem cell as other epithelial cell types and originate embryonically from the endoderm. These cells turn over at a slower rate than other epithelial cell types. In contrast, the cells that compose the enteric nervous system are neurons, derived from neural crest **(answer a)**. There is little cell replacement except in the glial populations **(answer d)**. The enteric nervous system, particularly the myenteric (or Auerbach's) plexus, is responsible for the intrinsic rhythmicity of the gut and peristalsis **(answer c)**. The enteroendocrine cells function in local paracrine regulation of the mucosa (e.g., acid secretion in the stomach, mucosal growth, small intestinal secretion, and turnover).

205. The answer is b. (*Kierszenbaum, p 395. Avery, pp 285–287. Moore and Dalley, pp 1098, 1100.*) Piercing of the tongue can result in complaints of pain, numbness, and loss of taste when eating. The loss of taste is associated with damage to the taste buds, which are shown in the photomicrograph. Taste from the anterior two-thirds of the tongue as shown in the accompanying photomicrograph are innervated by the VIIth (facial) cranial nerve. The Vth (trigeminal) cranial nerve **(answer a)** is responsible for transmitting general sensation from the anterior two-thirds of the tongue. The taste buds from the posterior one-third of the tongue are innervated by the IXth (glossopharyngeal) cranial nerve **(answer c)** specifically by the chorda tympani. The Xth (vagus) cranial nerve (**answer d**) innervates taste buds on the epiglottis and palate. The XIIth (hypoglossal) cranial nerve innervates the intrinsic musculature of the tongue (**answer e**).

206. The answer is e. (*Kasper, pp 231–232, 300, 449. Junqueira, p 282.*) Hirschsprung's disease (congenital megacolon) and Chagas' disease have different etiologies, but both inhibit intestinal motility by affecting the myenteric (Auerbach's) plexus located between the layers of the muscularis externa (layer **e**) in the figure. The submucosal (Meissner's) plexus is more involved in regulation of lumenal size and, therefore, will affect defecation, but will be less involved in peristalsis. Vascular smooth muscle, the muscularis mucosa, and enteroendocrine cells do not play a major role in the regulation of peristalsis, which is observed even after removal of the gut and placement in a nutrient solution. Hirschsprung's disease, also known as aganglionic megacolon, results from failure of normal migration of neural crest cells to the colon, resulting in an aganglionic segment. Although both the myenteric and submucosal plexuses are affected, the primary regulator of intrinsic gut rhythmicity is the myenteric plexus. Chagas' disease is caused by the protozoan *Trypanosoma cruzi*. Severe infection results in extensive damage to the myenteric neurons.

The wall of the GI tract contains four layers: mucosa, submucosa, muscularis externa, and serosa. The structure labeled **a** in the photomicrograph is the lamina propria, a loose connective tissue layer immediately beneath the epithelium. Also part of the mucosa is a double layer of smooth muscle cells (layer **b**) comprising the muscularis mucosa. In the photomicrograph, an inner circular and outer longitudinal layer of smooth muscle cells is discernible. A thick layer of dense irregular connective tissue, the submucosa (layer **d**), separates the muscularis mucosae from the muscularis externa. The structure labeled c is a nest of parasympathetic postganglionic neurons forming part of Meissner's plexus. The muscularis externa (labeled layer **e**) generally consists of inner circular and outer longitudinal layers of smooth-muscle cells. Slight variations in these components may occur in specific organs of the GI tract. The respiratory, urinary, integumentary, and reproductive systems differ from the gastrointestinal system in their epithelia and arrangement of underlying tissue.

207. The answer is a. (*Avery, pp 306–310. Guyton, pp 740–741.*) The woman in the scenario suffers from Sjögren's syndrome, which like other autoimmune diseases (presence of ANA and RF), is much more common in women than men. The striated ducts resorb Na^+ and secrete K^+ (**answer b**) from the isotonic saliva converting it to a hypotonic state. Na^+-independent chloride-bicarbonate anion exchangers appear to be involved in these processes by generating ion fluxes into the salivary secretion. The striated duct is the primary region for electrolyte transport in the salivary gland duct system. The primary secretion produced by the acinar cells is comprised of amylase, mucus, and ions in the same concentrations as those of the extracellular fluid. In the duct system, Na^+ is actively absorbed from the lumen of the ducts, Cl^- is passively absorbed [although the tight junctions between striated duct cells inhibit Cl^- from following Na^+ (**answer c**)]. HCO_3^- is secreted (**answer d**); Ca^{2+} transport is not a factor (**e**). The result is a hypotonic sodium and chloride concentration and a hypertonic potassium concentration.

208. The answer is b. (*Guyton, pp 739–741, 746–749, 855–856.*) The autonomic nervous system is the primary regulator of salivary gland function in contradistinction to the pancreas, which is regulated primarily by hormones [(cholecystokinin and secretin (**answers d and e**)]. Parasympathetic fibers carry neural signals that originate in the salivatory nuclei of the medulla and pons. The sympathetic nervous system originates from the superior cervical ganglion of the sympathetic chain and stimulates acinar enzyme production. Elevated aldosterone levels affect the amount and ionic concentration of the saliva, resulting in decreased NaCl secretion and increased K^+ concentration (**answer c**). Cholecystokinin (pancreozymin) and secretin are the hormones that regulate acinar and ductal secretions, respectively, in the exocrine pancreas. Antidiuretic hormone can modulate salivary gland production (**answer a**).

209. The answer is b. (*Young, p 25. Junqueira, pp 31–32, 49, 330–331, 333–334.*) The disease described in the scenario is type I (hepatorenal, von Gierke) glycogenosis caused by a defect in glucose-6-phosphatase, resulting in accumulation of glucose-6 phosphate and glycogen in the liver. The cytoplasmic inclusions labeled with the arrows in the transmission electron micrograph are glycogen. The hepatocyte, under the regulation of insulin and glucagon, stores glucose in its polymerized form of glycogen. In electron micrographs, glycogen appears as scattered dark particles with an approximate diameter of 15–25 nm. Lipid droplets appear as spherical, homogeneous structures of varying density and diameter, although their diameter is considerably larger than that of the glycogen granules. Ribosomes (**answer e**) are found on the rough endoplasmic reticulum or as free structures, in which case they are not found in clusters like glycogen. Mitochondria (**answer c**) contain distinctive cristae and are much larger (0.5–1.0 μm in diameter) than glycogen. Chylomicra (**answer a**) are located at the basal surface of the hepatocytes and are less dense than glycogen. Secretory granules (**answer d**) would also show polarity in their location.

210. The answer is c. *(Junqueira, pp 325, 328–329, 331.)* The bile canaliculi are labeled with arrows in the scanning electron micrograph. They comprise the space between the lateral surfaces of adjacent hepatocytes. Microvilli line the bile canaliculi and are visible protruding into the lumen. The membranes between the cells are connected by tight (zonula occludentes) and gap junctions, neither of which are visible in the photomicrograph. The zonula occludentes prevent material from passing between the hepatocytes and desmosomes, and when they are present between cells, function as spot welds.

211. The answer is e. *(Young, pp 283–284. Junqueira, pp 321–323, 407–411.)* The organ in the photomicrograph is the pancreas, and the cells labeled are the islets of Langerhans. The pancreas functions as both an exocrine (secretion of pancreatic juice) and endocrine (secretion of insulin and glucagon) gland. The islets (**A**) have a heterogeneous distribution within the pancreas (i.e., they decrease from the tail to the head of the gland) and may be used to distinguish the pancreas from the parotid gland. The submandibular and sublingual glands can be ruled out because of the purely serous nature of the acini within the exocrine portion of the gland. The centroacinar cells (**B**) are modified intralobular duct cells, specifically from the intercalated duct, and are present in the lumen of each acinus. The duct (**C**) can be distinguished by the presence of a cuboidal epithelium, the absence of blood and blood cells from the lumen, and the absence of a characteristic vascular wall. A pancreatic artery (**D**) and a vein (**E**) are shown within the interlobular connective tissue (**F**).

212. The answer is a. *(Junqueira, pp 281–282, 311.)* Photomicrographs A and B show two distinctly different types of epithelium: stratified squamous epithelium of the anus (top panel) and crypts (without villi) of the rectum (lower panel). The anus has anal valves and an absence of the muscularis mucosa. The esophageal-cardiac junction also represents a junction between stratified squamous and simple columnar epithelium, but the cardiac portion of the stomach forms the mucus-secreting cardiac glands with *no* goblet cells (**answer b**). The junction of the stomach (pylorus) and duodenum represents the juncture of two simple columnar epithelia, the pylorus containing the short (compared with fundus) pyloric glands and the duodenum with crypts and villi as well as the submucosal Brunner's glands (**answer d**). Skin is keratinized (**answer c**). The cervical mucosa contains extensive cervical glands, and the vaginal epithelium is keratinized. In vagina and cervix, the GI tract pattern [epithelium, connective tissue (CT), muscle, CT, muscle, CT] is *not* present (**answer e**).

213. The answer is b. (*Young, p 261. Junqueira, pp 290–295, 298–300.*) The patient in the scenario is suffering from celiac disease, an allergic response to gliadin. The result is villous atrophy and crypt and Brunner gland (the structures labeled with the asterisks in the photomicrograph) hyperplasia. The presence of the mucus and bicarbonate (HCO_3^-) secreting Brunner's glands in the submucosal layer of the small intestine is an identifying feature of the duodenum. The Brunner's gland secretions function to neutralize the acidic pH of the stomach and establish the appropriate pH for function of the enzymes in the pancreatic juice. Parietal cells are unique to the stomach and synthesize acid (**answer a**) and intrinsic factor (required for vitamin B_{12} absorption from the small intestine). Chief cells in the fundic glands produce pepsinogen (**answer c**) that is activated by acid to form pepsin. Paneth cells in the base of the crypts make lysozyme (**answer d**) and modulate the flora of the small intestine. Enterokinase (**answer e**) is made by the duodenal mucosa and is instrumental in the conversion of pancreatic zymogens to their active form (e.g., trypsinogen to trypsin).

214. The answer is a. (*Young, p 282. Junqueira, p 337. Moore and Dalley, pp 232–235.*) The photomicrograph illustrates the structure of the gallbladder that stores and concentrates the bile. Gallbladder inflammation can lead to pain referred to the top of the right shoulder. Diaphragmatic problems may be felt in the neck (**answer b**), stomach problems may refer to the spine between the scapulae (**answer c**), kidney pain may be felt in the groin area (**answer d**), and intestinal dysfunction may be felt in the middle or low back. Umbilical pain is typically referred from the appendix (**answer e**).

Although the finger-like extensions of the gallbladder resemble villi, they represent changes that occur in the mucosa with increasing age. The thinness of the wall is the notable characteristic of the gallbladder. The bile is synthesized by hepatocytes and transported from the liver to the gallbladder.

215. The answer is a. *(Junqueira, pp 76, 78–79, 263, 265, 298–302, 310.)* The transmission electron micrograph is taken from the small intestinal epithelium. Intraepithelial lymphocytes (labeled with the asterisks) are lymphocytes that have crossed the basal lamina. The intraepithelial lymphocytes may respond to antigen in the lumen of the small bowel. In the Peyer's patches of the ileum lymphocytes in the lamina propria may respond to antigen that has been sampled from the lumen and transported by M cells in the Peyer's patches. Enterocytes are the absorptive cells of the gut and possess numerous microvilli on their apical surfaces. Goblet cells synthesize and secrete mucins (**answer b**). Paneth cells and enteroendocrine cells contain granules, but secrete lysozyme [regulation of flora (**answer e**)] and endocrine peptides (**answer d**), respectively. Mast cells synthesize and secrete histamine and heparin (**answer c**).

216. The answer is b. *(Kasper, pp 238–240. Guyton, pp 800–801. Young, pp 274–279. Junqueira, pp 329–330, 332–333, 334–335.)* The structure labeled with the arrow is a bile duct and would contain elevated levels of bilirubin following hemolytic jaundice. Hemolytic jaundice is associated predominantly with unconjugated hyperbilirubinemia. The overproduction of bilirubin occurs because of accelerated intravascular erythrocyte destruction or resorption of a large hematoma. When hepatic uptake and excretion of urobilinogen are impaired or the production of bilirubin is greatly increased (e.g., with hemolysis), daily urinary urobilinogen excretion may increase significantly. In contrast, cholestasis [arrested flow of bile due to obstruction of the bile ducts (intrahepatic)] or extrahepatic biliary obstruction interferes with the intestinal phase of bilirubin metabolism and leads to significantly decreased production and urinary excretion of urobilinogen. Diapedesis of lymphocytes across the endothelium of the postcapillary high endothelial venules of lymphoid organs (e.g., lymph nodes) increases during inflammation.

Bile is formed by the hepatocytes and is released into bile canaliculi, which are located between the lateral surfaces of adjacent hepatocytes. The direction of flow is from the hepatocytes toward the bile duct, which drains bile from the liver on its path to the gallbladder, where the bile is stored and concentrated. The hepatic artery and hepatic portal vein (shown in the photomicrograph) plus the bile duct comprise the portal triad. Blood flows from the triad (hepatic artery, portal vein, and bile duct) toward the central vein, whereas bile flows in the opposite direction toward the triad.

Bile is synthesized by hepatocytes using the smooth endoplasmic reticulum (SER) and consists of bile acids and bilirubin. Bile acids are 90% recycled from the distal small and large intestinal lumen and 10% newly synthesized by conjugation of cholic acid, glycine, and taurine in the SER. Bilirubin is the breakdown product of hemoglobin derived from the action of Kupffer cells in hepatic sinusoids and other macrophages, particularly those lining the sinusoids of the spleen where degradation of RBCs is prominent.

217. The answer is a. *(Junqueira, pp 334–335. Kasper, pp 1817–1820. Kumar, pp 885–888.)* Commonly, initial low levels of glucuronyl (glucuronysl) transferase in the underdeveloped smooth endoplasmic reticulum of hepatocytes in the newborn, result in jaundice (neonatal unconjugated hyperbilirubinemia); less commonly, this enzyme is genetically lacking. The neonatal small intestinal epithelium also has an increased capacity for absorption of unconjugated bilirubin, which contributes to the elevated serum levels.

Bilirubin, a product of iron-free heme, is liberated during the destruction of old erythrocytes by the mononuclear macrophages of the spleen and, to a lesser extent, of the liver and bone marrow. The hepatic portal system brings splenic bilirubin to the liver, where it is made soluble for excretion by conjugation with glucuronic acid. Increased plasma levels of bilirubin (hyperbilirubinemia) result from increased bilirubin turnover, impaired uptake of bilirubin, or decreased conjugation of bilirubin. Increased bilirubin turnover occurs in Dubin-Johnson and Rotor's syndromes, in which there is impairment of the transfer and excretion of bilirubin glucuronide into the bile canaliculi. In Gilbert's syndrome, there is impaired uptake of bilirubin into the hepatocyte and a defect in glucuronyl transferase. In Crigler-Najjar syndrome, a defect in glucuronyl transferase occurs in the neonate.

The ability of mature hepatocytes to take up and conjugate bilirubin may be exceeded by abnormal increases in erythrocyte destruction (hemolytic jaundice) or by hepatocellular damage (functional jaundice), such as in hepatitis. Finally, obstruction of the duct system between the liver and duodenum (usually of the common bile duct in the adult and rarely from aplasia of the duct system in infants) results in a backup of bilirubin (obstructive jaundice, see question 218 and feedback).

218. The answer is d. (*Kaspeer, pp 1881–1882, 1898–1899. Kumar, pp 928–931. Junqueira, pp 334–335. Guyton, pp 800–801.*) The pattern of elevated liver enzymes, alkaline phosphatase, and bilirubin are consistent with obstructive jaundice (see table below). The presence of pain (in the right upper quadrant radiating to the shoulder) after eating a meal consisting of fried foods makes gallstones the most probable diagnosis. Similar pain often occurs in these patients when they have not eaten for long periods of time and then have a large meal. The pain is caused by the obstruction of the cystic duct or common bile duct that produces increased lumenal pressure within the bile vessels, which cannot be compensated for by cholecytokinin-induced contractions. The pain usually lasts for one to four hours as a steady, aching feeling. A mnemonic device for gallstones is 4F (F,F,F,F): female, forty, fat, and fertile.

Enzyme	Obstructive	Parenchymal
Liver enzymes (AST and ALT)	↑	↑↑↑
Alkaline phosphatase	↑↑↑	↑
Bilirubin	↑↑↑	↑↑↑

219. The answer is d. (*Junqueira, pp 283–285. Kumar, p 774. Kasper, p 2327.*) The patient in the scenario suffers from type II dentinogenesis imperfecta, an autosomal dominant disorder caused by mutation in the DSPP gene. The result is defective dentin, discoloration of the translucent teeth (blue-gray or yellow-brown color). Those teeth are weaker than normal, making them prone to rapid decay, wear, breakage, and loss. Type II dentinogenesis imperfecta occurs about 1 in 6000–8000 births. Type I occurs in conjunction with osteogenesis imperfecta with mutations in type I collagen; children with type I have typical blue sclerae with defects in bone and dentin.

The structure labeled **B** is dentin, which consists of mineralized collagen synthesized by odontoblasts. Odontoblasts are derived from the neural crest. The pulp of a mature tooth (labeled **D** in the diagram) consists primarily of loose connective tissue rich in vessels and nerves. Odontoblasts lie at the edge of the pulp cavity and secrete collagen and other molecules, which mineralize to become dentin **(B)**. Mineralization of the matrix occurs around the odontoblast processes and forms dentinal tubules. Ameloblasts, which are ectodermal derivatives, lay down an organic matrix and secrete enamel, initially onto the surface of the dentin. As hydroxyapatite crystals form at the apices of ameloblast (Tomes') processes, rods of enamel grow peripherally, and the ameloblasts resorb the organic matrix so that the enamel layer **(A)** is almost entirely mineral. It contains *no* collagen, but has unique proteins such as the amelogenins and enamelins.

On eruption of the tooth, enamel deposition is complete and the ameloblasts are shed. Cementum **(E)** has a composition similar to that of bone, is produced by cells similar in appearance to osteocytes, and covers the dentin of the root. The periodontal ligament **(C)** consists of coarse collagenous fibers running between the alveolar bone and the cementum of the tooth and separates the tooth from the alveolar socket. Although the periodontal ligament suspends and supports each tooth, the ligament permits physiologic movement within the limits provided by the elasticity of the tissue. It is a site of inflammation in diabetic patients and is affected in scurvy (recall the image of the 18th century British sailor).

220. The answer is a. (*Young, pp 254–257. Junqueira, p 294. Kumar, pp 639–642.*) The woman in the scenario suffers from pernicious anemia resulting from autoantibodies to the parietal cells, which are responsible for the production of intrinsic factor as well as HCl. The abnormal stage I Schilling test is indicative of a deficiency in intrinsic factor. Chief cells and parietal cells are found in the fundus **(region A)**. Chief cells synthesize pepsinogen and parietal cells produce HCl and intrinsic factor. The gastric (fundic) glands contain mucous cells, chief cells, and parietal cells. Intrinsic factor is required for absorption of vitamin B_{12} from the small intestine. The diagram shows the anatomic relationship between the esophagus, stomach, and duodenum. The esophagus **(C)** joins the stomach in the cardiac region **(D)**. The pylorus **(F)** contains shorter glands with deeper pits than those of the fundus and body. Those glands contain more mucous cells and many gastrin-secreting enteroendocrine cells. Food entering the pylorus stimulates the release of gastrin that stimulates HCl production by the parietal cells. The pylorus connects with the duodenum **(G)**, which contains the mucus and bicarbonate-neutralizing secretion of the Brunner's glands. The wall of the stomach consists of the mucosa (epithelium, lamina propria, and muscularis mucosa), submucosa, muscularis externa, and serosa **(B)** lined by a mesothelium.

221. The answer is e. *(Kasper, pp 755, 910–911. Kierszenbaum, pp 427–429. Alberts, pp 856, 1427–1428, 1437.)* Cholera toxin causes secretory diarrhea through the ADP-ribosylation of G_s of the GTP-binding protein, which leads to elevated cyclic AMP and the opening of the chloride channel **(answers c & d).** The exit of chloride through the open channels is followed by the passage of sodium and water. The result can be dehydration, which can be offset by intravenous feeding or oral rehydration therapy. Pancreatic secretion is regulated by hormones. Secretin regulates ductal secretion, whereas cholecystokinin **(answer b)** regulates the release of enzymes (amylase, lipase, DNAse, RNAse, and the other enzymes that compose the pancreatic juice). A number of pancreatic secretions are released into the pancreatic duct system as zymogens (inactive precursors). They are activated only when they arrive in the small intestinal lumen. Enterokinase, a brush border enterocyte enzyme, converts trypsinogen to trypsin **(answer a).** Trypsin and enterokinase are responsible for the activation of chymotrypsinogen, proelastase, and procarboxypeptidase A and B to their active forms: chymotrypsin, elastase, and carboxypeptidase A and B. These hormones are *not* related to cholera-induced diarrhea.

222. The answer is a. *(Kierszenbaum, pp 427–429. Kumar, pp 844–845. Kapser, pp 222–223.)* The area shown in the photomicrograph is the glycocalyx (brush border consisting of microvilli) of the small intestinal epithelium. It is the location of the brush border enzymes including lactase. The patient in the scenario is suffering from lactase deficiency which often has an adult onset since lactase activity decreases after childhood. The absence of lactase or reduced lactase activity results in passage of undigested lactose into the colon. Colonic bacteria carry out fermentation of the lactose to organic acids and hydrogen. The bloating, cramping, and abdominal pain are due to the breakdown of lactose and production of the hydrogen gas. The microvilli are also the site of the glucose/galactose transporter (**answers b and c**). However, the glucose/galactose transporter is *not* the site of the deficiency in lactose intolerance. Other brush border enzymes include the other monosaccharidases and enterokinase, which is important for cleavage of pancreatic zymogens (e.g., trypsinogen) to their active form.

Digestion of lipids occurs through the action of bile (from the liver and bile duct) and lipase (from the pancreas). Bile serves to emulsify the lipid to form micelles, whereas lipase breaks down the lipid from triglycerides to fatty acids, glycerol, and monoglycerides (**answers d and e**). Those three breakdown products diffuse freely across the microvilli to enter the apical portion of the enterocyte by passive diffusion. Triglycerides are resynthesized in the smooth endoplasmic reticulum. Proteins are synthesized in the RER and are combined with sugar and lipid portions in the Golgi to form glycoproteins and lipoproteins. Those two types of molecules form the coverings of the triglyceride cores of the chylomicra. The chylomicra are released at the basolateral membranes by exocytosis into the lacteals. From the lacteals, the chylomicra travel into the cisterna chyli and eventually into the venous system by way of the thoracic duct. Digestion of fat occurs to a greater extent in the duodenum and jejunum than in the ileum.

Sugars are broken down by amylase in the oral cavity, with continued digestion by brush border monosaccharidases. Proteins are broken down by pepsinogen in the stomach with continued breakdown in the small intestine by the enzymes of the pancreatic juice (e.g., trypsin, chymotrypsin, and carboxypeptidases). The products of protein digestion are amino acids that are actively transported by transporters also located in the brush border.

Endocrine Glands

Questions

DIRECTIONS: Each item below contains a question or incomplete statement followed by suggested responses. Select the **one best** response to each question.

223. The adrenal cortex influences the secretion of the adrenal medulla by means of which of the following?

a. Secretion of aldosterone into the intra-adrenal circulation
b. Secretion of glucocorticoids into the intra-adrenal circulation
c. Autonomic neural connections
d. Secretion of monoamine oxidase into the portal circulation
e. Secretion of androgens into the intrarenal circulation

224. A pheochromocytoma is a common tumor of the adrenal medulla. In the presence of this tumor, which of the following symptoms would most likely be observed?

a. Hypotension
b. Hypoglycemia
c. Hirsutism
d. Decreased metabolic rate
e. Paroxysms

225. Which of the following applies to the gland shown in the photomicrograph and labeled with the arrow in the MRI below?

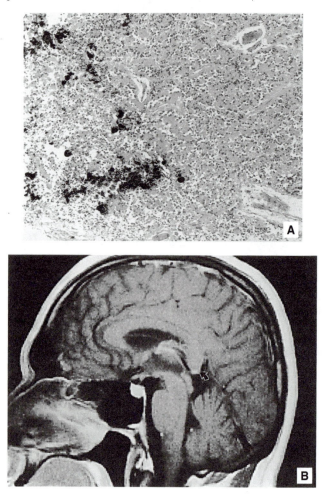

a.   It arises as an outgrowth of the midbrain
b.   It influences the rhymicity of other endocrine organs
c.   It contains many melanocytes
d.   It is innervated by preganglionic sympathetic fibers
e.   It secretes melanocyte-stimulating hormone (MSH)

226. During the physical examination of a newborn child, it is observed that the genitalia are female, but masculinized. The genotype is determined to be 46,XX. Which of the following is the most likely cause of this condition?

a. Androgen insensitivity
b. Decreased blood ACTH levels
c. Atrophy of the zona reticularis
d. A defect in the cortisol pathway
e. Hypersecretion of vasopressin

227. A 33-year-old woman visits the office of her family medicine physician. Her chief complaint is nervousness. She describes her nervousness as increasing over the past 6 weeks. She says that her children and husband describe her as atypically "easy to anger." She says that she now easily loses her temper and often cries for little or no apparent reason, and she has developed a tremor in her right arm. She has lost 22 lb since her last office visit 9 months ago and indicates that she has not changed her diet. She describes herself as always "hot." You observe that her eyes protrude and appear red and inflamed, and she describes her eyes as feeling "dry." Your examination reveals asthenia, tachycardia, and pretibial myxedema. A biopsy of the organ shown below shows an increase in lymphoid cells. An array of tests is completed. To which of the following would you expect to detect autoantibodies within this organ?

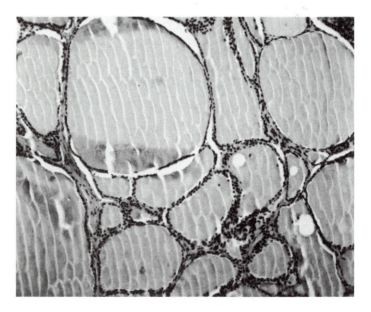

a. C cells
b. Parathyroid principal cells
c. Thyrotropin-releasing factor receptors
d. Thyroglobulin and thyroid peroxidase
e. TSH receptors

228. Which of the following cells or parts of the pituitary are derived embryologically from neuroectoderm?

a. Gonadotrophs
b. Pars intermedia
c. Pars tuberalis
d. Herring bodies
e. Lactotrophs

229. A pituitary adenoma is likely to result in which of the following?

a. Cushing's syndrome
b. Deficiency in T3 and T4
c. Diabetes insipidus
d. Osteoporosis
e. Stunted growth or dwarfism

230. A tumor in the specific region denoted by the asterisks will most likely cause which of the following?

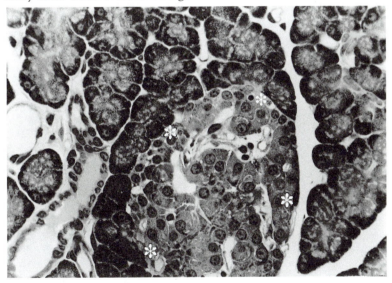

a. Diabetes
b. Hypoglycemia
c. Elevated blood pressure
d. Decreased blood pressure
e. Increased bone resorption

231. Refer to the photomicrograph below in answering this question. The low-magnification micrograph (**A**) and is from the same organ as the high-magnification micrograph (**B**).

A 30-year-old woman presents with chronic fatigue that has worsened during the past months. She has muscle weakness and describes a loss of appetite with a 15-lb weight loss since her last visit. She admits to having "no appetite and eating less," but "craves salty foods" when she is able to eat. She is nauseous much of the time and sometimes vomits after eating. Her bowel movements are loose with frequent diarrhea. Her blood pressure is low and she becomes dizzy when standing. It is the middle of winter in Kansas and she has a healthy tan. The darkening of her skin is most visible in her skin folds and at her elbows, knees and knuckles. She describes being "irritable and depressed" and has had very irregular menstrual periods over the 6 months, which she attributes to early menopause. However, she reports *no* "hot flashes." Which of the following would occur in the regions of a biopsy specimen labeled in the accompanying photomicrograph?

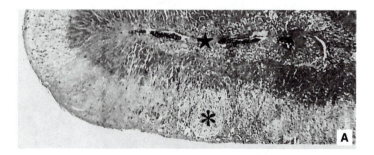

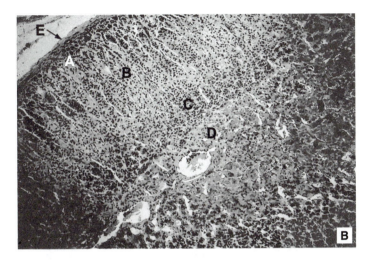

a. Hypertrophy of zone A only
b. Hypertrophy of zones A, B, and C only
c. Hypotrophy of zones A, B, and C only
d. Hypotrophy of zones A, B, C, and D only
e. Hypertrophy of zones A and B only

232. The region labeled C is not a good candidate for transplantation compared with other endocrine glands for which of the following reasons?

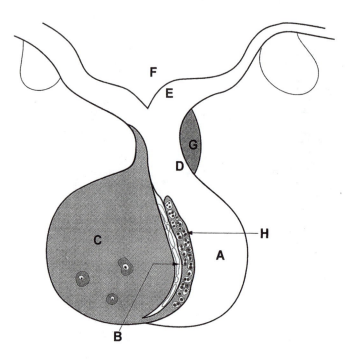

a. More severe rejection of neurally related tissue occurs compared with other endocrine organs
b. Its hormonal source is unavailable after its axonal connections to the hypothalamus are disrupted
c. It lacks function when separated from the hypothalamohypophyseal portal system
d. Neogenesis of blood vessels will not occur at the transplant site
e. The vascular wall of the superior hypophyseal arteries is unique

233. A 45-year-old woman, who works as a corporate executive, presents with the primary complaint of "always being tired." She comments that she has been tired for 4 months even though she is sleeping more. She complains of being unable to finish household chores and "dragging at work." She indicates that she is often constipated and is intolerant to cold. She is continuously turning the thermostats in the house and work to higher temperatures, to the dismay of family members and coworkers, respectively. She also complains that her skin is very dry; use of lotions and creams have not helped the dryness. A biopsy of the organ shown in question 227 indicates dense lymphocytic infiltration with germinal centers throughout the parenchyma. A battery of tests is carried out. You would expect which of the following?

a. Elevated TSH levels in the serum
b. Elevated T3 and T4 levels in the serum
c. Autoantibodies to the thyroid hormone receptor
d. Elevated calcitonin levels
e. Elevated glucocorticoid levels

234. Measuring T3 levels does not necessarily accurately depict the thyroid's ability to secrete T3 for which of the following reasons?

a. T3 is bound to thyroid-hormone binding proteins
b. The liver and kidney convert T4 to T3 peripherally
c. T3 and T4 are regulated by two different anterior pituitary hormones
d. Thyrotrophs produce T3
e. T4 and T3 immunoassays cross-react in immunoassays

Endocrine Glands

Answers

223. The answer is b. (*Kasper, pp 2127–2129. Junqueira, pp 400–402, 406.*) Metabolism in the adrenal medulla is regulated by glucocorticoids because they induce the enzyme phenylethanolamine-N-methyltransferase, which catalyzes the methylation of norepinephrine to epinephrine. Most of the blood supply entering the medulla passes through the cortex. Glucocorticoids synthesized in the zona fasciculata of the adrenal are released into the sinusoids and enter the medulla **(answers a and e)**. The adrenal gland is not usually considered a classic portal system although there are similarities. Monoamine oxidase is a mitochondrial enzyme that regulates the storage of catecholamines in peripheral sympathetic nerve endings **(answers c and d)**. The adrenal gland functions as two separate glands. The adrenal cortex is derived from mesoderm and the adrenal medulla from neural crest. The blood supply to the adrenal is derived from three adrenal arteries: (1) the superior adrenal (suprarenal) from the inferior phrenic, (2) the middle adrenal from the aorta, and (3) the inferior adrenal from the renal artery.

224. The answer is e. (*Kasper, pp 234, 2136, 2148. Junqueira, p 407. Kumar, pp 1219–1221.*) Patients with a pheochromocytoma often have paroxysms that are the hallmark of this tumor. These are seizure-like catecholamine-induced attacks that include headache, profuse sweating, palpitations, and overall anxiety. Pheochromocytoma is a common tumor of the adrenal medulla that leads to an excess of norepinephrine, which causes hypertension and hyperglycemia. Vasoconstriction of arterioles occurs in conjunction with the increased blood pressure. Epinephrine (e.g., cortisol and growth hormone) have anti-insulin effects, thus causing hyperglycemia.

225. The answer is b. (*Junqueira, p 417. Kumar, pp 1223–1224.*) The photomicrograph and the MRI illustrate the structure of the pineal gland, or *epiphysis cerebri*, which arises as an outgrowth of the diencephalon **(answer a)**. The pinealocytes secrete melatonin in response to the light-dark cycle and influence the rhythmicity of other endocrine organs. In a sense, the pineal, therefore, functions as a biologic clock. The pineal contains two main cell types: pinealocytes and neuroglia [the latter appear to be modified astrocytes (answer c)]. The pineal is innervated by postganglionic sympathetic fibers in a fashion similar to other glands in the head and neck region (e.g., salivary glands). The adrenal medulla is innervated by preganglionic sympathetic fibers (answer d). Corticotrophs in the anterior pituitary produce MSH. The pineal does not contain melanocytes or secrete MSH (answer e). There are age-related changes in the pineal in which the number of concretions and the degree of calcification of the "brain sand" increase. The pineal can be identified and used as a landmark in radiologic procedures by its calcification.

226. The answer is d. *(Sadler, pp 252–253. Kumar, pp 1211–1214. Moore and Persaud, Developing, pp 304, 307, 318.)* The newborn described is genotypically female and suffers from adrenogenital syndrome, also known as congenital virilizing hyperplasia, in which there is a deficiency in the pathway that leads to cortisol synthesis. The inability to synthesize cortisol in turn leads to production of high levels of ACTH and ACTH-releasing factor from the hypothalamus (answer b). The result is hypertrophy of the fetal adrenal cortex, which is a critical fetal structure that produces dehydroepiandrosterone. The excessive production of androgens by the fetal adrenal leads to masculinization of the female genitalia. Increased secretion of cortisol cannot occur because of the metabolic defect in this pathway; therefore, negative feedback control is not functional. The fetal cortex is part of maternal-feto-placental unit because dehydroepiandrosterone is used by the placenta to produce estradiol. The fetal adrenal cortex involutes following birth, causing an overall reduction in the size of the adrenal. The adult cortex (zona glomerulosa, zona fasciculata, and zona reticularis) replaces the fetal adrenal cortex. The zona fasciculata and zona reticularis produce androgens after birth (answer c). Vasopressin [(AVP) also known as antidiuretic hormone (ADH)] is released by the posterior pituitary and regulates fluid balance. ADH increases the permeability of the collecting duct through an aquaporin-mediated mechanism (answer e). Androgen insensitivity is the cause of testicular feminization and is not a factor in the adrenogenital syndrome (answer a).

227. The answer is e. *(Junqueira, pp 423–428. Kumar, pp 1172–1173. Moore and Persaud, Developing, pp 215–217.)* The patient is suffering from Graves' disease, an autoimmune disease that occurs much more frequently in women than in men. Graves' disease accounts for approximately 85% of diagnosed hyperthyroidism. Patients with Graves' disease produce autoantibodies to TSH receptors. CD8$^+$-T cells are also generated against the TSH receptors, leading to their destruction. The result is an increase in TSH produced by the anterior pituitary with a concomitant increase in thyroid hormone production [T4 (tetraiodothyronine, thyroxine) and T3 (tetraiodothyronine)] from the thyroid. The elevated thyroid hormone secretion leads to the nervousness, weight loss, and extreme mood changes experienced by the patient.

The thyroid gland is shown in the photomicrograph and is most often confused histologically with lactating mammary gland, which differs from the thyroid in the presence of an elaborate duct system. The thyroid is composed of follicles filled with colloidal material and surrounded by follicular cells with a cuboidal-to-columnar epithelium. The C cells are found outside the follicular cells and produce calcitonin, synthesized by the interfollicular "C" (parafollicular) cells derived embryologically from the ultimobranchial bodies (fourth and possibly fifth pair of branchial pouches). Calcitonin decreases elevated serum calcium levels by transiently inhibiting osteoclastic activity through receptors on osteoclasts. In Graves' disease there are no autoantibodies to the C cells (**answer a**). Destruction of C cells would lead to an absence of calcitonin and high serum calcium levels. Autoantibodies to principal cells of the parathyroid (**answer b**) would lead to decreased serum calcium levels as parathyroid hormone (PTH) synthesis and secretion would be reduced. PTH increases osteoclastic resorption and also stimulates Ca^{2+} uptake from the gut and Ca^{2+} reabsorption by the kidneys. The thyroid gland is under the direct regulation of TSH (thyrotropin) production by the anterior pituitary, which in turn is regulated by TSH-releasing factor (TSH-RF) released from the hypothalamus. TSH-RF is transported by the hypothalamic-hypophyseal (pituitary)-portal system to the anterior pituitary. Autoantibodies to TSH-RF (**answer c**) would result in elevated TSH and T3 and T4, but the receptors would be located in the anterior pituitary on thyrotrophs. Autoantibodies to thyroglobulin and thyroid peroxidase result in Hashimoto's thyroiditis [**answer d** (see question 233)].

Asthenia is loss of strength and tachycardia is accelerated heart rate. Pretibial myxedema presents as an orange-peel-like rash on the shins in some patients with Graves' disease.

The thyroid follicular epithelial cells import iodide and amino acids from the capillary lumen. The follicular cells synthesize thyroglobulin from

Other tumors of the islets of Langerhans include insulinomas in which elevated levels of insulin are secreted into the bloodstream. The result is hypoglycemia as blood sugar levels drop. Insulin removes sugar from the blood and, in the liver, either stores it as glycogen or metabolizes it through glycolysis. Insulin inhibits glycogen phosphorylase (which catalyzes the breakdown of glycogen to form glucose) and activates glycogen synthase in both muscle and liver resulting in increased storage of glycogen.

231. The answer is c. (*Kasper, pp 2141–2143. Junqueira, pp 366, 389, 407. Kumar, pp 1215–1216.*) The woman in the scenario suffers from Addison's disease, in which there is a progressive destruction (hypotrophy) of the adrenal cortex (zones A, B, and C). The result in the patient is asthenia (lack of strength, overall weakness, and fatigue), anorexia, nausea, vomiting, weight loss, hypotension, and low blood sugar. The hyperpigmentation results from elevated ACTH stimulation of melanocytes. The photomicrographs show the histology of the adrenal gland [cortex (✳) and medulla (– ✳ –)], which releases stress-related hormones [i.e., glucocorticoids and catecholamines (norepinephrine and epinephrine)]. The adrenal cortex originates from the intermediate mesoderm, whereas the adrenal medulla forms from neural crest. Adrenocortical cells are under the influence of corticotrophs in the anterior pituitary. Adrenocortical cells import cholesterol and acetate and produce the hormones shown in the table below. The zona glomerulosa (**A**) is found immediately beneath the capsule (**E**) and is followed by the zona fasciculata (**B**) and zona reticularis (**C**) as one moves toward the medulla (**D**). However, in all zones the cells do not store appreciable quantities of hormones, there is an absence of secretory granules, and the steroid hormones are released by diffusion through the plasma membrane without use of the exocytotic process used by most glands, including the adrenal medulla. The cells of the adrenal medulla (**D**) may be considered as modified postganglionic sympathetic neurons. Adrenal medullary cells synthesize and secrete norepinephrine, epinephrine, and enkephalins in response to stimulation of preganglionic sympathetic fibers that travel through the abdomen in the splanchnic nerves and innervate the gland. The adrenal cortical hormones are viewed as essential for life because of their regulation of metabolism.

The adrenal hormones are listed in the table below.

Zone	Secretion	Target	Regulatory Factors
Zona glomerulosa	Mineralocorticoids (aldosterone)	Collecting tubules	Angiotensin II
Zona fasciculata	Glucocorticoids (cortisol, hydro-cortisone) and weak androgens	Gluconeogenesis by the liver	ACTH (adrenocortico-tropic hormone)
Zona reticularis	Glucocorticoids and weak androgens	Androgens are precursors of estradiol in the fetus	ACTH
Medulla	Norepinephrine and epinephrine	Preparation for "flight or fight"	Preganglionic sympathetic fibers from the splanchnic nerves

232. The answer is c. *(Young, pp 309–314. Moore and Persaud, Developing, pp 445–448. Junqueira, pp 392–399. Sadler, pp 300–301.)* The region of the pituitary labeled C is the pars distalis, which contains corticotrophs, thyrotrophs, lactotrophs, and gonadotrophs that synthesize trophic hormones which regulate other endocrine organs. The anterior pituitary is unique in that it depends on the presence of the hypothalamo-hypophyseal portal system. Releasing and inhibitory factors are transported from the cell bodies in the hypothalamus along axons into the median eminence, where the secretion is released into a primary capillary plexus. The hypothalamo-hypophyseal portal system carries blood from the primary plexus to the secondary plexus, which comprises the sinusoids of the pars distalis. This system brings the hypothalamic hormones into close proximity with the appropriate cell types in the pars distalis. For example, CTH-RF (corticotropin-releasing factor, CRH) is synthesized in the hypothalamus, released into the primary capillary plexus in the median eminence, and subsequently carried in the portal system to the secondary capillary plexus, where it interacts with corticotrophs in the pars distalis. The pars nervosa is the neurally connected portion of the pituitary and contains the dilated axons of hypothalamic cell bodies that produce vasopressin and oxytocin.

The region labeled **A** is the posterior pituitary that stores oxytocin and vasopressin in dilated axonal terminals. Overall, the pituitary is derived from the ectoderm of the oral cavity (Rathke's pouch) and the floor of the diencephalon. The anterior **(C)** and intermediate **(H)** lobes and pars tuberalis **(G)** are derived from the oral cavity, whereas the remainder of the pituitary [pars nervosa **(A)** and the pituitary stalk **(D)**] is derived from a neuroepithelial origin. The cleft of Rathke's pouch **(B)** represents the lumen of the structure formed originally from the oral cavity. The pars distalis **(C)** contains acidophils and basophils regulated by stimulatory and inhibitory hormones produced by the hypothalamus. In the pars nervosa **(A)**, the major cell type present is the pituicyte, a supportive glial cell. Axons that originate in the supraoptic and paraventricular nuclei of the hypothalamus descend into the pars nervosa. Oxytocin (regulating the milk ejection reflex) and vasopressin [(AVP) also known as antidiuretic hormone (ADH) regulates collecting duct permeability] are stored in dilated endings in the pars nervosa called Herring bodies. Those secretions are, therefore, synthesized in the hypothalamus and stored in the pars nervosa. Structure **E** is the median eminence; F represents the cavity of the third ventricle.

233. The answer is a. (*Kasper, pp 2109–2111. Greenspan, pp 81, 91–92, 257–258. Kierszenbaum, p 504. Kumar, pp 1169–1171.*) The patient is suffering from Hashimoto's thyroiditis in which there is extensive infiltration of the thyroid gland. Autoantibodies develop to thyroglobulin and thyroid peroxidase, an iodine transporter and/or the TSH receptor. In cases where there are autoantibodies to TSH receptor, the TSH receptor activity is blocked, resulting in hypothyroidism compared to the hyperthyroidism, which occurs in Graves' disease (see question 227). The antibodies are to a different site on the receptor, resulting in the different overall effect. $CD8^+$ T cells are also directed against that site. T3 and T4 levels may be elevated early in the disease **(answer b)** process due to disruption of the follicles and release of hormones; however, the overall effect is hypothyroidism. Destruction of thyroid hormone receptors **(answer c)** would lead to hyperthyroidism. Calcitonin is secreted by the C cells in the thyroid and is not affected by the thyroiditis **(answer d)**. Glucocorticoid levels are not elevated **(answer e)**.

234. The answer is b. (*Kasper, pp 2104–2107. Kumar, p 1165.*) T4 (thyroxine) is the primary serum thyroid hormone and is produced only by the thyroid gland. In contrast, only about 20% of T_3 (triiodothyronine) is produced by the thyroid gland. T3 is formed in the liver and kidney by the action of a specific enzyme, 5'-deiodinase enzyme that converts T_4 to T_3. That enzyme also converts T4 to metabolically inactive thyroid hormone, rT_3 (reverse T_3). T_3 is three to five times more physiologically active than T_4. Both T_4 and T_3 are bound to thyroxine-binding globulin (TBG), transthyretin, and albumin **(answer a)**, with only about 1% of free circulating hormone. Levels of available binding proteins affect measurable levels of total T_4 and T_3. When those binding proteins are found in high concentrations, total T_4 and T_3 levels are also high, but free T4 and T3 values remain normal. The free fractions of T_4 and T_3 are responsible for the feedback mechanism at the level of the hypothalamus and the thyrotrophs in the anterior pituitary. T_3 and T_4 are regulated by TSH from the thyrotrophs **(answers c and d)**. There is some cross-reactivity of all immunoassays **(answer e)**, but that is not the reason for the possible inaccuracy of extrapolating from serum T_3 levels to thyroid function.

Reproductive Systems

Questions

DIRECTIONS: Each item below contains a question or incomplete statement followed by suggested responses. Select the **one best** response to each question.

235. Elevated estrogen levels during the menstrual cycle result in which of the following?

a. Decrease LH levels
b. Downregulate FSH receptors on granulosa cells
c. Increase FSH levels
d. Increase the ciliation of the epithelial cells of the oviduct
e. Decrease synthesis and storage of glycogen in the vaginal epithelium

236. A patient biopsy is reviewed by a pathologist. She diagnoses the tumor as originating from the cells delineated with the star. The tumor would most likely produce which of the following?

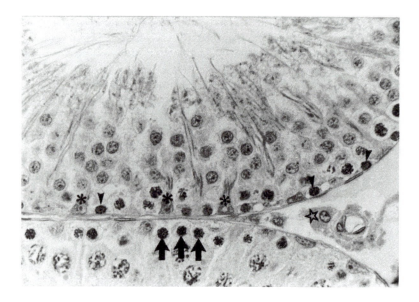

a. Calcitonin
b. Progesterone
c. Androgens
d. FSH
e. Parathyroid hormone

237. The structure or structures labeled B in the photomicrograph from the reproductive system below is which of the following?

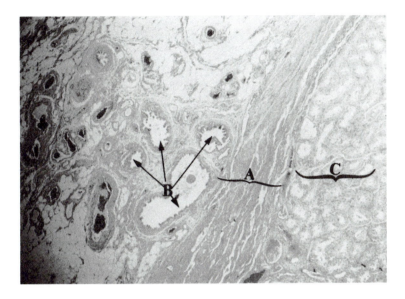

a. Rete testis
b. Efferent ductules
c. Seminiferous tubules
d. Vas deferens
e. Oviduct

238. The function of the organ shown in the photomicrograph below is which of the following?

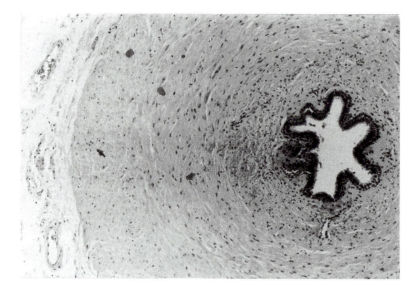

a. Passage of urine and sperm in the male
b. Passage of urine from the urethra to the vestibule in the female
c. Passage of urine from the bladder to the urethrae in males and females
d. Passage of sperm from the epididymis to the urethra
e. Storage of sperm and absorption of fluid

239. What organ is pictured below?

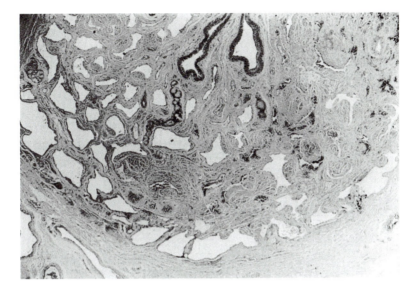

a. Female urethra
b. Male urethra
c. Oviduct
d. Ureter
e. Seminal vesicle

240. Malignancies most frequently arise from which portion of the organ shown in the photomicrograph below?

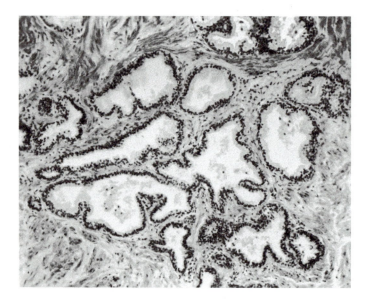

a. Lactiferous duct
b. Periurethral glands
c. Outer peripheral glands
d. Germ cells
e. Mammary alveoli

241. Naturally occurring, nonpathologic cervical eversions ("erosions") are usually naturally corrected by reepithelialization. These eversions are most prevalent in which one of the following reproductive classifications of women?

a. Prepubertal female
b. Postpubertal, premenopausal, nulliparous female
c. Premenopausal, multiparous female
d. Menopausal, nulliparous female
e. Late postmenopausal female

242. The organ shown in this photomicrograph is responsible for production of which of the following?

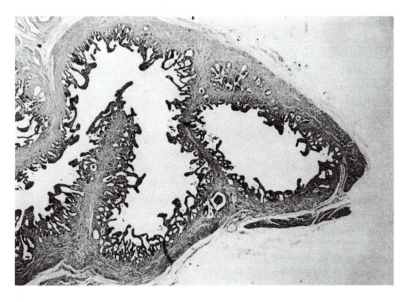

a. Spermine and fibrolysin
b. T3 and T4
c. Proteins that coagulate semen
d. Acid phosphatase
e. Milk

243. The organ in the photomicrograph performs which of the following functions?

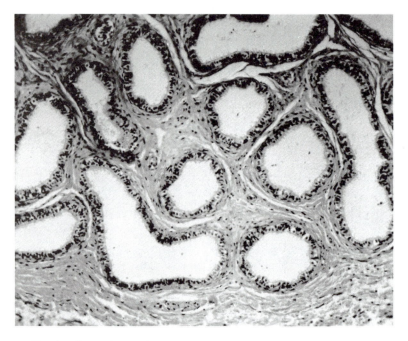

a. The site of spermiogenesis
b. Production of fructose and prostaglandins
c. Phagocytosis of sperm
d. The site of implantation
e. The site of milk production

244. Which of the following is independent of testosterone or other androgens?

a. Secretion from the prostatic epithelium
b. The function of the prostatic glands
c. Development of the penis from an indifferent phallus
d. Spermatogenesis
e. Fetal testis development from an indifferent gonad

245. A 26-year-old woman is in her last trimester of a normal pregnancy. Synthesis of milk by her mammary glands specifically requires which of the following?

a. Oxytocin from the neurohypophysis
b. Prolactin from the corpus luteum
c. The influence of vasopressin
d. Placental lactogen
e. Neurohumoral reflexes

246. The urologist may describe the reattachment of a severed vas deferens (vasovasostomy) as successful, more than 90% of the time. However, it is unsuccessful from the patients' point of view since a much lower percentage of these men can father a child. The difference in success rate is due to which of the following?

a. Spermatogonia are exposed to humoral factors
b. Genetic recombination in haploid sperm creates novel antigens
c. Cryptorchid testes are often incapable of producing fertile sperm
d. Vasectomy prevents phagocytosis of sperm by macrophages
e. Sperm coated with autoimmune antibodies are unable to fertilize an egg

247. A 29-year-old woman is trying to become pregnant. She presents with irregular menstrual cycles and heavy, prolonged, irregular uterine bleeding and undergoes an endometrial biopsy. The biopsy has the appearance shown in the photomicrograph below. Which of the following is characteristic of this stage of the menstrual cycle?

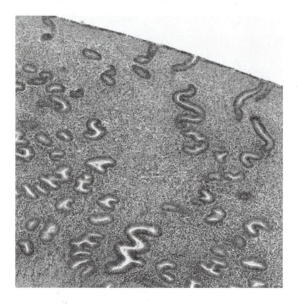

a. It precedes ovulation
b. It depends on progesterone secretion by the corpus luteum
c. It coincides with the development of ovarian follicles
d. It coincides with a rapid drop in estrogen levels
e. It produces ischemia and necrosis of the stratum functionale

248. The low pH in the vagina is maintained by which of the following?

a. A proton pump similar to that of parietal cells and osteoclasts
b. Acid secretion derived from intracellular carbonic acid
c. Secretion of lactic acid by the stratified squamous epithelium
d. Bacterial metabolism of glycogen to form lactic acid
e. Synthesis and accumulation of acid hydrolases in the epithelium

249. A 33-year-old woman with an average menstrual cycle of 28 days comes in for a routine Pap smear. It has been 35 days since the start of her last menstrual period, and a vaginal smear reveals clumps of basophilic cells. As her physician, you suspect which of the following?

a. She will begin menstruating in a few days
b. She will ovulate within a few days
c. Her serum progesterone levels are very low
d. There are detectable levels of hCG in her serum and urine
e. She is undergoing menopause

250. If the hormone necessary for maintenance of this structure in the photomicrograph below were absent 12 to 14 days after ovulation in a human female, which of the following would be the result?

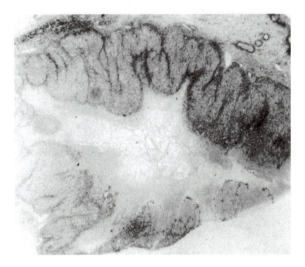

a. The absence of the structure
b. The absence of muscularization
c. Maintenance of the uterine epithelium for implantation beyond 14 days after ovulation
d. Pregnancy
e. The formation of a corpus albicans from the structure

251. The accompanying diagram shows a cross section of a developing human endometrium and myometrium. Hormonal ratios control the development of which of the labeled vessels?

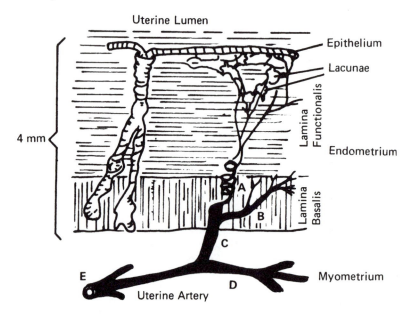

a. A
b. B
c. C
d. D
e. E

252. Cells in the layers labeled A and C in the figure below secrete plasminogen activator and collagenase that is required for which of the following?

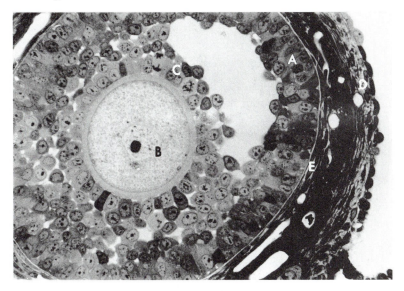

a. Dissolution of the zona pellucida to facilitate sperm penetration
b. pH regulation within the antral cavity
c. Breakdown of the basement membrane between the thecal and granulosa layers, facilitating ovulation
d. Diffusion of androgens between the thecal and granulosa cells
e. Facilitation of follicular atresia through breakdown of the basement membrane between the theca interna and externa

253. Secretions from the organ shown below carry out which of the following functions?

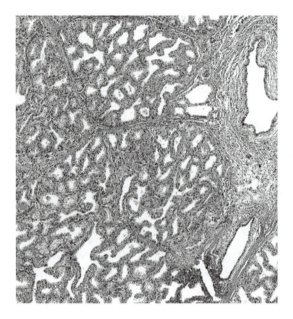

a. Regulation of metabolism
b. Transfer of maternal antibodies to the suckling neonate
c. Removal of waste products during gestation
d. Facilitate clotting of ejaculated semen in the female
e. Enhancement of sperm function

Reproductive Systems

Answers

235. The answer is d. *(Junqueira, pp 427–428. Guyton, pp 930–933. Kierszenbaum, pp 571–573.)* Estrogen levels increase during the maturation of ovarian follicles, which results in a concomitant increase in ciliation and height of the oviductal lining cells. Increases in the number of cilia serve to facilitate movement of the ovum. Increased estrogen levels also decrease FSH levels and cause an LH surge **(answers a and c)**. Elevated estrogen levels result in increased secretion of lytic enzymes, prostaglandins, plasminogen activator, and collagenase to facilitate the rupture of the ovarian wall and the release of the ovum and the attached corona radiata. Following ovulation, during the luteal phase of the cycle, the theca and granulosa cells are transformed into the corpus luteum under the influence of LH. Ovulation occurs near the middle of the menstrual cycle and is associated with an increase in basal body temperature that appears to be indirectly regulated by elevated estrogen levels, with IL-1 functioning as the endogenous pyrogen. Estrogen also upregulates FSH receptors on granulosa cell membranes and enhances synthesis and storage of glycogen in the vaginal epithelium **(answers b and e)**.

236. The answers is c. *(Young, pp 329–331. Junqueira, pp 420, 427.)* The cell marked with a star is a Leydig cell (i.e., interstitial cell) and is regulated by luteinizing hormone (LH), formerly known as interstitial cell–stimulating hormone (ICSH), secreted by gonadotrophs in the anterior pituitary. Leydig cells are located between seminiferous tubules and are responsible for the production of testosterone. The star delineates a cluster of Leydig cells, found between the seminiferous tubules. The Leydig cells normally synthesize and release testosterone in response to LH that is produced by gonadotrophs in the anterior pituitary. Leydig cell tumors develop in males between 20 and 60 years of age and produce androgens, estrogens, and sometimes glucocorticoids. Calcitonin is synthesized by C cells in the thyroid **(answer a)**. Progesterone **(answer b)** is synthesized by corpora lutea under the influence of LH. FSH (follicle- stimulating hormone) plays a key physiological role in both males (spermatogenesis) and females (regulation of follicular growth) and is produced and released by gonadotrophs in the anterior pituitary **(answer d)**. FSH stimulates the maturation of ovarian follicles. FSH treatment of humans results in development of more than the usual number of mature follicles and an increased number of mature gametes. FSH is also critical for sperm production. It supports the function of Sertoli cells, which serve a nutritive role in sperm cell maturation. Parathyroid hormone (**answer e**) is synthesized and released from the principal cells of the parathyroid gland.

Sertoli cells (asterisks, *) function in a nutritive and supportive role somewhat analogous to the glial cells of the CNS. The Sertoli cells produce inhibin, which feeds back on the anterior pituitary and hypothalamus to regulate FSH release. Testosterone binds to androgen-binding protein (ABP), which is synthesized by the Sertoli cells. Testosterone is necessary for maintenance of spermatogenesis as well as the male ducts and accessory glands. ABP is regulated by FSH, testosterone, and inhibin. Sertoli cells have extensive tight (occluding) junctions between them that form the blood-testis barrier. Sertoli cells communicate with adjacent cells through gap junctions and extend from outside the blood-testis barrier (basal portion) to luminal (apical portion). During spermatogenesis, preleptotene spermatocytes cross from the basal to the adluminal compartment across the zonula occludens between adjacent Sertoli cells. Each Sertoli cell is, therefore, associated with multiple spermatogenic cells.

The testis is composed of seminiferous tubules containing a number of spermatogenic cells undergoing spermatogenesis and spermiogenesis. The cells labeled with the arrowheads are spermatogonia, the derivatives of the embryonic primordial germ cells. These cells comprise the basal layer and undergo mitosis (spermatocytogenesis) to form primary spermatocytes, which have distinctive clumped or coarse chromatin (marked by arrows). Secondary spermatocytes are formed during the first meiotic division and exist for only a short period of time because there is no lag period before entry into the second meiotic division that results in the formation of spermatids. The spermatids begin as round structures and elongate with the formation of the flagellum. This last part of seminiferous tubule function is the differentiation of sperm from spermatids (spermiogenesis) and is complete with the release of mature sperm into the lumen of the tubule.

237. The answer is b. (*Young, pp 329, 335.*) The photomicrograph is taken from an area that shows the ductuli efferentes (efferent ductules) (**B**) with their distinctive wavy epithelium in which adjoining cells are tall (ciliated) and short (nonciliated). Also shown are the seminiferous tubules **(C)** and the mediastinum testis containing the rete testis **(A)**. Sperm leave the seminiferous tubules through short tubuli recti into the straight tubules of the rete testis, which subsequently drain into the efferent ductules. For the vas deferens, see answer to question 238.

238. The answer is d. *(Young, p 336. Junqueira, pp 429–430.)* The organ shown in the figure is the vas deferens (ductus deferens). The vas deferens conducts sperm from the epididymis to the urethra. The thick muscular wall is unique in the presence of an inner longitudinal, a middle circular, and an outer longitudinal layer of smooth muscle. The ureter has two thin layers of muscle: inner longitudinal and outer circular **(answer c)**. The male and female urethra contain extensive vascular channels **(answers a and b)**. The epididymis consists of a connective tissue stroma and stores sperm, resorbs fluid, and produces sperm maturation factors **(answer e)**.

239. The answer is b. *(Young, pp 339–340. Junqueira, p 433.)* The photomicrograph shows the histology of the male (penile) urethra. It possesses a primarily pseudostratified columnar type of epithelium. The glands of Littré that produce mucus are also observed in the section. The thick-walled arteries of the penile and cavernous sinuses of penile erectile tissue are also a distinguishing feature of this organ. Helicine arteries supply the sinuses. Action of the parasympathetic nervous system mediates the dilation of these vessels during erection.

240. The answer is c. *(Young, pp 337–339. Junqueira, pp 429–431. Kasper, pp 1025–1033.)* The photomicrograph is from the prostate. Seventy percent of carcinomas of the prostate arise from the main (external gland), also known as the outer (peripheral) glands **(answer b)**. The prostate consists of three parts: (1) a small mucosal (inner periurethral) gland, (2) a transition zone that consists of a submucosal (outer periurethral) gland, and (3) a peripheral portion known as the main, or external, gland. Because of the peripheral location, most prostatic carcinomas (primarily adenocarcinomas) remain undiagnosed until the later symptoms of back pain or blockage of the urethra are detected. Digital rectal examination can identify some tumors earlier. Benign prostatic hypertrophy, also known as benign nodular hyperplasia, occurs in the mucosal and submucosal glands, which are rarely sites of carcinoma. Benign hyperplasia causes urethral obstruction in its early stages because of its location in the mucosal and submucosal glands surrounding the urethra. The main gland is sensitive to androgens, whereas the periurethral glands are sensitive to androgens and estrogens. Acid phosphatase and prostatic-specific antigen (PSA) levels are used in the diagnosis of prostatic carcinoma and its metastasis.

Carcinoma of the breast occurs in about 1 of 10 females in the United States. By definition, a carcinoma is ductal in origin (**answers a and e**). Carcinoma of the breast metastasizes to the brain, lungs, and bones. The easy access of tumor cells to the extensive axillary blood supply and lymphatic drainage facilitates the spread of the cancer into the blood and lymph supplies. Self-examination and mammography are urged in an attempt to increase early diagnosis, which has reduced mortality of this disease.

Germ cell tumors (**answer d**) of the testes (testicular neoplasms) are classified as seminomas (germinomas) of pure germ cells and more heterogeneous cell types (e.g., teratomas and embryonal carcinomas).

241. The answer is c. (*Rubin, pp 942–943.*) To a minor extent, the uterine cervical stroma changes during each reproductive cycle; however, during pregnancy (especially parturition) there is a thinning of the uterine stroma. This results in eversions (mistakenly called "erosions"), which are sites of exposed uterine columnar epithelium in the acidic, vaginal milieu. These sites often become reepithelialized as stratified epithelium (squamous metaplasia) and are believed to be the location of cancerous transformation in the cervix. As part of the process of reepithelialization, the openings of cervical mucous glands are obliterated, which results in the formation of nabothian cysts.

242. The answer is c. (*Young, pp 337–339. Junqueira, pp 429, 431.*) The organ shown in the light micrograph is the seminal vesicle that produces fructose, ascorbic acid, prostaglandins, and proteins responsible for semen coagulation. The seminal vesicle produces about 50% of the seminal fluid on a volume basis and comprises most of the ejaculate. The wall consists of smooth muscle and the mucosa of anastomosing "villus-like" folds. In comparison, the prostate (**answers a and d**) is composed of 15 to 30 tubuloalveolar glands surrounded by fibromuscular tissue with concretions in the lumina. The prostate secretes a thin, opalescent fluid that contributes primarily to the first part of the ejaculate and includes acid phosphatase, spermine (a polyamine), fibrolysin, amylase, and zinc. Spermine oxidation results in the musky odor of semen, and fibrolysin is responsible for the liquefaction of semen after ejaculation. Acid phosphatase and prostatic-specific antigen are important for the diagnosis of metastases. The thyroid synthesizes T_3 and T_4 **(answer b)**; the lactating mammary gland produces milk **(answer e)**.

243. The answer is c. *(Young, pp 329, 336, 341, 357, 368–371. Junqueira, pp 429, 430.)* The figure is a light micrograph of the epididymis which functions in the storage, maturation, and phagocytosis of sperm. In addition, the epididymis is involved in the absorption of testicular fluid and the secretion of glycoproteins involved in the inhibition of capacitation. The epithelium of the epididymis is pseudostratified with stereocilia (long microvilli), and the wall contains extensive connective tissue. The seminal vesicle **(answer b)** produces fructose and prostaglandins and contains a thick smooth muscle layer. Sperm are often found in the lumina. Spermiogenesis occurs in the testes **(answer a)**. Milk production occurs in the mammary gland **(answer e)**, which contains alveoli and lactiferous ducts. Implantation occurs in the uterus **(answer d)**, which is lined by a simple columnar epithelium with endometrial glands that differ in arrangement, depending on the phase of the cycle (long and straight in the proliferative phases and S-shaped in the secretory phase). The myometrium, composed of smooth muscle, is hormone-sensitive and undergoes both hypertrophy and hyperplasia during pregnancy and atrophy after menopause, resulting in a shrinking of the uterus in postmenopausal women.

244. The answer is e. *(Kierszenbaum, p 533. Junqueira, pp 426–427. Sadler, pp 240–242. Moore and Persaud, pp 325–326.)* The development of the testis from an indifferent gonad depends on the presence of the testis-determining factor, a gene on the short arm of the Y chromosome. During fetal development, the production of androgens by the developing testis results in masculinization of the indifferent gonadal ducts and the indifferent genitalia **(answer c)**. In the absence of androgens, female genitalia and female ducts (vagina, oviducts, and uterus) develop. In the mature male, testosterone is required for the initiation and maintenance of spermatogenesis as well as the structural and functional integrity of the accessory glands and ducts of the male reproductive system (**answers a, b and d**). Testosterone is bound to androgen-binding protein (ABP), which is synthesized by the Sertoli cells under the influence of follicle-stimulating hormone (FSH). ABP is important for both the storage and delivery of androgens in the male ducts and accessory glands.

245. The answer is d. *(Junqueira, pp 453–454. Kierszenbaum, pp 490, 601–605. Strauss and Barbieri, pp 307–310.)* The mammary gland enlarges during pregnancy in response to several hormones, including prolactin synthesized by the anterior pituitary [*not* by the corpus luteum (**answer b**)], estrogen and progesterone synthesized by the corpus luteum, and placental lactogen. The alveoli at the end of the duct system respond to those hormones by cell proliferation, which increases the size of the mammary glands. Growth continues throughout pregnancy; however, secretion is most notable late in pregnancy. Milk is synthesized in the alveoli and is stored in their lumina before passage through the lactiferous ducts to the nipples. Secretion of milk lipids occurs by an apocrine mechanism whereby some apical cytoplasm is included with the secretory product. In comparison, milk proteins, such as the caseins, are secreted by exocytosis. Oxytocin is required for the release of milk from the mammary gland through the action of the myoepithelial cells that surround the alveoli and proximal (closer to the alveolus) portions of the duct system. Oxytocin is not required for milk synthesis (**answer a**). Arginine Vasopressin [AVP, Antidiuretic hormone (ADH)] binds to receptors in the collecting tubules of the kidney and promotes resorption of water into the circulation (**answer c**). AVP stimulates water resorption by stimulating insertion of aquaporins (water channels) into the membranes of kidney tubules. These channels transport solute-free water through collecting duct cells and into blood, leading to a decrease in plasma osmolarity and an increase osmolarity of urine. Neurohumoral reflexes are involved in the suckling-milk ejection response (**answer e**).

246. The answer is e. *(Kasper, p 281.)* Attempts to counteract or repair the effects of a vasectomy (vasovasostomy) are often unsuccessful because of the development of antisperm antibodies. This lack of success occurs despite the fact that 90% of the patients undergoing vasovasostomy have sperm return to the ejaculate. In the case of vasectomy, sperm that have leaked from the male reproductive tract are viewed as foreign by immune surveillance and antibodies develop. The phagocytosis of sperm by macrophages plays a role in the development of antisperm antibodies that occurs following the ligation or removal of a segment of the vas deferens **(answer d)**. Sperm are immunologically foreign because of a number of factors.

Spermatogenesis begins at puberty long after the development of self-recognition in the immune system **(answer b)**. The blood-testis barrier protects developing sperm from exposure to systemic factors **(answer a)**. The basal compartment containing the spermatogonia and preleptotene spermatocytes is exposed to plasma; however, the adluminal compartment, which contains primary and secondary spermatocytes, spermatids, and testicular sperm, prevents these antigens from entering the blood. The inability of cryptorchid testes to produce fertile sperm is related to the higher temperature in the abdomen than in the normal scrotal location **(answer c)**.

247. The answer is b. (*Ross and Pawlina, p 787. Young, pp 341, 351–355. Junqueira, pp 444–451. Kierszenbaum, p 578.*) The secretory phase of the menstrual cycle depends on progesterone secretion and follows the proliferative (follicular) phase. The menstrual phase occurs after the secretory phase. During the follicular phase (approximately days 4 to 16), estrogen produced by the ovaries drives cell proliferation in the base of endometrial glands and the uterine stroma. The proliferative phase culminates with ovulation. The secretory phase (approximately days 16 to 25) is characterized by high progesterone levels from the corpus luteum, a tortuous appearance of the uterine glands, and apocrine secretion by the gland cells. During this phase, maximum endometrial thickness occurs. The menstrual phase (approximately days 26 to 30) is characterized by decreased glandular secretion and eventual glandular degeneration because of decreased production of both progesterone and estrogen by the theca lutein cells. Contraction of coiled arteries and arterioles leads to ischemia and necrosis of the stratum functionale. The events of the menstrual cycle are shown in the figure on the next page.

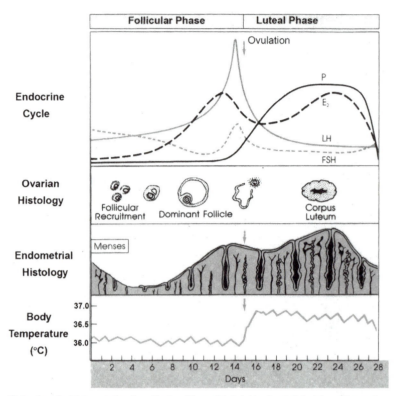

(*Reproduced, with permission, from Kasper DL, et al (eds.). Harrison's Principles of Internal Medicine, 16th ed. New York, NY: McGraw-Hill, 2005: 2201.*)

248. The answer is d. (*Young, pp 341, 359. Junqueira, pp 449, 459, 463–464. Kierszenbaum, p 582.*) The low (4.0) pH of the vagina is maintained by bacterial metabolism of glycogen to form lactic acid. The vagina is characterized by a stratified squamous epithelium that contains large accumulations of glycogen. Glycogen is released into the vaginal lumen and is subsequently metabolized to lactic acid by commensal lactobacilli. The low pH inhibits growth of a variety of microorganisms, but not sexually transmitted pathogens, such as Trichomonas vaginalis. Treatment for vaginal infections usually includes acidified carriers to reestablish a more acidic pH like that usually seen in mid-menstrual cycle.

249. The answer is d. *(Young, p 358. Junqueira, p 451. Strauss and Barbieri, pp 262–270.)* The patient described in this question is probably pregnant. The delay in menstruation coupled with the presence of basophilic cells in a vaginal smear are clues. Ovulation is the midpoint of the cycle and should be more than a few days away **(answers a and b)**. She is relatively young for the onset of menopause and there are no other symptoms **(answer e)**. The vaginal epithelium varies little with the normal menstrual cycle. Exfoliative cytology can be used to diagnose cancer and to determine if the epithelium is under stimulation of estrogen and progesterone. The presence of basophilic cells in the smear with the Pap-staining method would indicate the presence of both estrogen and progesterone **(answer c)**. The data suggest the maintenance of the corpus luteum (i.e., pregnancy).

250. The answer is e. *(Ross and pawlina, pp 781–782. Young, pp 347, 352. Junqueira, pp 439–440. Kierszenbaum, p 572.)* The structure in the photomicrograph is a corpus luteum. In the absence of the hormones necessary for maintenance of the corpus luteum [luteinizing hormone (LH) or human chorionic gonadotropin (hCG)], the corpus luteum regresses to form a corpus albicans, which consists primarily of fibrous connective tissue. Without LH or hCG, the uterine epithelium, which has undergone glandular proliferation in preparation for implantation, collapses and degenerates as part of menstruation. The corpus luteum forms from the granulosa and theca layers of the follicle following ovulation. The luteal phase is the second half of the menstrual period and follows the follicular phase during which follicles mature. The corpus luteum synthesizes progesterone in response to high LH levels. In each reproductive cycle, the production of LH stimulates development and maintenance of the corpus luteum, which is well formed by 12 to 14 days following ovulation. In the case of fertilization and subsequent implantation, the corpus luteum of pregnancy is maintained by human chorionic gonadotropin (hCG) produced by the embryo.

251. The answer is a. *(Young, pp 349–352. Ross and Pawlina, p 791. Junqueira, pp 444–446.)* The spiral arteries of the endometrium (labeled **A** in the diagram accompanying the question) depend on specific estrogen/progesterone ratios for their development. They pass through the basalis layer of the endometrium into the functional zone, and their distal ends are subject to degeneration with each menses. The straight arteries **(B)** are not subject to these hormonal changes. In the proliferative phase, the endometrium is only

1- to 3-mm thick, and the glands are straight, with the spiral arteries only slightly coiled. This diagram of the early secretory phase shows an edematous endometrium that is 4-mm thick, with glands that are large, beginning to sacculate in the deeper mucosa, and coiled for their entire length. In the late secretory phase, the endometrium becomes 6- to 7-mm thick.

252. The answer is c. (*Young, pp 342–346, 352. Kierszenbaum, pp 565–568, 570. Junqueira, pp 436–439.*) The cells labeled **A** and **C** in the photomicrograph of the Graafian follicle are granulosa cells that produce plasminogen activator and collagenase. Those molecules, along with plasmin and prostaglandins, facilitate the rupture of the ovarian follicle, leading to ovulation. The increase in LH in midcycle induces production of collagenase and plasminogen activator. Those proteases facilitate ovulation by initiating connective tissue remodeling, including the breakdown of the basement membrane between thecal and granulosa layers. Connective tissue remodeling is involved in the process of follicular atresia. This process occurs throughout life and involves the death of follicular cells as well as oocytes, but there is no basement membrane between the theca interna and externa. In fact, there is an absence of a clear delineation between the theca interna and externa. Development of ovarian follicles begins with a primordial follicle that consists of flattened follicular cells surrounding a primary oocyte. During the follicular phase, those cells undergo mitosis to form multiple granulosa layers (primary follicle) in response to elevated levels of FSH and LH from the anterior pituitary. A glycoproteinaceous coat surrounds the oocyte and is called the zona pellucida. The connective tissue around the follicle differentiates into two layers: theca externa (**D**) and theca interna (**E**). The theca externa is closest to the ovarian stroma and consists of a highly vascular connective tissue. The theca interna synthesizes androgens (e.g., androstenedione) in response to LH. Androgens are converted to estradiol by the action of an aromatase enzyme synthesized by the granulosa cells under the influence of FSH. Increased levels of estrogen from the ovary feed back to decrease FSH secretion from gonadotrophs in the anterior pituitary. *Liquor folliculi* is produced by the granulosa cells and is secreted between the cells. When cavities are first formed by the development of follicular fluid between the cells, the follicle is called secondary. When the antrum is completely formed, the follicle is called a mature (Graafian) follicle, and the antrum is completely filled with liquor folliculi. The granulosa cells form two structures. The corona radiata (**C**) represents those granulosa cells that remain attached to the zona pellucida. The cumulus oophorus (*not* labeled) represents those granulosa cells that surround the oocyte (**B**) and connect it to the wall. Structure **A** is the membrana granulosa.

253. The answer is b. (*Kumar, pp 1120–1121. Junqueira, pp 452–453.*) Lactating mammary gland is shown in the photomicrograph. It synthesizes milk including antibodies from IgA secreting plasma cells in the connective tissue of the gland. The lactating mammary gland differs histologically from the thyroid gland (**answer a**) in the presence of lactiferous ducts for exocrine secretion compared to the endocrine secretion of the thyroid. The placenta removes waste products during gestation (**answer c**); secretions from the seminal vesicle [fructose, prostaglandins and other proteins, (**answer d**)] facilitate clotting of ejaculated semen; and prostatic secretions (zinc, citric acid, antibiotic-like molecules, and enzymes) enhance sperm function (**answer e**).

Urinary System

Questions

DIRECTIONS: Each item below contains a question or incomplete statement followed by suggested responses. Select the **one best** response to each question.

254. Acetazolamide, a member of the sulfonamide family of antibacterial drugs, blocks carbonic anhydrase activity. Which of the following would most likely occur after treatment with acetazolamide?

a. Metabolic alkalosis
b. Increased excretion of hydrogen ions from the kidney
c. Decreased bicarbonate in the pancreatic juice
d. Increased bone resorption
e. Increased acid production by parietal cells

255. In the accompanying transmission electron micrograph of the renal corpuscle, which of the following is the function of the cell marked with an asterisk?

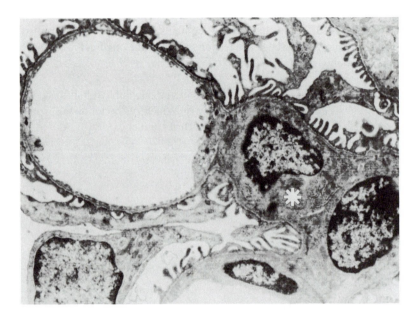

a. Synthesizes extracellular matrix for support of the capillary wall
b. Exerts an antithrombogenic effect
c. Forms the visceral layer of Bowman's capsule
d. Separates the urinary space and the blood in the capillaries
e. Forms the filtration slits through the interdigitations of the pedicels

256. A 15-year-old boy presents with hematuria, hearing loss, lens dislocation, and cataracts. Genetic analysis shows a mutation of the COL4A5 gene. A renal biopsy is performed. In which area labeled A–E on the accompanying electron micrograph would you expect to see the primary site of damage?

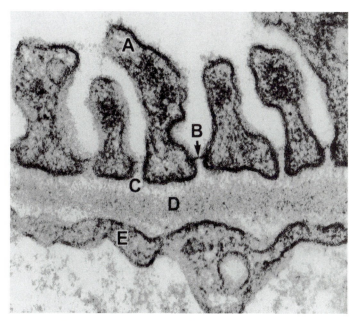

(Electron micrograph courtesy of Dr. Dale R. Abrahamson.)

a. Area A
b. Area B
c. Area C
d. Area D
e. Area E

257. A 14-year-old girl presents in the pediatric nephrology clinic with fatigue, malaise, anorexia, abdominal pain, and fever. She reports a loss of 6 lb in the last 2 months. Serum gamma globulin as well as the immunoglobulins: IgG, IgA, and IgM are all elevated. She is diagnosed with bilateral photophobia as a result of nongranulomatous uveitis. Her serum creatinine is 1.4 mg/dL (normal: 0.6 to 1.2 mg/dL) and urinalysis of glucose and protein are 2⁺ on dipstick test and are confirmed by the laboratory at 8.0 g/dL and 0.95 g/dL, respectively. A renal biopsy is prepared for light and electron microscopy. Lymphocytes, plasma cells, and eosinophils are found within infiltrates with pathological change in the tubular basement membrane. The cell most affected is shown in the accompanying transmission electron micrograph. Which of the following is a correct statement about this cell?

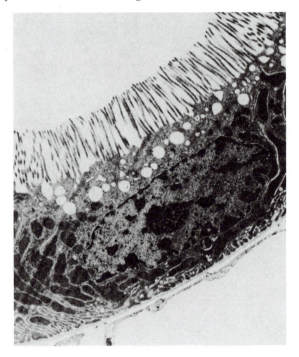

a. Impermeable to water despite the presence of ADH
b. The site of the countercurrent multiplier
c. The site of action of aldosterone
d. The source of renin
e. The primary site for the reduction of the tubular fluid volume

258. The arrows in the accompanying scanning electron micrograph of the renal glomerulus indicate which of the following?

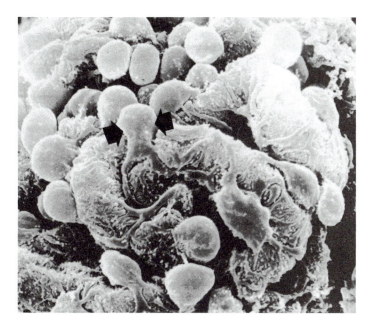

a. A red blood cell
b. A podocyte
c. An endothelial cell
d. A parietal cell
e. The macula densa

259. In a patient with diabetes mellitus of 30 years' duration, complications related to kidney function may include which of the following?

a. Enhanced selectivity of the filtration barrier
b. Decreased permeability to plasma proteins
c. Increased glomerular filtration rate
d. Decreased secretion of aldosterone
e. Glycation of proteins in the basal lamina

260. Which of the following is found exclusively in the renal medulla?

a. Proximal convoluted tubules
b. Distal convoluted tubules
c. Collecting ducts
d. Afferent arterioles
e. Thin loops of Henle

Urinary System

Answers

254. The answer is c. *(Kierszenbaum, pp 124, 389, 413, 456. Junqueira, pp 294, 296, 353.)* Carbonic anhydrase is a critical enzyme that plays an essential role in a number of cells by catalyzing the hydration of carbon dioxide and the dehydration of bicarbonate. In the pancreas, blocking carbonic anhydrase results in a reduction in secretion of bicarbonate into the pancreatic juice by the pancreatic duct cells. Blockage of carbonic anhydrase results in metabolic acidosis not alkalosis **(answer a)** because of the decrease in renal tubular excretion of hydrogen ions from the kidney **(answer b)**. In osteoclasts, blockage of carbonic anhydrase would result in decreased bone resorption **(answer d)**. In parietal cells blocking carbonic anhydrase activity results in the reduction in protons moving toward the lumen and bicarbonate toward the blood **(answer e)**.

255. The answer is a. *(Kierszenbaum, pp 375, 377. Junqueira, pp 373–379.)* The cell labeled in the transmission electron micrograph of the renal corpuscle is a mesangial cell that synthesizes extracellular matrix including the basement membrane of the glomerulus for the support of the capillary wall. Mesangial cells are morphologically similar to pericytes found in association with other systemic blood vessels. The mesangial cells surround glomerular capillaries as illustrated in this electron micrograph. Other proposed functions for the mesangial cells include phagocytosis and regulation of glomerular blood flow. Mesangial cells synthesize cyclooxygenase-2 [Cox-2 (a critical enzyme in prostaglandin synthesis)] and nitric oxide and are therefore involved in vasoactive regulation. Like endothelial cells they synthesize endothelin. Endothelial cells are anti-thrombogenic **(answer b)**. An endothelial cell within a glomerular capillary is also shown below the mesangial cell. A podocyte with its processes in close association with the glomerular capillary is observed below the mesangial cell. The podocytes form the visceral layer of the Bowman's capsule **(answer c)** and possess processes that interdigitate to form the pedicels **(answer e)**. The outer layer of the Bowman's capsule is formed by parietal cells, one of which is located in the lower left corner of the micrograph. The urinary space and the blood are separated by the glomerular basement membrane **(answer d)**

formed from the fusion of the capillary and podocyte-produced basal laminae.

256. The answer is d. (*Kierszenbaum, pp 373–375. Junqueira, pp 373–374, 379. Kumar, p 988.*) The genetic mutation in COL4A5 leads to a defect in the α-chains that comprise type IV collagen found in the lamina densa labeled **A** on the electron micrograph of the basement membrane in the accompanying electron micrograph of the basal lamina. The glomerular basement membrane will therefore show abnormal splitting and thinning in the lamina densa and overall thickening. The hematuria results from breakdown of the basal lamina allowing the passage of red blood cells and eventually protein (proteinuria). The patient suffers from Alport's syndrome resulting from a mutation of the α5 chain of type IV collagen. Remember that type IV collagen consists of three alpha chains forming a triple helix. The noncollagenous C-terminal (NC1) and the 7S N-terminal are particularly important for the cross-linking of type IV collagen. The cross-linking forms the scaffolding of the basement membrane necessary for the normal filtration properties of the basal lamina. Proliferation of mesangial cells and increased production of mesangial matrix are typical of later stages of Alport's syndrome when glomerulonephritis is a prominent feature of the disease.

The glomerular filtration barrier consists of the pedicel (**A**) of the podocyte, the basal lamina (**C** = lamina rara, **D** = lamina densa) synthesized by the podocyte, and the endothelial cell (**E**). The podocyte consists of a "cell body" of cytoplasm with long processes that encircle the glomerular basement membrane. The filtration slits are labeled **B**. The filtration slits are located between adjacent pedicels (foot processes of the podocytes). The remainder of the filtration barrier is formed by the glomerular basement membrane, which contains type IV collagen and heparan sulfate. At high magnification there are three distinct layers within the glomerular basement membrane: (1) an electron-dense lamina densa (type IV collagen) in the center surrounded by (2) the lamina rara externa on the glomerular side and by (3) the lamina rara interna on the capillary endothelial side.

The glomerular filtration barrier is a physical and charge barrier that exhibits selectivity based on molecular size and charge. The presence of collagen type IV in the lamina densa of the basement membrane presents a physical barrier to the passage of large proteins from the blood to the urinary space. Glycosaminoglycans, particularly heparan sulfate, produce a polyanionic charge that binds cationic molecules. The foot processes are coated with a glycoprotein called podocalyxin, which is rich in sialic acid and provides mutual repulsion to maintain the structure of the filtration slits. It also possesses a large polyanionic charge for repulsion of large anionic proteins. Patients with a mutation in the gene encoding for nephrin suffer from proteinuria resulting in extensive edema. This syndrome is known as congenital nephritic syndrome. Nephrin is the key protein comprising the slit diaphragm; it functions to inhibit the passage of molecules through the filtration slits. It is an integral membrane protein, which is anchored by other proteins to the cytoskeleton of the pedicel of the podocyte.

257. The answer is e. *(Junqueira, pp 385–386, 392–393. Kumar, pp 996–1004.)* Tubulointerstitial nephritis uveitis (TINU) is an autoimmune disease in which autoantibodies are targeted against the renal tubular cells. The transmission electron micrograph illustrates a proximal convoluted tubule cell, the primary site for reduction of the tubular fluid volume by reabsorption from the glomerular filtrate. The elaborate microvilli at the apical surface and the extensive endocytic vacuoles are "designed" for protein reabsorption and are the distinguishing features of proximal convoluted tubule cells. Numerous mitochondria, within basal folds, provide energy for transport. In the distal tubule, there are very few microvilli.

The afferent arterioles contain the juxtaglomerular cells, modified arterial smooth muscle cells that produce renin **(answer d)**, a major factor in blood pressure regulation. The thin loop of Henle is responsible for the production of the countercurrent multiplier **(answer b)**, which allows the kidneys to produce a hyperosmotic medulla. The multiplier moves Na^+ and Cl^- out of the ascending limb (which is impermeable to water) and into the medullary interstitial fluid. Subsequently, the descending limb, which is permeable to water, takes up the Na^+ and Cl^- from the interstitium. The vasa rectae adjust their osmolarity to that of the medulla.

The distal convoluted tubule (DCT) has the highest concentration of Na^+, K^+-ATPase. The DCT pumps Na^+ against a concentration gradient and is relatively impermeable to water, leading to the production of a hypotonic tubular fluid. The distal tubules empty into the connecting and collecting ducts, which are permeable to water under the regulation of ADH **(answer a).**

ADH stimulation increases collecting duct permeability to water, allowing the production of hyperosmotic urine. Without ADH, the urine leaving the kidney would be hypo-osmotic. The collecting duct principal cells are the ADH responsive cells and contain fewer mitochondria and basal infoldings than occur in the cells of the distal convoluted tubule. Aldosterone **(answer c)** also acts on the principal cells and secondarily on the thick ascending limb of Henle to increase reabsorption of Nacl.

258. The answer is b. *(Kierszenbaum, pp 526–527. Junqueira, pp 373, 375, 377–380.)* The arrows on the scanning electron micrograph illustrate a podocyte. The podocytes surround the glomerular capillaries. The spaces between the foot processes (pedicels) form the filtration slits, an important part of the filtration barrier of the kidney. The macula densa is a portion of the distal tubule that is specialized for determination of distal tubular osmolarity.

259. The answer is e. *(Kasper, pp 1688–1689. Kumar, pp 990–992. Kierszenbaum, pp 370–373. Junqueira, pp 373–374, 379.)* In patients who have suffered from diabetes mellitus for many years glycation (nonenzymatic addition of sugar to proteins and other molecules) occurs in response to high blood glucose levels. The critical renal changes are the thickening of the glomerular basement membrane, elimination of the separation of laminae rarae and densa, loss of anionic repulsion of sugar groups, and obliteration of the filtration slits. These renal changes are known as nephrotic syndrome and lead to loss of selectivity of the filtration barrier **(answer a)** and increased permeability to proteins **(answer b)**. This causes the loss of protein from the blood to the urine (proteinuria). The liver adjusts to the proteinuria by producing more proteins (e.g., albumin). After continued proteinuria, the liver is unable to produce sufficient protein, which results in hypoalbuminemia leading to an overall decrease in osmotic pressure. Edema then occurs as fluid leaves the vasculature to enter the tissues. The movement of fluid from the vasculature to the tissues results in reduced plasma volume and decreased glomerular filtration rate [GFR **(answer c)**]. The overall effect is further edema because of compensatory release of aldosterone **(answer d)** coupled with reduced GFR and the already existing edema.

Glycation results in the production of advanced glycation end-products (AGE, see figure on the next page), which alters the properties of the glomerular basement membrane. The cellular receptor for AGE is called RAGE and is a multiligand member of the immunoglobulin superfamily of cell surface molecules. In addition, to its role in diabetes, RAGE interacts with molecular pathways that regulate homeostasis, development, and inflammation and plays a role in pathological conditions such as Alzheimer's disease and diabetes mellitus. Binding of a ligand to RAGE activates key cell signaling pathways, such as p21 (ras), MAP kinases, and NF-kappa-B (NFκB), thereby reprogramming cellular characteristics. The interactions and terminology are further complicated by the presence of ENRAGE (extracellular newly identified RAGE-binding protein) that interacts with cellular RAGE on endothelial cells, macrophages, lymphocytes, and other cells to activate proinflammatory mediators. Interactions between AGE, RAGE, and ENRAGE may explain many diabetic complications including delayed wound healing. AGE derivatization is probably nonspecific and involves not only basal lamina-specific molecules, but also a vast array of extracellular and intracellular proteins (transcription factors, structural proteins, and membrane transporters). Hence, cellular coordination/communication becomes slowly but progressively hampered in the kidney and other organs.

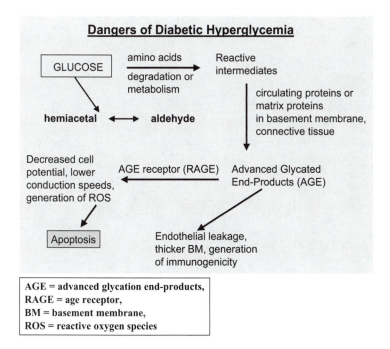

260. The answer is e. *(Junqueira, pp 374–377.)* Only the thin loops of Henle are found exclusively in the medulla. The collecting ducts are found in both the cortex and medulla of the kidney **(answer c)**. Cortical collecting ducts are found in the medullary rays, whereas medullary collecting ducts are found in the medulla and lead into the papillary duct. The convoluted portions of the proximal and distal tubules are found exclusively in the cortex **(answers a and b)**. Afferent arterioles **(answer d)** are found adjacent to the vascular pole of the glomeruli within the cortex.

Eye and Ear

Questions

DIRECTIONS: Each item below contains a question or incomplete statement followed by suggested responses. Select the **one best** response to each question.

261. In the surgical procedure known as LASIK, the shape of the cornea may be flattened. This will result in which of the following?

a. Decreased refraction of light by the cornea
b. A decreased amount of light entering through the cornea
c. Conversion of the cornea from a "stationary" to an "adjustable" form of refraction
d. Maintenance of the lens in a more flattened state
e. Focusing of light on the retina at a point other than the fovea

262. Retinal detachment most commonly results from which of the following?

a. Local swelling in specific retinal layers
b. Leakage of blood from the inner retinal capillaries
c. Fluid accumulation between the retina and the retinal pigment epithelium (RPE)
d. Impaired pumping of water toward the photoreceptors by the RPE
e. Increased phagocytosis of outer segments by the RPE cells

263. Visual transduction involves which of the following?

a. Inactivation of phosphodiesterase
b. Increase in cGMP levels
c. Conversion of all-*trans*-retinal to 11-*cis* retinal
d. closing of a Na^+ channel
e. Depolarization of the rod cell membrane

264. The retinal pigment epithelium (RPE) is characterized by which of the following?

a. The presence of the photoreceptor (rod and cone) perikarya
b. Phagocytosis of worn-out components of photoreceptor cells
c. Origin from the inner layer of the optic cup during embryonic development
d. Presence of amacrine cells
e. Synthesis of vitreous humor

265. Which of the following occurs in diabetic retinopathy?

a. Reduction in the thickness of the basal lamina of small retinal vessels
b. Microaneurysms
c. Decreased capillary permeability
d. Increased retinal blood flow
e. Loss of phagocytic ability of the pigmented epithelium

266. Which of the following statements describes the structure labeled B in the figure below?

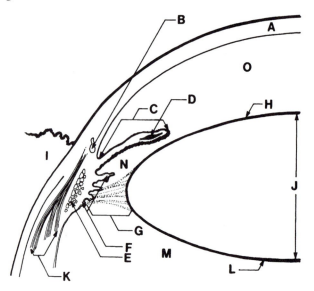

a. It is responsible for the production of aqueous humor
b. It is the site of outflow of vitreous humor from the posterior chamber
c. It is the site of blockage in glaucoma
d. It is involved in the regulation of accommodation
e. It is the major corneal artery

267. Data from the photoreceptors are integrated in which of the following?

a. Outer segment of the rod
b. Inner segment of the rod
c. Ganglion cell layer
d. Inner nuclear layer of the retina
e. Outer plexiform layer of the retina

268. The direction in which vestibular hair cell stereocilia are deflected is important for which of the following reasons?

a. Differentiates between type I and type II hair cells
b. Determines whether cells are depolarized or hyperpolarized
c. Determines whether linear or angular acceleration is detected
d. Determines the direction of blood flow in the stria vascularis
e. Is determined by the frequency of the sound

269. Which of the following is directly involved in sound transduction?

a. Release of neurotransmitter onto the afferent endings of cranial nerve VIII
b. Shearing motion of the tympanic membrane against hair cell stereocilia
c. Movement of the tectorial membrane resulting in hair cell depolarization
d. Equalization of the pressure in the middle ear and nasopharynx by the Eustachian tube
e. Vibration at the round window via the stapes

270. Perilymph is located in which of the following structures?

a. Utricle
b. Saccule
c. Semicircular canals
d. Scala media
e. Scala tympani

271. In the structure shown below, the structure labeled D is responsible for which of the following?

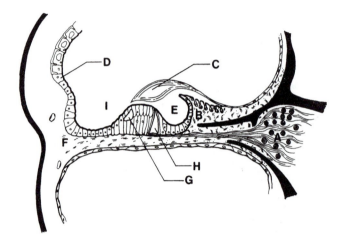

a. Transduction of the sound to a nerve impulse
b. Support of the organ of Corti
c. The characteristic ionic composition of the perilymph
d. Forms the tectorial membrane
e. The characteristic ionic composition of the endolymph

272. Which of the following is the function of the vestibular membrane?

a. Maintain the gradient between the endolymph and the perilymph
b. Maintain communication between the tympanic and vestibular cavities
c. Transmit sound to the oval window
d. Maintain the concentration gradient necessary for sensory transduction
e. Dampen the action of the auditory ossicles

273. Detection of angular acceleration is accomplished by which of the following structures?

a. Maculae of the utricle and saccule
b. Hair cells of the organ of Corti
c. Cristae ampullaris of the semicircular canals
d. Interdental cells
e. Pillar cells

Eye and Ear

Answers

261. The answer is a. *(Kasper, p 162.)* LASIK has largely replaced radial, or refractive, keratotomy. Both methods can be used to decrease the refraction of light by the cornea. LASIK alters corneal (not lens) anatomy to create a new shape that is more flattened in the center and higher at the periphery of the cornea. This occurs because intraocular pressure will cause a reshaping of the cornea due to induced weakness produced by the laser removal of tissue. The purpose of the procedure is to reduce myopia to eliminate the need for corrective lenses. The reduction in curvature of the central portion of the cornea results in decreased refractive power of the cornea. The removal of tissue and the degree of correction required is estimated by computer simulations.

262. The answer is c. *(Newell, pp 322–324. Vaughan, pp 172–173, 187–189.)* Retinal detachment is the result of the accumulation of fluid between the retina and the RPE. In one type of detachment, rhegmatogenous retinal detachment, fluid accumulates after a break occurs in the retina. Detachments without breaks in the retina are called nonrhegmatogenous, or serous, detachments. Vitreous degeneration usually is a prerequisite for retinal detachment that results in the breaking of the retina. The breakdown of the vitreous produces traction on the retina, which may already possess an inherent area of weakness. The site of retinal detachment is the area between the inner and outer layers of the embryonic optic cup and represents a relatively weak area of adherence between the retinal and RPE layers.

263. The answer is d. *(Junqueira, pp 456–458, 466. Kierszenbaum, pp 244–245.)* Visual transduction involves closing of the Na^+ channel in rod cells in response to photons of light. Rhodopsin is the visual pigment found in the outer segments of rod cells and is composed of retinal, a vitamin A derivative, bound to opsin. When photons strike rhodopsin, 11-*cis*-retinal is isomerized to 11-trans-retinal resulting in bleaching, which represents the dissociation of retinal from opsin. The conformationally-altered opsin then acts on transducin, a G protein that couples bleaching to cGMP through the action of a phosphodiesterase enzyme that cleaves cGMP to GMP. Breakdown of cGMP results in the closing of the gated Na^+ channels, a reduction in permeability to Na^+, and hyperpolarization of the cell membrane. The signal spreads to the inner segment and through gap junctions to nearby photoreceptor cells. In the presence of cGMP, the Na^+ channel remains open; in its absence, the channel closes and the cell hyperpolarizes. Therefore, the rods and cones differ from other receptors in that hyperpolarization of the cell membranes occurs rather than the depolarization that occurs in other neural systems. Closing the channel slows down the release of the visual transmitter.

264. The answer is b. *(Junqueira, pp 462–467.)* The retinal pigment epithelium (RPE) is a single layer of cells that phagocytose old components of photoreceptor cells. It is derived from the outer layer of the optic cup and is continuous from the ora serrata retinae to the optic nerve. Microvilli are prominent on the apical surfaces of the RPE and play an important role in the maintenance of the blood-retinal barrier. In addition, the RPE synthesizes melanin and stores vitamin A for the photoreceptor cells. Rod and cone perikarya and amacrine cells are found in the photosensitive retina derived from the inner layer of the optic cup.

265. The answer is b. *(Kumar, pp 1437–1440. Kasper, pp 2163–2164. Newell, pp 507–510. Vaughan, pp 191–194. Kierszenbaum, pp 526–527.)* Retinopathy is one of the major complications of diabetes mellitus. In diabetic retinopathy pathologic changes usually begin with thickening of the basement membrane of small retinal vessels. The abnormal vessels develop microaneurysms, which leak and hemorrhage with resultant ischemia of the retinal tissue. New vessels proliferate in response to ischemia and production of angiogenic factors. Loss of phagocytic capacity of the RPE occurs in retinal dystrophy, but is not a characteristic of diabetic retinopathy. Retinopathy also occurs with prematurity when retinal vascularization is disturbed.

266. The answer is c. *(Junqueira, pp 456–463.)* The structure labeled B is the sinus venosus sclerae (canal of Schlemm), which carries aqueous humor to the scleral veins and the systemic vasculature. Blockage of the canal of Schlemm, the trabecular meshwork, or the scleral veins results in glaucoma. The overall figure shows the region of the iridocorneal angle and other associated structures in the eye. This region is extremely important in the production and outflow of the aqueous humor and in the distribution of zonule fibers to the lens. The iris **(C)** contains both sphincter **(D)** and dilator muscles, which work in opposition to one another and are innervated by parasympathetic and sympathetic fibers, respectively. The center of the iris is a "hole," the pupil.

The ciliary body contains the ciliary muscles (**E** and **K**). The ciliary muscles stretch the choroid and relax the lens, which is essential for the process of lens accommodation. The ciliary processes (**F**) extend from the ciliary body and produce aqueous humor. They are also the origin of the zonule fibers (**G**), which are similar in structure to elastic fibers and are important for anchorage of the lens. The zonule fibers are involved in accommodation. When the ciliary muscles contract, causing forward displacement of the ciliary body, the tension on the zonule fibers is reduced, which leads to an increase in lens thickness and maintenance of focus. The aqueous humor produced by the ciliary processes (**F**) is transported into the posterior chamber (**N**) and flows into the anterior chamber (**O**) through the pupil. Outflow from the anterior chamber occurs through the trabecular meshwork at the iridocorneal angle and flows through the canal of Schlemm.

The cornea (**A**) forms the transparent, avascular anterior portion of the eye. The outer anterior surface of the cornea is covered by an epithelium. Beneath the epithelium is Bowman's membrane, the corneal stroma, Descemet's membrane, and the endothelium (at the posterior surface of the cornea), which lines the anterior boundary of the anterior chamber.

The lens (**J**) is formed embryologically from a thickening of the surface ectoderm called the lens placode, which eventually forms a lens vesicle. Lens fiber production continues throughout life with no turnover. The lens is surrounded by a capsule and an underlying epithelium (**H** and **L**). The three compartments of the eye include the posterior and anterior chambers, which are filled with aqueous humor, and the vitreous body (**M**), which is filled with a gel consisting of hydrated hyaluronic acid and other glycosaminoglycans.

The conjunctiva is the mucosa, or lining, of the eyelid and is labeled **I** in the figure.

267. The answer is d. *(Junqueira, pp 462–466.)* The inner nuclear layer is responsible for the integration of data from adjacent photoreceptors. The retina consists of 10 layers:

1. The retinal pigment epithelium (RPE) is derived from the outer wall of the optic cup. The RPE functions in the phagocytosis of rod disks.

2. The photoreceptor layer consisting of the rods and cones is the outer layer of the retina.

3. The outer limiting membrane is formed by the junctional complexes between Müller's cells and the membranes of photoreceptor cells.

4. The outer nuclear layer contains the nuclei of rod and cone cells and the surrounding cytoplasm (perikarya).

5. The outer plexiform layer contains rod and cone synapses as well as the cell processes of bipolar, horizontal, and photoreceptor cells.

6. The inner nuclear (bipolar) layer is composed of the nuclei and perikarya of the bipolar and amacrine cells as well as the nuclei of Müller's cells.

7. The inner plexiform layer consists of amacrine cells dispersed between the processes of bipolar and ganglion cells. This layer is responsible for modulation of signals from the ganglion to the photoreceptor cells.

8. The ganglion cell layer contains the ganglion cells separated by the cytoplasm of astrocyte-like glia (Müller's cells).

9. The nerve fiber layer consists of axons of the ganglion cells that will form the optic nerve.

10. The internal limiting membrane is located between the vitreous body and the retina. The photoreceptors are of two types: rods and cones. The nuclei of the rods and cones are found in the outer nuclear layer and extend across the outer limiting membrane in one direction and toward the outer plexiform layer in the other direction. The outer segment is the photon-sensitive portion of the rod and cone and contains membranous disks. Rhodopsin is composed of opsin and retinal. It is responsible for transduction of light (photons) into hyperpolarization of the cell membrane. Rhodopsin is present in the disks of the outer segment of the rod. The inner segment contains numerous mitochondria, glycogen, and protein synthetic apparatus. Rods are responsible for night vision, whereas the cones are responsible for color vision, which is best resolved at the fovea. The fovea, which is the center of the macula, is composed exclusively of cones and is the site of optimal resolution.

The choroid is a highly vascular layer that consists of three parts: stroma, choriocapillaris, and Bruch's membrane. Blood supply to the retina is derived from the choriocapillaris of the choroid. The sclera is a layer of relatively avascular dense connective tissue.

268. The answer is b. (*Kandel, pp 597, 614–615, 803.*) The vestibular hair cells are the sensory transduction system of the inner ear and are responsible for the conversion of mechanical energy into an electrical signal for cranial nerve VIII. These cells are called hair cells because their surface contains stereocilia. These are modified microvilli that contain a large number of actin filaments and extend from the surface of the cell. The stereocilia are different lengths and are arranged in order by size with a large kinocilium at one end. The arrangement of the stereocilia is very important because bending in one direction (i.e., toward the kinocilium) depolarizes the cell and increases the rate of nervous discharge, whereas bending them in the other direction (i.e., away from the kinocilium) results in hyperpolarization and decreased neural discharge. The classification of type of hair cell (I or II) is based on the pattern of efferent and afferent innervation.

269. The answer is c. (*Junqueira, pp 471–475.*)Movement of the tectorial membrane results in hair cell depolarization and the release of neurotransmitter onto afferent endings of the auditory cranial nerve leads to initiation of an action potential. Sound waves are directed toward the tympanic membrane by the pinna and the external auditory canal of the external ear. The vibration of the tympanic membrane is transmitted to the oval window by way of the ossicles of the middle ear. Induction of waves in the perilymph results in the movement of the basilar and vestibular membranes toward the scala tympani and causes the round window to bulge outward. The movement of the hair cells is facilitated because the tectorial membrane is rigid and the pillar cells form a pivot. The stabilization of the pressure between the middle ear and the nasopharynx is *not* directly related to the mechanism of sound transmission.

270. The answer is e. (*Junqueira, pp 471–474.*) The scala tympani contains perilymph. Endolymph is similar to extracellular fluid (high K^+, low Na^+). It is found in the utricle, saccule, semicircular canals, and scala media (cochlear duct), which are parts of the membranous labyrinth (**answers a, b, c and d**). Endolymph is synthesized by the highly vascular stria vascularis in the lateral wall of the scala media. The endolymphatic sac and duct are responsible for absorption of endolymph and the endocytosis of molecules from the endolymph.

271. The answer is e. *(Young, pp 398–401. Junqueira, pp 471–474.)* The stria vascularis **(D)** is found in the lateral wall of the cochlear duct (scala media, I) and is responsible for the ionic composition of the endolymph. The organ of Corti is found within the cochlear duct and contains the hair cells that are responsible for transduction of the sound to a nerve impulse. It rests on the basilar membrane, which separates it from the epithelial lining of the tympanic cavity. The inner tunnel **(H)** of the organ of Corti separates the outer from the inner hair cells. The outer hair cells possess microvilli that are attached to the tectorial membrane **(C)**. In contrast, the inner hair cells are unattached. Supportive cells include the phalangeal and pillar cells, which are not labeled on the figure. The spiral lamina is a bony structure that protrudes from the modiolus. The spiral limbus **(B)** is a connective tissue structure superior to the unattached edge of the spiral lamina. Along the outer wall of the canal of the organ of Corti is a thickened projection of periosteum known as the spiral ligament **(F)**. The spiral ganglion is labeled **A** on the figure and contains bipolar cells. Peripheral processes of spiral ganglion cells reach the organ of Corti, whereas central processes terminate in nuclei located in the medulla. The internal spiral tunnel is labeled **E** in the figure.

272. The answer is a. *(Junqueira, pp 471–474.)* The vestibular membrane, also known as Reissner's membrane, maintains the gradient between the endolymph of the scala media and the perilymph of the vestibular cavity. The middle ear contains the auditory ossicles, which transmit sound to the oval window and, therefore, serve in the conduction of sound waves to the perilymph. The helicotrema represents the opening that allows communication of the tympanic and vestibular cavities. The epithelium possesses extensive occluding junctions, which serve to maintain the concentration gradient that is essential for sensory transduction. The movement of the middle ear bones is dampened by the stapedius and tensor tympani when an individual is exposed to a loud noise.

273. The answer is c. *(Junqueira, pp 471–474. Sadler, pp 317–320. Moore and Persaud, pp 476–478.)* The semicircular canals, which extend from the utricle, contain the cristae ampullares and detect angular acceleration. The utricle represents the dorsal portion of the otocyst-derived inner ear; the saccule represents the ventral portion. Both the utricle and saccule contain maculae that detect linear acceleration **(answer a)**. The maculae of the utricle and saccule are perpendicular to one another. These maculae contain type I and type II hair cells, which differ in their innervation. The hair cells have stereocilia and a kinocilium embedded in a membrane that contains otoconia (statoconia) composed of calcium carbonate. The stereocilia and kinocilia are embedded in the cupola, which does not contain the otoconia found in the maculae. The endolymph turns right when the head turns left and vice versa. Movement stimulates the stereocilia and induces depolarization **(answer b)**. The interdental cells **(answer d)** produce the tectorial membrane, which is essential for the development of the shearing force in the process of sound transduction in the organ of Corti. It detects sound vibration and is responsive to variation in the frequency of sound waves. There are 2 types of pillar cells: inner and outer. The pillar cells along with Deiter's cells provide cellular mechanical coupling between the mechanosensory hair cells and the basilar membrane **(answer e)**.

Head and Neck

Questions

DIRECTIONS: Each item below contains a question or incomplete statement followed by suggested responses. Select the **one best** response to each question.

274. When you examine the "corneal reflex" in a patient, you touch the cornea with the wisp of cotton that causes the eyelid of the touched eye to rapidly shut. Thus, as with most reflexes, you are testing both the afferent information that is carried back to the central nervous system and the reflex motor response. What specific cranial nerve branches are responsible for both the afferent and efferent parts of the corneal reflex?

a. Short ciliary nerve (CN III); zygomatic and temporal branches of the facial nerve (CN VII)
b. Short ciliary nerve (CN III); oculomotor nerve (CN III)
c. Long ciliary nerve (CN V^1); zygomatic branches of the facial nerve (CN VII)
d. Long ciliary nerve (CN V^1); infraorbital branch of the trigeminal nerve (CN V^2)
e. Infraorbital nerve (CN V^2); zygomatic branches of the facial nerve (CN VII)

275. A 79-year-old man is brought to your office by his wife because he "keeps running into things" on his right side. His wife also states that he seems to ignore objects on his right. You test his vision in each eye and determine that your patient cannot see anything in the right visual field of either eye. You order a head MRI because you suspect which of the following?

a. A pituitary tumor compressing his optic chiasm
b. A tumor in the medial wall of the right orbit compressing the optic nerve
c. An aneurysm of the left middle cerebral artery compressing the left optic tract
d. A tumor in the middle cranial fossa compressing the right optic tract
e. An aneurysm in the arterial supply to the visual cortex

276. A carcinoma in the medial portion of the lower lip is most likely to first metastasize via which of the following lymph nodes?

a. Submandibular
b. Parotid
c. Superficial cervical
d. Submental
e. Buccal

277. The central nervous system floats in cerebrospinal fluid. This fluid is largely produced in the choroid plexus within the ventricular system and should have a pressure of less than 20 cm of water. The arachnoid villi allow cerebrospinal fluid to pass between which of the following two spaces?

a. Choroid plexus and subdural space
b. Subarachnoid space and subdural space
c. Subarachnoid space and superior sagittal sinus
d. Subdural space and cavernous sinus
e. Superior sagittal sinus and jugular vein

278. A tumor in the infratemporal fossa may gain entrance to the orbit through which of the following?

a. The optic canal (foramen)
b. The inferior orbital fissure
c. The pterygoid canal
d. The ethmoidal sinuses
e. The superior orbital fissure

279. A 28-year-old man is treated in an emergency room for a superficial gash on his forehead. The wound is bleeding profusely, but examination reveals no fracture. While the wound is being sutured, he relates that while he was using an electric razor, he remembers becoming dizzy and then waking up on the floor with blood everywhere. The physician suspects a hypersensitive cardiac reflex. The patient's epicranial aponeurosis (galea aponeurotica) is penetrated, resulting in severe gaping of the wound. The structure overlying the epicranial aponeurosis is which of the following?

a. A layer containing blood vessels
b. Bone
c. The dura mater
d. The periosteum (pericranium)
e. The tendon of the epicranial muscles (occipitofrontalis)

280. Which pair of venous structures contributes to the confluence of dural sinuses on the interior surface of the occipital bone?

a. Sigmoid and transverse sinuses
b. Inferior sagittal and cavernous sinuses
c. Occipital and straight sinuses
d. Transverse and inferior petrosal sinuses
e. Superior petrosal and occipital sinuses

281. A 19-year-old teenager comes into the emergency room (ER) at 5:00 PM with cotton in his nose and blood running down the front of his T-shirt nearly to his belt. He was in the ER the night before. The previous night, gauze soaked in procoagulant had stopped the problem, but not now. No history of trauma was reported. Upon removing the blood soaked gauze, blood pumped from an artery on Kiesselbach's area, on the nasal septum, just superior and posterior to the external nasal aperture. An ENT was called in to cauterize the boy's nose. There are four major blood vessels that normally supply blood to Kiesselbach's area. Describe how, for at least two of the arteries, you could have the boy apply pressure elsewhere (not directly on the pulsating artery) that may successfully cut off blood to the pulsating artery, while the ENT cauterizes the blood vessel.

a. Hold both sides of the bridged of the nose at the apex from the exterior.
b. Hold both sides of the upper lip between his fingers.
c. Hold both sides of the nose at the junction of the nasal bones with the lateral nasal cartilages.
d. Apply pressure from the oral cavity over the incisive foramen.
e. a and b
f. b and d

282. Which of the following is the most direct route for spread of infection from the paranasal sinuses to the cavernous sinus of the dura mater?

a. Pterygoid venous plexus
b. Superior ophthalmic vein
c. Frontal emissary vein
d. Basilar venous plexus
e. Parietal emissary vein

283. Most skeletal elements of the face, for example, bone and cartilages are derived from which of the following?

a. Cranial intermediate mesoderm
b. Cervical somites
c. Neural crest cells migrating from the cranial neural tube
d. The somatic layer of cranial lateral plate mesoderm
e. The splanchnic layer of cranial lateral plate mesoderm

284. A 53-year-old woman has a paralysis of the right side of her face that produces an expressionless and drooping appearance. She is unable to close her right eye, has difficulty chewing and drinking, perceives sounds as annoyingly intense in her right ear, and experiences some pain in her right external auditory meatus. Physical examination reveals loss of the blink reflex in the right eye on stimulation of either cornea and loss of taste from the anterior two-thirds of the tongue on the right. Lacrimation appears normal in the right eye, the jaw-jerk reflex is normal, and there appears to be no problem with balance. The inability to close the right eye is the result of involvement of which of the following?

a. Zygomatic branch of the facial nerve
b. Buccal branch of the trigeminal nerve
c. Levator palpebrae superioris muscle
d. Superior tarsal muscle (of Müller)
e. Orbital portion of the orbicularis oculi muscle

285. A 62-year-old rock and roller fell out of a palm tree while vacationing in Fiji. He had climbed the tree and had fallen while trying to reach one of the coconuts. He didn't think he had broken any bones in the fall. While he felt fine the day of the fall, the next morning he awoke with a bad headache and was relatively incoherent. At the Fiji emergency room both frontal and lateral skull plain films showed no evidence of any fracture but during the physical exam papilledema was noted especially in one eye. He was flown to New Zealand where head CT findings were consistent with which of the following diagnoses?

a. epidural hematoma
b. subdural hematoma
c. pituitary tumor
d. Grave's disease
e. trigeminal neuralgia

286. A 55-year-old man was brought into the hospital with a severe burn on his left hand. The man had placed his hand on the hot burner of an electric stove, but had not sensed anything wrong until he smelled burning flesh. Neurologic examination revealed loss of pain and temperature sensation over dermatomes C4 through T6 bilaterally. However, pain and temperature were perceived bilaterally both above C4 and below T6. Discriminative touch was present in unburned dermatomes on the left and in the right extremity. Although the left hand was too damaged to accurately assess muscle function, weakness and wasting of small muscles of the right hand was noted. Muscle strength and reflexes were otherwise normal. Pain and temperature sensations from the extremities ascend in the spinal cord in which of the following?

a. Intermediolateral cell column
b. Cuneate fasciculus
c. Lateral spinothalamic tract
d. Dorsal columns
e. Fasciculus gracilis

287. You deliver a full-term baby boy who is otherwise normal, but has a left cleft of the upper lip that extends upward toward the left nostril and left anterior cleft of the primary palate just deep to the cleft lip. You explain to the mother that these defects are most likely due to a failure of which of the following?

a. Mandibular process to fuse with the lateral nasal process
b. Mandibular process to fuse with the medial nasal process
c. Maxillary process to fuse with the lateral nasal process
d. Maxillary process to fuse with the medial nasal process
e. Lateral and medial nasal processes to fuse with each other

288. A sudden extreme pain that shoots along the left side of the jaw and up anterior to the ear and along the side of the head is most likely due to which of the following?

a. Ménière's disease
b. Horner's syndrome
c. Tic douloureux (trigeminal neuralgia)
d. Wry neck
e. Craniosynostosis

289. A 9-year-old girl is brought to your pediatric office by her mother because the girl has been complaining about how sore her throat is, and the mother has noticed that she has started to snore loudly at night. You examine the girl's mouth and oral pharynx and you immediately discover the likely source of the problem to be extremely large palatine tonsils. You suggest surgical removal of the tonsils, but you do explain that there is a small risk of the surgery, which may result in which of the following?

a. Loss in the ability to taste salt in the anterior two-thirds of the tongue
b. Loss in the ability to protrude her tongue, thus limiting her ability to lick an ice cream cone
c. Weakness in the ability to open her mouth fully when eating an apple due to damage to the innervation to the lateral pterygoid muscle
d. Loss in the ability to taste in the posterior one-third of the tongue and perhaps some difficulty in swallowing
e. Weakened ability to move her jaw from side to side because of loss in innervation of the medial pterygoid muscle

290. The course of the vertebral arteries is best described by which of the following statements?

a. They arise from the common carotid artery on the left and the brachiocephalic artery on the right
b. They enter the cranium via the anterior condylar canals
c. They enter the cranium via the posterior condylar canals
d. They pass through the transverse processes of several cervical vertebrae
e. They directly give rise to the posterior cerebral arteries

291. A 43-year-old mother of two watching her son play baseball has been hit in the side of the head with a foul ball that came from another field. She had been knocked unconscious for a few seconds and was taken to the emergency room of a local hospital by her husband. At the emergency room in addition to observing a growing "goose egg" over her right temporal region, examination of her fundi with an ophthalmoscope showed subtle papilledema. She was immediately sent for frontal and lateral skull films, which showed a fracture in the frontal bone near the pterion. Head CT showed an accumulation of blood near the fracture on both sides of the frontal bone, but anterior to the coronal suture. What is the most likely diagnosis given to the on call neurosurgeon to bring him into the hospital on a Saturday afternoon?

a. Extracranial hematoma
b. Extracranial and epidural hematomas
c. Extracranial and subdural hematomas
d. Subarachnoid hemorrhage
e. Extracranial hematoma and subarachnoid hemorrhage

292. One of your patients boxes semiprofessionally. One time he was almost knocked out by a right "hook" to the head and for about a week he had frequent headaches and a very runny nose, which finally stopped running by itself. However, he was never able to smell with his left nostril again. What is the most likely site of injury that explains the symptoms?

a. Fracture at the cribriform plate
b. Fracture of the lacrimal bones
c. Fracture of the nasal bones
d. A Le Fort II fracture
e. A Le Fort III fracture

293. A 72-year-old man presents in the emergency room with dizziness and nystagmus. Examination reveals a loss of pain and temperature sensation over the right side of the face and the left side of the body. The patient exhibits ataxia and intention tremor on the right in both the upper and lower extremities and is unable to perform either the finger-to-nose or heel-to-shin tasks on the right. In addition, he is hoarse and demonstrates pupillary constriction and drooping of the eyelid on the right. Finally, the right side of his face is drier than the left. Following vascular blockage, necrotic damage in which of the following would explain the patient's hoarseness?

a. Nucleus ambiguus
b. Lateral spinothalamic tract
c. Spinal nucleus of CN V
d. Descending sympathetic pathways
e. Inferior cerebellar peduncle

294. In dislocation of the jaw, displacement of the articular disk beyond the articular tubercle of the temporomandibular joint results from spasm or excessive contraction of which of the following muscles?

a. Buccinator
b. Lateral pterygoid
c. Medial pterygoid
d. Masseter
e. Temporalis

295. You are viewing at the anterior neck of a 24-year old male medical student.

He has reddish spot (in circle) that is in the center of a slightly raised area just anterior to his sternocleidomastoid muscle about one and a half inches superior to his jugular notch. He has had this reddish raised area for as long as he can remember. If you push on it, it feels attached to something that extends superiorly from this location. At times it leaks a little clear fluid after he has been heavily exercising for long periods of time. What do you think this congenital anomaly is?

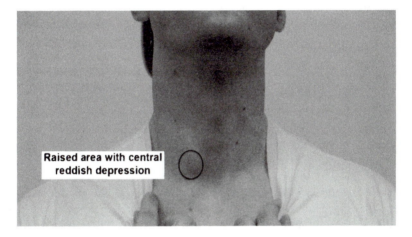

Raised area with central reddish depression

a. Glossopharyngeal fistula
b. An internal branchial sinus
c. A branchial fistula
d. A hyperactive sebaceous gland
e. Spina bifida occulta
f. Thyroglossal duct cyst

296. A 63-year-old woman was brought into the emergency room by her son, who suspected she had suffered a stroke the previous night. Subsequent examination revealed spastic hemiplegia on the left side with hyperreflexia and a positive Babinski's sign. The left side of the patient's face was paralyzed below the eye, and the right eye was turned out and down. The right pupil made direct and consensual responses to light, but the left pupil was fixed and unresponsive. There were no apparent sensory deficits. Which is the most likely location of the lesion?

a. Left motor cortex
b. Right sensory cortex
c. Right midbrain
d. Left thalamus
e. Right thalamus

297. A 75-year-old man was rushed to the hospital from his retirement community when he suddenly became confused and could not speak but could grunt and moan. The patient could follow simple commands and did recognize his wife and children although he could *not* name them or speak to them. Additional immediate examination revealed weakness of the right upper extremity. Several days later, a more comprehensive examination revealed weakness and paralysis of the right hand and arm with increased biceps and triceps reflexes. Paralysis and weakness were also present on the lower right side of the face. Pain, temperature, and touch modalities were mildly decreased over the right arm, hand, and face, and proprioception was reduced in the right hand. The patient had regained the ability to articulate a few simple words with great difficulty, but could *not* repeat even simple two or three word phrases. Which artery or major branch of a large artery suffered the occlusion that produced the observed symptoms?

a. Anterior choroidal artery
b. Middle cerebral artery
c. Posterior communicating artery
d. Ophthalmic artery
e. Anterior cerebral artery

298. A 53-year-old banker develops paralysis on the right side of the face, which produces an expressionless and drooping appearance. He is unable to close the right eye and also has difficulty chewing and drinking. Examination shows loss of blink reflex in the right eye to stimulation of either right or left cornea. Lacrimation appears normal on the right side, but salivation is diminished and taste is absent on the anterior right side of the tongue. There is no complaint of hyperacusis. Audition and balance appear to be normal. Where is the lesion located?

a. In the brain and involves the nucleus of the facial nerve and superior salivatory nucleus
b. Within the internal auditory meatus
c. At the geniculate ganglion
d. In the facial canal just distal to the genu of the facial nerve
e. Just proximal to the stylomastoid foramen

299. The dark structure in the midbrain indicated by the arrow in this midsagittal MRI represents a passage for which of the following?

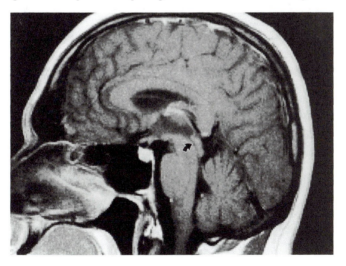

a. Venous blood
b. Arterial blood (in the basilar artery)
c. Neurons of the corticospinal tract
d. Cerebrospinal fluid
e. Spinothalamic (sensory) fibers

300. As an ENT you are about to remove a pair of enlarged palatine tonsils from an 11-year-old boy who has suffered with their repeated infection for about 3 years. The palatine tonsils are located between the anterior and posterior palatine (faucial) folds. The muscles that form these folds are, respectively, which of the following?

a. Levator veli palatini and tensor veli palatini
b. Palatoglossus and palatopharyngeus
c. Palatopharyngeus and salpingopharyngeus
d. Styloglossus and stylopharyngeus
e. Superior constrictor and middle constrictor

301. Which of the following is true of neural tube development?

a. Closure of the neural tube proceeds in a craniocaudal sequence
b. The basic organization of the neural tube features peripheral neuronal cell bodies and centrally located myelinated processes
c. The primitive neurectoderm cells of the neural tube give rise to both neurons and all glial components
d. During development, neuronal and glial precursors are born near the central canal and migrate to the periphery
e. Mature neurons migrate out of the spinal cord to form the sensory ganglia

302. An 87-year-old man had been sitting on the toilet when suddenly he fell to the left side against an adjacent wall. Fortunately his wife was in the adjoining bedroom and had heard him hit his head against the tile wall and found him partially wedged against the wall. His wife left him to call 911, and then went back to him. While he was conscious, he had difficulty speaking and had little control of his left side, though he had some movement. The paramedics arrived and lifted him from his stuck position and gave him oxygen during the ambulance ride, hooked up ECG leads, and found normal heart rhythm and patterns. By the time he got to the emergency room, he was a little more responsive and had slurred speech. A head CT was immediately performed and was read as normal other than slight shrinkage of the brain, typical of an 87-year old. He then reported he had a bad headache and stiff neck. There was no papilledema, so a spinal tap was performed since they didn't know whether to start tissue plasminogen activator (TPA) treatment or not. The spinal tap was quickly performed and had some blood within all four tubes collected, so TPA was *not* initiated. Which of the following is the most likely diagnosis?

a. Subarachnoid hemorrhagic stroke, which had stopped by the time the CT, was performed
b. Ischemic stroke, which had opened by the time the CT was performed
c. Subdural hematoma
d. Epidural hematoma
e. Alzheimer's dementia

303. A patient is observed to suffer from hypoglossal hemiplegia. There is atrophy of the tongue on the right side and deviation of the protruded tongue to the right. In addition, the patient exhibits upper motor neuron paralysis of the left side of the body. Deviation of the tongue toward the right involves which of the following?

a. Left nucleus ambiguus
b. Left pyramidal tract caudal to the decussation
c. Right hypoglossal nerve
d. Right nucleus ambiguus
e. Right pyramidal tract rostral to the decussation

304. A woman is found to have internal (medially directed) strabismus of the left eye, paralysis of the muscles of facial expression on the left side, hyperacusis (louder perception of sounds) of the left ear, and loss of taste from the anterior two-thirds of the tongue on the left. Her mouth is somewhat drier than normal. In addition, there is a lack of tearing in her left eye, and a blink reflex cannot be elicited from the stimulation of either the right or the left cornea. She has upper motor neuron paralysis of the right side of her body. Internal strabismus (deviation of the eye medially) results from paralysis of which of the following cranial nerves?

a. Cranial nerve II
b. Cranial nerve III
c. Cranial nerve IV
d. Cranial nerve V
e. Cranial nerve VI

305. During a neck dissection, the styloid process is used as a landmark. Which of the following statements correctly pertains to one of the four structures that attach to the styloid process?

a. The stylohyoid muscle attaches to the lesser horn of the hyoid bone
b. The styloglossus muscle acts to protrude the tongue
c. The stylohyoid ligament attaches to the lingula of the mandible
d. Distally the stylopharyngeus muscle is split by the digastric muscle

306. A very concerned mother brings her teenager into your pediatric office. The teenager awoke in the morning with a large swollen mass that filled part of his upper eyelid and medial forehead just above his left eye. His eyelid was so swollen he could barely keep it open. His history reveals that he suffers from indoor allergies and a head cold of about a week's length. During your physical examination you note purulent nasal discharge and extreme tenderness to percussion over his paranasal sinuses. The large swollen mass in his eyelid and forehead is quite pliable. You prescribe intravenous antibiotics and give which of the following explanations to the very concerned mother and the teenager?

a. He suffers from trigeminal neuralgia that affects the ophthalmic portion of cranial nerve V
b. He suffers from tic douloureux that affects the ophthalmic portion of cranial nerve V
c. He suffers from sinusitis, which has eroded through the wall on the frontal sinus, and since the frontalis muscle is not attached to bone, allowed pus to leak into the upper eyelid
d. He has Bell's palsy, which is generally caused by herpes simplex virus infection of the facial nerve within the facial canal that caused the loss of ability to raise the upper eyelid and thus allow fluid to accumulate within it
e. He suffers from a sty, which is an inflammation of Meibomian or tarsal glands, which lies on the inner surface of the eyelid

307. During a prenatal ultrasound, images suggest that the fetus has a defective spinal cord. Alpha-fetoprotein (AFP) levels are two standard deviations above normal. The mother elects to deliver the child via a C-section so as to reduce the chances of damaging any protruding spinal cord and meninges. After birth, ultrasound is used to determine that the covering of the spinal cord, along with the intact spinal cord, forms a saclike projection through a dorsal defect in the vertebral column. What would you call this condition?

a. Rachischisis
b. Anencephaly
c. Meningocele
d. Meningomyelocele
e. Hydrocephaly

308. A teenage baseball player was hit in the base of the skull by a loose bat. He is hoarse and complains of difficulty swallowing. The cranial x-ray indicates a basal skull fracture that passes through the jugular foramen. The examining physician notes a large hematoma behind the ear on the injured side. If the nerves passing through the jugular foramen were severed as a result of the cranial fracture, which of the following muscles would remain functional?

a. Palatoglossus muscle
b. Sternomastoid muscle
c. Styloglossus muscle
d. Stylopharyngeus muscle
e. Trapezius muscle

309. Like all endocrine glands, the thyroid is highly vascular. The thyroid gland normally receives its blood supply, in part, from branches off which of the following?

a. Internal carotid artery
b. Lingual artery
c. Subclavian artery
d. Transverse cervical artery
e. Vertebral artery

310. Muscle relaxants are used routinely during anesthesia with resultant closure of the vocal folds. Laryngeal intubation by the anesthesiologist is necessary because which of the following muscle(s) is/are unable to keep the glottis open?

a. Cricothyroid muscle
b. Lateral cricoarytenoid muscles
c. Posterior cricoarytenoid muscles
d. Thyroarytenoid muscle
e. Transverse arytenoid muscles

311. The image below is a midsagittal CT of the head. Which of the following are structures 8 and 9?

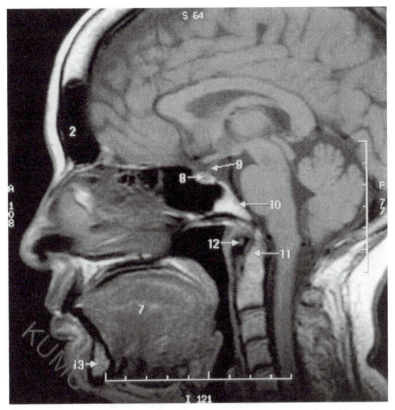

(Image 1302-003, used with permission from the Radiological Anatomy web site, University of Kansas, School of Medicine, http://classes.kumc.edu/som/radanatomy/.)

a. Optic chiasm and optic tract
b. Anterior and posterior pituitary
c. Pituitary gland and infundibular stalk
d. Ethmoid and sphenoid air sinus

312. If a patient had a motor vehicle accident that fractured the base of the skull and caused compression of the structure that passes through foramen 42 which of the following would be the resulting deficit?

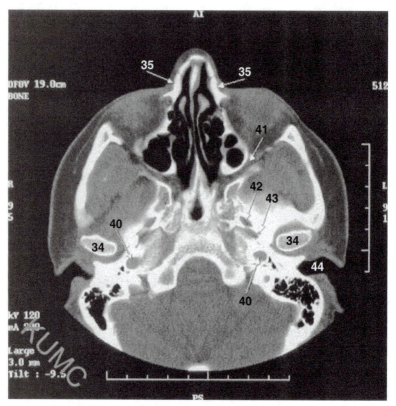

(*Image 1205-028, used with permission from the Radiological Anatomy web site, University of Kansas, School of Medicine, http://classes.kumc.edu/som/radanatomy/.*)

a. Weakened facial expression on the left side
b. Weakened ability to chew on the left side
c. Weakened ability to turn head
d. Weakened voice
e. Weakened ability to shrug shoulders

313. A 32-year-old woman was brought into the emergency room from a car accident. She was conscious, but had been knocked unconscious for a couple of minutes by the forces of a car that had run a stop sign, broadsiding her. You note that she complains of a stiff neck and tilts her head slightly to the right. While performing a cranial nerve exam, you note that her left eye has difficulty moving inferiorly from a fully adducted horizontal position, as when she looks down at her feet. You would order a head CT with specific imaging of which of the following cranial nerves?

a. Right cranial nerve III
b. Left cranial nerve III
c. Right cranial nerve IV
d. Left cranial nerve IV
e. Left cranial nerve VI

314. An 85-year old woman comes into your family practice office because she says she is losing weight and she is having trouble chewing. Which of the following muscles is a pure elevator of the jaw?

a. Buccinator muscle
b. Geniohyoid muscle
c. Lateral pterygoid muscle
d. Medial pterygoid muscle
e. Posterior fibers of temporalis muscle

315. The parents of a 3-year-old at are their wit's end because he has had six middle ear infections. You explain that his eustachian (auditory) tube is *not* functioning correctly. You correctly explain that in order to treat recurrent middle-ear infections, pressure equalization (PE) tubes are sometimes placed at what location within the ear drum?

a. At the umbo of the tympanic membrane
b. At the attachment of the manubrium with the tympanic membrane
c. At the pars flaccida of the tympanic membrane where the fibrous layer is missing
d. In the inferior half of the tympanic membrane
e. In the eustachian tube to keep it open, because that is often the cause of the initial problem

316. Specific neurons supplying the head and neck region have their cell bodies located in ganglia. Cell bodies that bring about accommodation for near vision are located where?

a. Ciliary ganglion
b. Geniculate ganglion
c. Otic ganglion
d. Pterygopalatine (sphenopalatine) ganglion
e. Semilunar ganglion
f. Submandibular ganglion

317. A 63-year-old man is on your hospital service for workup of a stiff neck and the "worse headache" of his life and general malaise. Two days earlier, he had had a spinal tap, which was bloodless and consistent with viral meningitis. This morning on rounds you note that he seems to have to turn his whole head towards you when he looks at you as you enter his hospital room. While his headache is getting better, you notice that both his eyes have reduced ability to move laterally; rather he tends to turn his head. When you get out your ophthalmoscope and look at his fundi, there is no evidence of papilledema. You check his back at the site of his spinal tap that had been performed two days earlier and it seems OK. The rest of the cranial nerve exam is normal. Which of the following is the most likely cause of his reduced eye movement?

a. Viral meningitis
b. Stretching of cranial nerve VI
c. Excess cerebral spinal fluid that is stretching just cranial nerves III
d. Bilateral tumors at the superior orbital fissures
e. Normal stiffening process following hospitalization for couple of days

318. A 87-year-old man is having difficulty swallowing and often chokes on his food. You check his gag reflex by touching the posterior one-third of his tongue and palatine tonsil area. Which of the following cranial nerves provides the afferent limb of the gag reflex?

a. Cranial nerve I
b. Cranial nerve II
c. Cranial nerve III
d. Cranial nerve IV
e. Cranial nerve V
f. Cranial nerve VI
g. Cranial nerve VII
h. Cranial nerve VIII
i. Cranial nerve IX
j. Cranial nerve X
k. Cranial nerve XI
l. Cranial nerve XII

319. You are called to the room of a 93-year-old nursing home patient during morning rounds. She is quite upset because she has awoken with double vision and an inability to open her left eye completely. Your presence calms her down somewhat, and you start asking her questions as you perform a complete cranial nerve exam. Her left eye, under her drooping eyelid, is dilated and rotated down and out. It lacks the normal light reflex when you shine light in either eye. There is no evidence of papilledema in either eye. The rest of the cranial nerve exam is normal. Which of the following is the most likely explanation for this condition?

a. An aneurysm of the left posterior cerebral artery compressing cranial nerve III
b. An aneurysm of the right anterior cerebral artery compressing cranial nerve III
c. A tumor at the left optic canal
d. Glaucoma
e. A left parotid gland tumor compressing cranial nerve VII

320. A 73-year-old man presents because of repeated, biting of his tongue and cheek, and some difficulty chewing in general. You examine him and note that the left side of his tongue is somewhat swollen and that he has two different cuts on it. His left cheek is slightly less full over the angle of the mandible compared to the right side. During your physical exam you note that he has very little sensation over his left mandible and up along the side of his head, and on the left side of his tongue and that he has weakened ability to elevate his jaw on the left side. Taste sensation on his tongue is normal. He also complains of a slightly dry mouth on the left side. The rest of his cranial nerve exam is normal. You send him for a head CT because you suspect which of the following?

a. A tumor at the left superior orbital fissure
b. A tumor blocking the left foramen rotundum
c. A tumor blocking left foramen ovale
d. A tumor blocking the left internal acoustic meatus
e. A tumor blocking the right internal acoustic meatus

321. A 43-year-old man comes to your office presenting with left-sided maxillary tooth pain of one week's duration. Because he thought it might have been one of his maxillary fillings (the newer plastic polymers) he visited his dentist first, but his dentist could not find any dental problems. You tap on his maxillae and elicit sharp pain when you tap on the left but not right side of his face. While he does not think he has any allergies he admits that his girlfriend has recently bought a cat that lives inside. You send him for a sinus series because you suspect which of the following?

a. Sphenoid sinusitis
b. Anterior ethmoidal sinusitis
c. Posterior ethmoidal sinusitis
d. Maxillary sinusitis
e. Frontal sinusitis

322. When performing a cardiac catheterization of the right heart chambers you need to remember that the carotid sheath contains which of the following?

a. Internal carotid artery (lateral), internal jugular vein (medial), and sympathetic chain
b. Internal carotid artery (medial), external jugular vein (lateral), and sympathetic chain
c. Internal carotid artery (medial), external jugular vein (lateral), and phrenic nerve
d. Internal carotid artery (lateral), internal jugular vein (medial), and phrenic nerve
e. Internal carotid artery (medial), internal jugular vein (lateral), and the vagus nerve

323. You witness a choking incident in a restaurant. The Heimlich maneuver is unsuccessful at removing the food from the pharynx. The victim is having extreme difficulty breathing and starts to pass out. Where are you most likely to produce an emergency airway?

a. In the midline just superior to the hyoid bone
b. In the midline just inferior to the hyoid bone
c. At the laryngeal notch
d. At the junction between the thyroid cartilage and cricoid cartilage
e. At tracheal ring 2 to 3 below the cricoid cartilage

324. Within the figure below of a cross section of an embryo, which of the following structures will become the auditory tube?

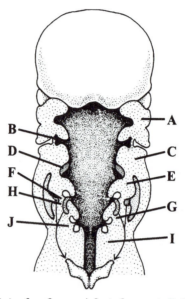

(Reproduced, with permission, from Sweeney L. Basic Concepts in Embryology: A Student's Survival Guide. New York, McGraw-Hill, 1998.)

a. A
b. B
c. C
d. D
e. E
f. F
g. G
h. H
i. I
j. J

325. A 68-year-old woman presents to your ENT clinic because of a small lump on the right side of her face just anterior to her ear. At first you thought it might be just an enlarged lymph node, but careful examination of her ear and scalp doesn't show any signs of pimples or infections in the area. The small lump appears to be within the superficial portion of the parotid salivary gland, anterior to the external ear, yet posterior to the masseter muscle. You perform a needle biopsy of the lump and send it for pathological assessment. The pathology report comes back as suspicious for parotid gland cancer (pleomorphic adenoma). You tell your patient that the tumor needs to be surgically removed and that one of the risk of the surgical resection is . . . .

a. that she may lose her ability to taste on the right side of her tongue
b. that she may lose her ability to chew on the right side of her month
c. that she may develop right sided facial muscle paralysis
d. that she may lose the ability to move the right side of her tongue .
e. that she may develop increased sensitivity to sounds on the right side

326. A 53-year-old woman comes to your office with a hearing problem. About 2 months ago she first noticed that she did not hear in her left ear as well as she used to. Within the last 2 weeks she has also had some "ringing" in her left ear. About a month ago she had a couple of days of dizziness and felt sick but that seemed to pass. She has had more recent and numerous headaches, always on the left side. When you perform a complete cranial nerve exam all cranial nerves are fine except you note a little weakness in her left facial muscles. You send her for a head MRI because you are concerned about which of the following?

a. she has conductive hearing loss
b. Meniere's disease
c. acoustic neuroma
d. tic douloureux

327. A 13-month-old baby boy is brought into your pediatric office by his concerned mother. The boy is just beginning to talk and seems to have difficulty speaking some sounds. The mother had also noted that his tongue seems "sort of stuck in his mouth" compared to her two older children. When you examine the baby and look in his mouth, you agree with the mom that his tongue seems to be stuck in the floor of his mouth. You correctly explain which of the following to the mother?

a. The hypoglossal nerves that control the tongue must have never developed
b. That the problem could likely be corrected by cutting the lingual frenulum
c. That the problem could likely be corrected by shortening the posterior belly of the digastric muscle
d. That the problem could likely be corrected by cutting the pterygomandibular raphe
e. That the problem could likely not be corrected and the speech therapy is the best option

328. A 19-year-old man comes into your office in extreme pain holding a handkerchief over his right eye. He explains to you that he was accidentally struck in the eye with a pool cue and the he can't see anything other than a milky white cloud in that eye. You carefully exam his right eye and note that while there appears to be a scratch on the cornea, the anterior chamber of the eye has partially filled with blood, but the eye has not ruptured. You use a tonometer and determine that the intraocular pressure is normal. You tell the patient that it is important to avoid any other blows to the head since the retina is at increased risk for detachment and to return to the office the next day to redetermine if the intraocular pressure has risen. You explain to the patient that the anterior chamber of the eye, where his blood is, is normally filled with a clear fluid called aqueous humor, which is produced at the ciliary process. The abnormal red blood cells in the aqueous humor may plug the normal site of drainage, leading to excessive intraocular pressure if left untreated. Where in the anterior chamber of the eye does aqueous humor normally drain?

a. Trabecular meshwork that leads to the scleral venous sinus (canal of Schlemm)
b. Ciliary muscle which has zonular fibers (suspensory ligament of the lens) attached to it
c. Ciliary process
d. Lens

Head and Neck

Answers

274. The answer is c. *(Moore and Dalley, p 973.)* The long ciliary (CN V1) nerve carries pain information from the eye, which causes the eye to close due to firing of the orbicular oculi, a muscle of facial expression innervated by the zygomatic branch of the facial nerve (CN VII). Short ciliary nerves **(answers a and b),** by definition, have traveled through the ciliary ganglia (some have synapsed) and therefore are postganglionic parasympathetic fibers, which will innervate the intraocular eye muscles for accommodation of the iris and pupil. The infraorbital branch of CN V_2 **(answers d and e),** while sensory, does not innervate the eye, but does innervate the skin and lower eyelid, but not the cornea of the eye.

275. The answer is c. *(Moore and Dalley, pp 1134–1135.)* Information from the nasal retinal field crosses the midline at the optic chiasm; thus images from the right visual fields strike the left retinal fields of both eyes and from the right eye cross at the optic chiasm (see figure on next page).

The images that strike the left temporal retina (from the right visual field) of the left eye stay on the left and join the nasal retinal field of the right eye in the left optic tract. An aneurysm in the left middle cerebral artery, if large enough, would likely impinge on the left optic tract. A pituitary tumor **(answer a)** would likely compress the optic chiasm leading to a loss of the temporal visual fields in both eyes, or tunnel vision (or bitemporal hemianopsia). A tumor in the right orbit that compresses the right optic nerve **(answer b)** would just lead to loss of vision in the right eye. Compromise of the right optic tract **(answer d)** would lead to loss of left visual fields in both eyes. An aneurysm affecting the arterial supply to the occipital visual cortex **(answer e)** would be very unlikely to produce the symptoms described.

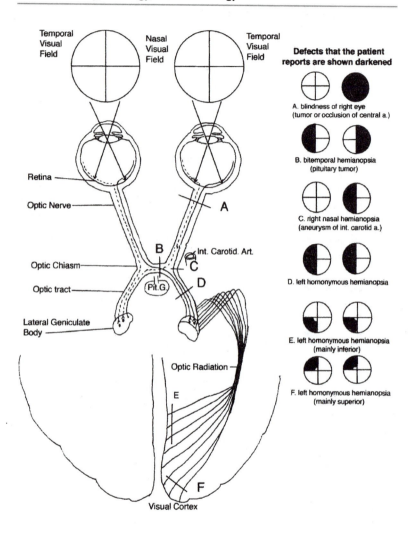

Temporal Visual Field

Nasal Visual Field

Temporal Visual Field

Defects that the patient reports are shown darkened

Retina

Optic Nerve

A

B

Int. Carotid. Art.

C

Optic Chiasm

D

Optic tract

Pit. G.

Lateral Geniculate Body

Optic Radiation

E

Visual Cortex

F

A. blindness of right eye (tumor or occlusion of central a.)

B. bitemporal hemianopsia (pituitary tumor)

C. right nasal hemianopsia (aneurysm of int. carotid a.)

D. left homonymous hemianopsia

E. left homonymous hemianopsia (mainly inferior)

F. left homonymous hemianopsia (mainly superior)

276. The answer is d. (*Moore and Dalley, pp 952, 990.*) Lymph from the medial portion of the lower lip preferentially drains through the submental nodes in the chin and metastases may first appear here. Lymph from the upper lip and lateral portions of the lower lip drains preferentially through the submandibular nodes (**answer a**) on the inferolateral aspect of the mandible. The parotid nodes (**answer b**) receive lymph from upper and lateral regions of the face including the forehead, eyelids, and middle ear. Superficial and deep cervical nodes (**answer c**) receive lymph from other nodes including the parotid and retroauricular. Buccal lymph nodes (**answer e**) drain the cheeks and sides of the nose.

277. The answer is c. *(Moore and Dalley, pp 919, 923–925.)* Cerebrospinal fluid formed in the choroid plexus circulates in the subarachnoid space and is absorbed by the venous sinuses through the arachnoid villi, some of which project into the superior sagittal sinus. Cerebrospinal fluid protects the nervous system from concussions and mechanical injuries and is important for metabolism. It circulates slowly through the ventricles of the brain and through the meshes of the subarachnoid space.

278. The answer is b. *(Moore and Dalley, pp 979–980.)* The infratemporal fossa communicates directly with the orbit via the inferior orbital fissure and the pterygopalatine fossa. The fissure normally carries branches of the maxillary nerve (V_2) and branches of the infraorbital vessels. The optic canal (**answer a**) and superior orbital fissure (**answer e**) open into the middle cranial fossa and carry the optic nerve (CN II) and the oculomotor (CN III), trochlear (CN IV), and abducent (CN VI) nerves, respectively. The pterygoid canal (**answer c**) connects the middle cranial fossa with the pterygopalatine fossa. The Vidian nerve traverses the pterygoid canal on its way to the pterygopalatine ganglion. The ethmoidal sinuses (**answer d**) are mucosa-lined cavities within the ethmoid and adjacent bones. They drain into the nasal cavity.

279. The answer is a. *(Moore and Dalley, pp 906–907.)* A mnemonic device for remembering the order in which the soft tissues overlie the cranium is SCALP: Skin, Connective tissue, Aponeurosis, Loose connective tissue, and Periosteum (**answer d**). The scalp proper is composed of the outer three layers, of which the connective tissue contains one of the richest cutaneous blood supplies of the body. The occipitofrontal muscle complex inserts into the epicranial aponeurosis, which forms the intermediate tendon of this digastric muscle (**answer e**). This structure, along with the underlying layer of loose connective tissue, accounts for the high degree of mobility of the scalp over the pericranium. If the aponeurosis is lacerated transversely, traction from the muscle bellies will cause considerable gaping of the wound. Secondary to trauma or infection, blood or pus may accumulate subjacent to the epicranial aponeurosis. Bone (**answer b**) is too deep, as is the dural mater (**answer c**).

280. The answer is c. (*Moore and Dalley, pp 910–913.*) The confluence of sinuses is formed by the superior sagittal sinus, both transverse sinuses, the occipital sinus, and the straight sinus. The inferior sagittal sinus (**answer b**) and the great cerebral vein join to form the straight sinus. The superior (**answer e**) and inferior petrosal sinuses (**answer d**) both drain the cavernous sinuses, the former connecting with the ipsilateral transverse sinus. The sigmoid sinus (**answer a**) is in between the transverse sinus and the origin of the internal jugular vein.

281. The answer is f. (*Moore and Dalley, pp 1018–1019.*) You may be able to reduce blood flow to Kiesselbach's area by holding both sides of the upper lip and also pressing on the incisive foramen. Kiesselbach's area on the nasal septum is just superior and posterior to the external nasal aperture. Many nosebleeds occur in this area since it is exposed to most of the incoming air. There are four blood vessels that supply blood to this area: 1) anterior ethmoid artery (a branch off the ophthalmic artery); 2) sphenopalatine artery (a branch off the maxillary artery that came through the sphenopalatine foramen; 3) greater palatine artery (a branch also off the maxillary artery, but has run through both the greater foramen and the incisive foramen to get to the nose); and 4) septal branch artery (a branch off the superior labial artery which comes off the facial artery). While the lay press often suggests holding the bridge of the nose (**answers a and e**), this would only block blood within the infratrochlear artery, which mainly serves the exterior dorsal surface of the nose. Holding (**answer c**) both sides of the nose at the junction of the nasal bones with the lateral nasal cartilages would tend to block blood flow within the external branch of the anterior ethmoid. This might actually increase the blood coming from an artery in Kiesselbach's area. Thus (**answer b**) holding both sides of the upper lip between his fingers will cut off blood to the septal branch of the superior labial artery and apply pressure from the oral cavity over the incisive foramen (**answer d**) would cut off blood coming from the greater palatine arteries. Note, it is difficult to stop blood within either the sphenoid palatine artery or anterior ethmoid arteries by applying any external pressure.

282. The answer is b. (*Moore and Dalley, pp 911–913.*) The superior ophthalmic vein drains the region of the paranasal sinuses and is directly connected with the cavernous sinus although blood flow is normally away from the brain. The pterygoid venous plexus (**answer a**) communicates with the cavernous sinus via the ophthalmic veins. The frontal emissary vein (**answer c**) communicates with the superior sagittal sinus via the foramen cecum. The basilar venous plexus (**answer d**) communicates with the inferior petrosal sinus. The parietal emissary vein (**answer e**) also communicates with the superior sagittal sinus.

283. The answer is c. (*Sander, pp 126–129.*) Neural crest cells from cranial regions of the neural tube migrate into the presumptive pharyngeal arches and give rise to many structures of both the viscerocranium and neurocrania. Intermediate mesoderm (**answer a**) never forms in the cranial region. Also, somites never develop past the initial stage (somitomere), but do give rise to some mesodermal derivatives of the head including the bones at the base of the skull (visceral chondrocranium). Cervical somites (**answer b**) only contribute minimally. In the cranial region, the lateral plate mesoderm forms a solid core. It is *not* divided into somatic (**answer d**) and splanchnic (**answer e**) portions separated by a coelom.

284. The answer is a. (*Moore and Dalley, pp 945–946.*) The palpebral portion of the orbicularis oculi muscle (innervated by the zygomatic branch of the facial nerve) produces the blink, whereas the orbital portion (**answer e**) is involved in "scrunching" the eye shut. The buccal branch of the facial nerve innervates muscles of facial expression (including the buccinator muscle) between the eye and the mouth, whereas the buccal branch of the trigeminal nerve (**answer b**) is sensory. The levator palpebrae superioris muscle (**answer c**), which elevates the upper eyelid, is innervated by the oculomotor nerve, whereas the involuntary superior tarsal muscle (**answer d**) is supplied by sympathetic nerves.

285. The answer is b. (*Moore and Dalley, pp 919–920, 967.*) The head CT findings were consistent with subdural hematoma. This is the most likely finding. Falls in older adults (while 62 many not be old for those young at heart) that do *not* produce skull fracture may still provide enough force to cause the brain to move in relationship to the meningeal layers causing bleeding inside the skull. (Older brains tend to shrink due to slow neuronal loss leaving more space for movement within the skull.) Subdural hematomas are often due to a tearing of cerebral veins as they enter the superior sagittal sinus. As the vein tears it often bleeds into to a potential space inside the dura mater, but outside the fluid impervious outer layer of the arachnoid mater. These are veins that bleed into this potential space, so bleeding is often slow to develop. Subdural hematomas are usually treated by drilling a small hole in the skull bones over the center of the hematoma and the blood clot is removed. Normally the initial tear of the vein repairs itself with time. Epidural hematomas (**answer a**) are rare if there are *no* skull fractures. A pituitary tumor (**answer c**) might affect vision, but normally does *not* cause papilledema. Grave's disease (**answer d**) may produce exophthalmus and would be present before the fall. Trigeminal neuralgias (**answer e**) are rarely produced by falls.

286. The answer is c. (*Moore and Dalley, pp 919–920, 967. Waxman, pp 66–67, 203.*) A lesion of the spinal canal that compresses the ventral commissure (syringomyelia) would interrupt ascending fibers crossing there, but would not interfere with already crossed fibers ascending in the lateral spinothalamic tracts. Pain and temperature sensation above and below the level of the cord lesion would be preserved. The cell bodies of first-order afferent (sensory) neurons are located in the dorsal root ganglia. Their central processes enter the spinal cord and ascend one segment before synapsing with a second-order neuron in the dorsal horn. The central processes of second-order neurons cross in the ventral white commissure to the opposite side of the cord and ascend in the lateral spinothalamic tract to the ventral posterior lateral nucleus of the thalamus where they synapse with third-order neurons, which relay the message to cortical neurons of the postcentral gyrus of the parietal lobe. Lesions occurring unilaterally in a peripheral nerve would result in an ipsilateral deficit, whereas lesions in a crossed ascending pathway, in the thalamus, or in the cortex would result in contralateral deficits.

287. The answer is d. (*Moore and Dalley, p 990. Sadler, pp 273–278.*) The lateral nasal process forms the alar region of the nose. Normally the maxillary process moves medially and fuses with the medial nasal process at the philtrum on both sides of the upper lip. The fact that the cleft involves both the lip and bony primary palate suggests failure of the maxillary process to fuse with the medial nasal process. The mandibular process (**answers a and b**) does *not* normally fuse with either the lateral or medial nasal processes (**answer c**). That would reduce the size of the mouth. The lateral and medial nasal processes (**answer e**) fuse to form a nostril separate from the oral cavity.

288. The answer is c. (*Moore and Dalley, pp 944, 1141.*) Tic douloureux or trigeminal neuralgia is a sudden pain about one of the branches of the trigeminal nerve (CN V). It is generally due to vascular compression by cerebral arteries on a portion of the trigeminal nerve that causes pain, especially during situations that cause increases in blood pressure. Ménière's disease (**answer a**) is generally associated with vertigo, nausea, or tinnitus, thought to be due to failure to maintain proper endolymphatic pressure. Horner's syndrome (**answer b**) is characterized by a ptosis of the upper eyelid, a miosis of the pupil and anhidrosis (reduced sweating), all a result of loss of head sympathetic innervation. Wry neck (**answer d**) may be due to tearing of the sternocleidomastoid muscle during the birthing process. Craniosynostosis (**answer e**) is an abnormal head shape often due to the premature replacement of a fibrous cranial suture with bone.

289. The answer is d. (*Moore and Dalley, p 1110.*) The palatine tonsil sits in the lateral wall of the oropharynx in the palatine arch posterior to the palatoglossus muscle and anterior to the palatopharyngeus muscle. The glossopharyngeal CN (IX) traverses the bed of the pelatine tonsil and carries afferent information to the brain regarding both general sensation and the special sense of taste from the posterior one-third of the tongue. The glossopharyngeal nerve is at risk for being cut during tonsillectomy. The ability to taste in the anterior two-thirds of the tongue (**answer a**) is *not* at risk because that information is carried by the lingual nerve, below the tongue. The ability to protrude your tongue (**answer b**) is provided by innervation from the hypoglossal nerve, which innervates all the intrinsic tongue muscles and lies below the tongue and is *not* a risk. The mandibular division of the trigeminal CN (V_3) does *not* course near the palatine arch and would *not* be at risk. It aids in the opening of the mouth (**answer c**) and movement of the mandible from side-to-side (**answer e**).

290. The answer is d. (*Moore and Dalley, pp 1077–1079.*) The vertebral arteries usually arise from the subclavian arteries (**not answer a**) and ascend through the transverse foramina of the sixth to the first cervical vertebrae, but not the seventh. They enter the cranium through the foramen magnum after which they join to form the basilar artery. The basilar artery terminates by bifurcating into the posterior cerebral arteries. The hypoglossal nerves (CN XII) leave the cranium via the anterior condylar (hypoglossal) canals (**answer b**), whereas the posterior condylar canals (**answer c**) transmit emissary veins. The vertebral arteries form the basilar artery which in turn feeds the posterior cerebral arteries (**answer e**).

291. The answer is b. (*Moore and Dalley, pp 919–920, 967.*) The most likely diagnosis is extracranial and epidural hematomas. The extracranial hematoma is the growing "goose egg" that was developing on the outside of her head. This condition is not life threatening. The physical findings of papilledema, frontal bone skull fracture and accumulating blood inside the cranial bones anterior to the cranial suture are all consistent with epidural hematoma. Most likely the frontal bone fractured, lacerating the frontal branch of the middle meningeal artery and veins which run in grooves near the pterion. The temporal region of the skull is particularly thin in this region and more prone to compression fractures. Subdural hematomas (**answer c**) rarely present in a limited area, rather they occupy one complete cerebral hemisphere as the arachnoid mater separates from the dura mater. It is unlikely that a spinal tap, if performed would contain blood [indication of subarachnid hemorrhage (**answers d and e**)].

292. The answer is a. (*Moore and Dalley, pp 1018, 1030–1031.*) A fracture through the cribriform plate would likely cause both a leaking of cerebrospinal fluid (CSF) out the nose (rhinorrhea) and headaches. In addition it would likely shear off the olfactory nerves that pass through the cribriform plate of the ethmoid bone, resulting in anosmia (inability to smell) on left side. The lacrimal bone (**answer b**) surrounds the nasal lacrimal duct and if fractured might lead to a runny nose, but this would *not* explain the lack of ability to smell. The nasal bone (**answer c**) froms the root of the nose is often broken in boxers, but would *not* necessary lead to a runny nose or continued headaches. Le Fort fractures (**answers d and e**) are fractures of the face involving the displacement of the maxillary and nasal region (type II) including displacement of the maxilla and zygomatic arch, thus displacing the maxillary teeth, nose and zygomatic arch (type III). Neither of the Le Fort fractures would fit with the symptoms.

293. The answer is a. *(Waxman, pp 86–91, 117–122.)* The nucleus ambiguus, along with special visceral efferent (SVE) components of CN IX, X, and XI, is a column of lower motor neurons that innervate muscles of the pharynx, larynx, and palate. Damage to this nucleus results in loss of the gag reflex, difficulty in swallowing, and hoarseness. The lateral spinothalamic tract **(answer b)** passes through the medulla and carries sensory information (pain and temperature) from the contralateral extremities and trunk. Similarly, the spinal tract of CN V **(answer c)** carries pain and temperature sensation from the ipsilateral face. Descending sympathetic pathways **(answer d)** course through the medulla to reach the intermediolateral cell column of the spinal gray matter. Damage to those fibers would result in loss of ability to dilate the pupil (meiosis), drooping eyelid (ptosis), and loss of sweating ipsilaterally (hemianhydrosis). Damage to nerve fibers passing to and from the cerebellum via the inferior cerebellar peduncle **(answer e)** would result in intention tremor and lack of coordination.

294. The answer is b. *(Moore and Dalley, pp 986–987.)* The temporalis, masseter, and medial and lateral pterygoid muscles are the muscles of mastication that attach to the mandible. The buccinator muscle **(answer a)**, which controls the contents of the mouth during mastication, is innervated by the facial CN VII. The lateral pterygoid muscles, acting bilaterally, protract the jaw and, acting unilaterally, rotate the jaw during chewing. Because the fibers of the superior head of the lateral pterygoid muscle insert onto the anterior aspect of the articular disk of the temporomandibular joint as well as onto the head of the mandible, spasm of this muscle, such as in a yawn, can result in dislocation of the mandible by pulling the disk anterior to the articular tubercle. Reduction is accomplished by pushing the mandible downward and back, so that the head of the mandible reenters the mandibular fossa. The temporalis **(answer e)**, medial pterygoid **(answer c)**, and masseter **(answer d)** muscles primarily elevate the jaw in molar occlusion.

295. The answer is c. *(Moore and Dalley, p 1111.)* This congenital anomaly is a branchial fistula. When the pharyngeal pouches persist, they may form connections to the exterior of the neck immediately anterior to the boundary of the sternocleidomastoid muscle. Since this weeps fluid it is most likely a fistula or external cyst (which was not one of the options). An internal branchial sinus **(answer b)** would only be a blind pouch off the pharynx and have no external connections. The internal opening for this fistula would most likely be within the bed of the palatine fossa (2nd pharyngeal pouch) or further inferiorly within the pharynx if is from the third or lower pharyngeal embryonic pouches. Persistent glossopharyngeal fistula **(answer a)** (opening of the embryonic glossopharyngeal duct) more rarely makes a connection to the surface ectoderm and like a thyroglossal duct cyst **(answer f)** would be a midline structure. A hyperactive sebaceous gland **(answer d)** would not secrete a clear fluid. Spina bifida occulta **(answer e)** is associated with a tuft of hairy skin over a defect in the posterior arch of the spinal cord.

296. The answer is c. (*Waxman, pp 993–994.*) The symptoms indicate that the lesion is at the level of the midbrain. The spastic paralysis, hyperreflexia, and positive Babinski reflect an upper motor neuron lesion. The corticobulbar and corticospinal tracts pass through the cerebral peduncles (basis pedunculi). Those originating in the right cortex will pass through the right peduncle and then cross to the contralateral side in the pyramidal decussation, resulting in left-side hemiplegia. It is of interest that the lower motor neurons innervating muscles of facial expression located below the eye receive upper motor neurons (corticobulbar tract) only from the contralateral cortex, whereas lower motor neurons innervating facial muscles above the eye (e.g., frontalis) receive input from both sides of the cortex. This explains why only the lower portion of the left face was paralyzed. The deficit in movement of the right eye indicates damage to the ipsilateral oculomotor nerve (CN III), which passes through the cerebral peduncle *en route* to the interpeduncular fossa. The "down and out" direction of the right eye is explained by unopposed contraction of the lateral rectus (CN VI) and superior oblique (CN IV) muscles. Because there were no sensory deficits, neither the thalamus **(answers d and e)** nor sensory cortex **(answers a and b)** were involved. The sensory tracts are arranged dorsolaterally in the midbrain and do *not* pass through the affected area.

297. The answer is b. (*Waxman, pp 169–170.*) The middle cerebral artery supplies a large portion of cerebral cortex, including portions of the frontal, parietal, and temporal lobes. These regions include the Broca's and Wernicke's areas and the precentral motor and postcentral sensory regions. Decreased blood flow in these regions explains the observed motor and sensory deficits. The anterior choroidal artery **(answer a)** is a branch of the internal carotid artery and is primarily distributed to the basal ganglia, hippocampus, and choroid plexus of the lateral ventricle. The posterior communicating artery (**answer c**) connects the internal carotid and vertebral arterial systems. The ophthalmic artery (**answer d**) is a direct branch of the internal carotid artery that enters the orbit along with the optic nerve. Although the anterior cerebral artery (**answer e**) has a wide distribution and anastomoses with branches of both the middle and posterior cerebral arteries, it primarily supplies medial and superior portions of the cortex.

298. The answer is d. (*Moore and Dalley, pp 1143–1145.*) The patient has facial paralysis, which indicates injury to the facial nerve. A problem in the internal auditory meatus (**answer b**) usually affects hearing and balance. That the superior salivatory nucleus (**answer a**) is normal is indicated by normal lacrimation. Hence, the lesion must be distal to the origin of the greater superficial nerve at the genu of the facial nerve (**answer c**). However, absence of hyperacusis indicates that the branch to the stapedius muscle is functioning normally, and this fact suggests that the lesion is close to the stylomastoid foramen. Loss of taste and diminished salivation locate the lesion proximal to the origin of the chorda tympani nerve. If the lesion were distal to the stylomastoid foramen (**answer e**), taste and salivation would have been normal, with facial paralysis as the only sign.

299. The answer is d. (*Moore and Dalley, pp 923–926.*) The arrow indicates the cerebral aqueduct, which is the narrow canal connecting the third and fourth ventricles. The cerebrospinal fluid produced in the lateral and third ventricles must reach the fourth ventricle to escape into the subarachnoid space through the foramina of Luschka and Magendie. Venous blood (**answer a**) would be dark regions along the superior sagiatal sinus for instance. The basilar artery (**answer b**) would be located for anteriorly, along the clivus. Neuronal tacts (**answers c and e**) would not appear dark in and MRI.

300. The answer is b. (*Moore and Dalley, p 997.*) The tensor veli palatini and levator veli palatini, which arise from opposite sides of the auditory tube and base of the skull, insert into the soft palate. They are innervated, respectively, by the trigeminal nerve and the pharyngeal branch of the vagus nerve. The anterior palatoglossal arch, or anterior faucial pillar, is formed by the mucosa overlying the palatoglossal muscle. The posterior faucial pillar, or palatopharyngeal arch, likewise is formed by the palatopharyngeus muscle. The palatoglossus and palatopharyngeus muscles insert into the tongue and pharynx, respectively, and both are innervated by the pharyngeal branch of the vagus nerve (CN X). The salpingopharyngeus muscle (**answer c**), also innervated by the pharyngeal branch of the vagus nerve, arises from the torus tubarius at the opening of the auditory tube and inserts into the pharyngeal musculature. The superior and middle pharyngeal constrictors (**answer e**) are innervated by the pharyngeal branch of the vagus nerve. The stylopharyngeus and styloglossus muscles (**answer d**) originate from the styloid process and insert onto the lesser horn of the hyoid and into the tongue, respectively. They are innervated by the glossopharyngeal and hypoglossal nerves, respectively. Levator veli palatini and tensor veli palatini muscles (**answer a**) are above the soft palate.

301. The answer is d. (*Sadler, pp 285–291.*) After closure of the neural tube, cells proliferate and establish three primitive layers: (1) the ventricular zone adjoining the central canal and ventricles; mitoses of neuronal and glial precursors continue in this zone; (2) a mantle zone consisting of cell bodies of neurons and glia that have migrated out of the ventricular zone; and (3) a marginal zone on the periphery containing the myelinated nerve processes characteristic of white matter. Closure of the neural tube begins near the midpoint of its length and proceeds in both directions simultaneously (thus not **answers a and c**). The neurectoderm of the neural tube will give rise to neurons and some glial cells (astrocytes, oligodendroglia, and ependymal cells), but the precursors of microglia (the monocyte-macrophage lineage) migrate into the nervous system from the blood (thus not **answer b**). The sensory ganglia are formed by neural crest cells that migrated before the development of mature neurons (**answer e**).

302. The answer is a. (*Moore and Dalley, pp 930–931.*) The most likely diagnosis is a subarachnoid hemorrhagic stroke, which had stopped by the time the CT, was performed. While most strokes present with sudden onset of neurological symptoms, the majority of stokes are ischemic (**answer b**) in nature due to blood clots blocking blood to the brain. In this man, however, he probably had a hemorrhagic stroke as a consequence of increased blood pressure due to straining, because of constipation. This is also consistent with his developing headache, stiff neck and blood within the CSF collected at the spinal tap. One would not want to give TPA to a patient with a hemorrhagic stroke because it would probably make conditions worse. The CT was normal because the blood vessel had spontaneously stopped bleeding and the amount of blood was too small to detect radiographically. Subdural hematoma (**answer c**), while common in the elderly, would *not* result in a bloody spinal tap. Epidural hematoma (**answer d**) would *not* result in a bloody spinal tap. Alzheimer's dementia (**answer e**) has nothing to do with this case.

303. The answer is c. (*Moore and Dalley, p 1154.*) Atrophy of the intrinsic musculature of the tongue on one side is due to a lesion of the ipsilateral hypoglossal nerve. Deviation of the tongue to the right on protrusion results from the unopposed action of the left genioglossus muscle, which is innervated by the left hypoglossal nerve. The hypoglossal nerve also innervates numerous other tongue muscles involved in deglutition. The question only asks about the cause of the tongue deviation so the other answers (**answers a, b, d, e**) are irrelevant.

304. The answer is e. (*Moore and Dalley, p 1142.*) The abducent nerve (CN VI) innervates the lateral rectus muscle. Remember, the "formula" LR_6SO_4. Lateral rectus is innervated by CN VI, superior oblique by CN IV and the remainder of the extrinsic eye muscles by CN III. Loss of innervation to the lateral rectus results in unopposed tension by the medial rectus, which produces internal strabismus. The oculomotor nerve (CN III) innervates the medial, superior, and inferior recti, the inferior oblique, and the levator palpebrae superioris muscles. Paralysis of this nerve (**answer b**) would result in lateral deviation of the eye (external strabismus) accompanied by ptosis (drooping eyelid). In addition, mydriasis (dilated pupil) results from loss of function of the parasympathetic component of the oculomotor nerve. Damage to the trochlear nerve (CN IV) results in paralysis of the superior oblique muscle with impaired ability to direct the eye downward and outward (**answer c**). The optic nerve (**answer a**) is responsible for receiving the special sense of sight. The trigeminal cranial nerve (**answer d**) carries pain information from the eye.

305. The answer is a. (*Moore and Dalley, p 1069.*) The stylohyoid muscle inserts onto the lesser horn of the hyoid bone (both derivatives of the second branchial arch) and raises that bone during swallowing. The distal tendon of the stylohyoid muscle is split by the digastric muscle (not **answer d**) passing through its trochlea attached to the lesser horn. The styloglossus muscle acts to retract the tongue (**answer b**). The spheno-mandibular ligament inserts onto the lingula of the mandibular foramen (**answer c**); the stylohyoid ligament inserts onto the lesser horn of the hyoid bone. The stylopharyngeus muscle inserts of the into the middle pharyngeal constrictor.

306. The answer is c. (*Moore and Dalley, p 1019.*) He suffers from sinusi-tis, which has eroded through the wall on the frontal sinus, and since the frontalis muscle is *not* attached to bone, allows pus to leak into the upper eyelid. Inflammation of the mucous membrane that lines the sinuses may sometimes lead to a build up of pus that can block the normal drainage pathways. If pressure builds, erosion of the bony wall of the sinus can occur. In this instance, the anterior wall of the frontal sinus was compromised and pus escaped into the forehead and into the upper eyelid, since the frontalis muscle, a normal barrier, attaches only into skin of the forehead. In order to allow movement, the skin of the eyelid is only attached to underlying struc-tures by loose areolar connective tissue, through which infections easily spread. Intravenous antibiotics were initiated. The swelling spontaneously reduced after the first week of treatment and no visible defects were noted 1 month later. Trigeminal neuralgia or tic douloureux (**answers a and b**) is characterized by sudden sharp pains over the distribution of one or more branches of the trigeminal nerve. Although pain is perceived within the ophthalmic division, the teenager would *not* suffer from sudden sharp twinges of pain, rather a dull constant pain from swollen tissue. Bell's palsy (**answer d**) is generally caused by a herpes simplex virus infection of the facial nerve within the facial canal that causes unilateral facial paral-ysis, which would limit one's ability to close the upper eyelid, *not* raise it. A sty (**answer e**) is an inflammation of the sebaceous gland, associated with each eyelash or cilia. A chalazion is an inflammation of a Meibomian or tarsal gland, which lies on the inner surface of the eyelid. This could cause a bulge in the upper eyelid but does *not* fit with the other clinical findings.

307. The answer is d. (*Sandler, p 294.*) In the family of conditions known as spina bifida, failure of the dural portions of the developing vertebrae may expose a portion of the spinal cord and its covering. This usually occurs near the caudal end of the neural tube. If there is no projection of the spinal cord or its covering through the bony defect, the condition is generally hidden (spina bifida occulta). However, it is termed spina bifida cystica when spinal material traverses the defect. In a meningocele (**answer c**), this is a saclike projection formed only by the meninges. If the projection contains neural material, it is a meningomyelocele, which is the case for this newborn. Rachischisis (**answer a**) is an extreme example of spina bifida cystica in which the neural folds underlying the vertebral defect fail to fuse, leaving an exposed neural plate. Anencephaly (**answer b**) occurs when the cranial neural tube fails to fuse, thus resulting in lack of formation of forebrain structures and a portion of the enclosing cranium. Hydrocephaly (**answer e**) results from blockage of the narrow passageways between the ventricles or between the ventricles and the subarachnoid space. Resultant swelling of the ventricles compresses the brain against the cranial vault and may cause serious mental deficits.

308. The answer is c. (*Moore and Dalley, pp 900, 1151–1153.*) The styloglossus muscle is innervated by the hypoglossal nerve, which leaves the posterior cranial fossa by way of the anterior condylar canal. In addition to the internal jugular vein, the jugular foramen contains the glossopharyngeal nerve (innervating the stylopharyngeus muscle) (**answer d**), the vagus nerve (innervating palatal (**answer a**), pharyngeal, and laryngeal musculature), and the spinal accessory nerve [innervating the sternocleidomastoid (**answer b**) and trapezius muscles (**answer e**)].

309. The answer is c. (*Moore and Dalley, pp 1083–1084.*) The inferior thyroid artery arises from the thyrocervical trunk, a branch of the subclavian artery. The superior thyroid artery arises from the external carotid artery. An inconsistent thyroid ima artery, when present, may arise from the aortic arch, the innominate artery, or the common carotid artery. There are no branches of the internal carotid artery (**answer a**) and infrequent branches of the common carotid artery in the neck. The transverse cervical artery (**answer d**) supplies the posterior triangle of the neck. The vertebral arteries (**answer e**) give off spinal and muscular branches in the neck. The lingual artery only supplies blood to the tongue (**answer b**).

310. The answer is c. (*Moore and Dalley, pp 1094–1099.*) The posterior cricoarytenoid muscles rotate the arytenoids laterally, which swings the vocal process of that cartilage outward to abduct the vocal cords and open the glottis. These are the sole abductors of the vocal folds. The lateral cricoarytenoid muscles (**answer b**) and the unpaired transverse arytenoid muscle (**answer e**) adduct the vocal folds. The thyroarytenoid muscle (**answer d**) and its innermost portion, the vocalis muscle, act to tense the cords. The cricothyroid muscle (**answer a**) lengthens the vocal cords.

311. The answer is c. (*Moore and Dalley, p 924.*) Structures 8 and 9 are the pituitary gland and infundibular stalk. You can see hints of the anterior and posterior pituitary (**answer b**). The infundibular stalk is inferior to the hypothalamus. The optic chiasm and optic tract (**answer a**) are partially visible slightly above the pituitary gland. The pituitary gland sits in the sella turcica which is surrounded by the large sphenoid air sinus (black region) just inferior to the pituitary gland (**answer d**). Cancers of the pituitary gland are often removed by operating through the nose and punching through the sphenoid air sinus, leaving the brain relatively undisturbed. Other labeled structures are as follows: 2, frontal sinus; 7, tongue genioglossus; 8, pituitary gland; 9, infundibular stalk; 10, clivus portion of the occipital bone; 11, odontoid process of axis (C2); 12, anterior arch of atlas (C1); and 13, mandible.

312. The answer is b. (*Moore and Dalley, p 900.*) Structure 42 is the foramen ovale. It transmits the mandibular division of the trigeminal cranial nerve (CN V3), which is responsible for innervating the muscles of mastication. The patient would also likely suffer from loss of sensation along the mandible due to loss of sensation within the mandibular division of the trigeminal cranial nerve. Weakened facial expressions (**answer a**) would result from compromising the stylomastoid foramen, which transmits part of the facial cranial nerve (CN VII) (not on this image). Weakened ability to turn one's head (**answer c**) and shrug (**answer e**) would be the result of damage to the accessory cranial nerve (CN XI), which exits the skull out the jugular foramen (not on this image). The vagus (**answer d**) cranial nerve (CN X) passes out the jugular foramen along with CN IX and XI. Structure 40 is the carotid canal. Other labeled structures are as follows: 34, condyle of the mandible; 35, frontal process of the maxilla; 41, inferior orbital fissure; 43, foramen spinosum; and 44, external auditory canal.

313. The answer is d. (*Moore and Dalley, p 1137.*) Cranial nerve IV has a long intracranial course, so it has an increased chance of injury from. The nerve originates from the trochlear nucleus in the midbrain and is the only cranial nerve to exit the brain on the dorsal rather than ventral surface. It exits the middle cranial fossa by passing out of the superior orbital fissure (along with CN III, V_1, and VI). The nerve also does *not* pass through the common tendineous ring to reach the superior oblique muscle, the only extraocular muscle to pass through a pulley, the trochlea. A patient with a cut CN IV tends to tilt her/his head towards the unaffected side (in this case to the right) [thus not **(answer c)**]. You examine individual extraocular muscle function by performing the "H" test (see High Yield Facts, page 67). To test the function of the superior oblique muscle (innervated by the trochlear nerve) you have the patient first look medial (adduction) and then inferior (towards the nose). Cranial nerve III **(answers a and b)** is involved with the bulk of the other extraocular eye movements and is normal. Cranial nerve VI **(answer e)** innervates the lateral rectus muscle, which is responsible for abducting each eye, and is normal in this patient.

314. The answer is d. (*Moore and Dalley, p 986.*) The medial pterygoid muscle, which originates on the medial side of the lateral pterygoid plate, and the masseter muscle, which originates from the zygomatic arch, pass medially and laterally to the ramus of the mandible to form a sling about the angle of the mandible. These muscles are powerful elevators of the jaw. The muscle bundles of the anterior portion of the temporalis muscle run nearly vertically into the coronoid process of the mandible, acting as a jaw elevator. The lateral pterygoid muscles **(answer c)** run from the lateral side of the pterygoid plate and from the infratemporal fossa to the head of the mandible and the articular disk of the temporomandibular joint. Contraction of the lateral pterygoid muscles bilaterally protrudes the jaw. Unilateral contraction swings the jaw toward the opposite side. The submental muscles, assisted by gravity, are the primary depressors of the jaw. These include the geniohyoid **(answer b)** and mylohyoid muscles as well as the anterior belly of the digastric muscle, all of which function in conjunction with the infrahyoid strap muscles. The posterior muscle bundles of the temporalis **(answer e)** originate over the temporal region and pass nearly horizontally into the coronoid process of the mandible and, therefore, function as jaw retractors. The buccinator muscle **(answer a)** fibers are horizontal between the maxilla and mandible so that they cannot act on the mandible. This is a muscle of facial expression and assists mastication by working with the tongue to keep food on the occlusive surfaces of the teeth.

315. The answer is d. (*Moore and Dalley, pp 1129–1130.*) The umbo (**answer a**) is where the tip of the manubrium of the malleus is attached to the tympanic membrane (**answer b**) and would *not* be a site of insertion of a pressure equalization tube; thus both answers a and b are wrong. The pars flaccida (**answer c**) of the tympanic membrane is near the course of the chorda tympani nerve which is therefore a dangerous location for incisions to place tubes. It would be difficult to place a tube within the eustachian tube (**answer e**), even though that is the site of the malfunction.

316. The answer is a. (*Moore and Dalley, pp 964–966, 1136–1137.*) The ciliary ganglion receives preganglionic parasympathetic nerves from the Edinger-Westphal nucleus (cranial nerve III) that synapse in the ciliary ganglion. Those collections of postganglionic parasympathetic nerve cell bodies innervate the sphincter pupillae muscles, which constrict the pupil, closing it during bright-light conditions. The geniculate ganglion (**answer b**) houses the pseudounipolar cell bodies that receive taste information from the presulcal (anterior 2/3) of the tongue. The otic ganglia (**answer c**) is a parasympathetic ganglia that contains postganglionic parasympathetic nerves to stimulate the parotid salivary gland (preganglionic fibers from cranial nerve IX). The pterygopalatine (sphenopalatine) ganglion (**answer d**) contains postganglionic parasympathetic nerves to stimulate the lacrimal gland and glands of the nose and paranasal sinuses (preganglionic parasympathetic fibers from cranial nerve VII). The semilunar (trigeminal) ganglion (**answer e**) contains pseudounipolar cell bodies that receive pain, touch and temperature information from the face via the trigeminal nerve. The submandibular ganglion (**answer f**) contains postganglionic parasympathetic nerves to stimulate the submandibular and sublingual salivary glands (preganglionic parasympathetic fibers from cranial nerve VII).

317. The answer is b. (*Moore and Dalley, pp 526–527, 925, 967, 1142.*) You order a head CT with specific imaging of cranial nerves VI. One of the consequences of a spinal tap can be continued leaking of cerebral spinal fluid (CSF) at the site of the tap since the meninges have been compromised. (If CSF continues to leak then autologous blood is injected at the site of the spinal tap to stimulate closing of the hole in the meninges.) This may lead to sliding of the brain down the foramen magnum, which is a rare consequence of spinal taps. Since cranial nerve VI exits the brain at the junction of the medulla and the pons and then enters the Dorello's dural cave along the clivus it cannot slide down with the brain and thus would be subjected to stretching. Stretching of the abducent nerve would likely lead to bilateral compromised ability to look laterally since *no* other cranial nerves can abduce the eyes. The viral meningitis (**answer a**) would *not* cause a selective loss of both abducent cranial nerves. Excess cerebral spinal fluid and cause CN VI palsy, but generally *not* CN III palsy (**answer c**). Bilateral tumors at the superior orbital fissures (**answer d**) would be both unlikely, and also would compromise other cranial nerves as well. Loss of the ability to look laterally is *not* part of a normal hospitalization (**answer e**).

318. The answer is i. (*Moore and Dalley, p 1149.*) The cranial nerve that provides the afferent limb of the gag reflex is the glossopharyngeal, IX cranial nerve. Cranial nerve IX provides general sensation from the posterior one-third of the tongue and palatine tonsil area. The response to touching this area is to contract the soft palate and pharynx in a protective manor or gag reflex. The motor aspects of this reflex are mainly mediated by the vagus, cranial nerve X.

319. The answer is a. (*Moore and Dalley, pp 973, 1137.*) This condition is most likely due to an aneurysm of the left posterior cerebral artery compressing cranial nerve III. The woman's symptoms, ptosis of the upper eyelid, an eye that is rotated down (because superior oblique muscle, innervated by CN IV is still functioning) and out (because the lateral rectus muscle, innervated by CN VI is still functioning) with a dilated pupil (because sympathetics, which innervate the dilator pupili muscles are still V_3 functioning) are all consistent with loss of function of cranial nerve III. An aneurysm in either the posterior cerebral or superior cerebellar artery often can compress cranial nerve III as it exits the midbrain. An aneursym of the right anterior cerebral artery (**answer b**) would be very unlikely to cause a problem for the left third cranial nerve. A tumor within the left optic canal (**answer c**) would effect the left optic nerve which passes through it. Cranial nerve III passes into the orbit through the superior orbital fissure along with CN IV, V_1, and VI. Neither glaucoma (**answer d**) nor parotid gland tumor (**answer e**) would present with those symptoms.

320. Answer is c. (*Moore and Dalley, pp 1130, 1139.*) You suspect a tumor is blocking left foramen ovale. The mandibular division of the trigeminal cranial nerve exits the skull through the foramen ovale. This division provides general sensation to the tongue (via the lingual nerve) and mandibular teeth (via the inferior alveolar nerve) and area over the mandible (via the buccal nerve). In addition the mandibular division of the trigeminal also innervates 8 muscles (the four muscles of mastication [temporalis, masseter, medial and lateral pterygoid muscles], two associated with the floor of the mouth [the mylohyoid and anterior belly of the digastric muscles] and two tensors [tensor tympani in the middle ear and tensor palati in the soft palate]). In addition preganglionic nerves from cranial nerve IX (via the lesser petrosal nerve) also pass through the foramen ovale on their way to stimulate the parotid salivary gland. A tumor at the superior orbital fissure (**answer a**) would affect eye movements and forehead sensation. A tumor at the foramen rotundum (**answer b**) would affect sensation under the eye on the face and maxillary teeth pain. A tumor at the internal acoustic meatus (**answers d and e**) would affect the facial nerve, hearing and balance.

321. The answer is d. (*Moore and Dalley, p 1022.*) You send him for a sinus series because you suspect he has maxillary sinusitis. The maxillary sinus is the most frequent site of sinusitis. This is likely due to the fact that its ostium is high on the medial wall of the sinus when erect, thus requiring ciliary action to drain the sinus when in the anatomical position. Lying on the right side of the head may help this patient drain his left maxillary sinus. The maxillary sinus ostium is generally large enough that a cannula can be threaded into the sinus and vacuum applied to help drain the sinus. Sphenoid sinus pain (**answer a**) is generally referred to the top of the skull near the vertex. Anterior (**answer b**) and posterior (**answer c**) ethmoidal sinus pain generally refers to areas around the eyes (either medial or lateral). Frontal sinusitis pain (**answer e**) generally presents over the frontal sinus and tapping on the forehead there will elicit pain.

322. The answer is e. (*Moore and Dalley, pp 1150, 1172–1173.*) The correct answer is the internal carotid artery (medial), internal jugular vein (lateral), and the vagus nerve. **Answers a** and **b** are *not* correct because the carotid sheath contains the vagus, *not* the sympathetic chain, *nor* the phrenic nerve **(answers c and d).** The internal carotid artery (which has a palpable pulse) is medial and the internal jugular vein, into which you insert your cardiac catheter, is just lateral within the carotid sheath.

323. The answer is d. (*Moore and Dalley, pp 1095–1096.*) The food is most likely stuck in the laryngeal pharynx, so you must produce an alternative airway below the glottis, which reflexly closes. Locations around the hyoid bone **(answers a and b)** and above the laryngeal notch **(answer c)** are above the blockage and would *not* get air into the lungs. The isthmus of the thyroid gland generally lies in front of the second and third tracheal ring **(answer e),** and because it is so highly vascular, it is *not* an ideal location for an emergency airway. An additional alternative location for an emergency airway would be the jugular notch, but is *not* preferred because of the occurrence of a thyroid ima artery below the isthmus, in a small percentage of the population.

324. The answers is b. (*Sadler, pp 262–264.*) A, C, E, G, and I denote the first, second, third, fourth, and sixth branchial arches, respectively. B, D, F, H, and J denote the first, second, dorsal third, ventral third, and fourth branchial pouches, respectively. See the following table.

| TABLE OF PRINCIPAL BRANCHIAL DERIVATIVES | |
Arch	Pouch
I	Mandible, Malleus, incus anterior part of tongue, muscles mastication, tensor tympani m., tensor veli palatini m., mylohyoid m., antr. belly of the digastric m., trigeminal nerve.	Auditory tube, middle-ear cavity
II	Lesser horn of the hyoid, styloid process, stapes m., muscles of facial expression, stapedius m. styloid hyoid m., post. belly of the digastric m., facial cranial n.	Tonsillar fossa
III	Greater horn of hyoid, posterior part of tongue, stylopharyngeus m. glossopharyngea cranial n.	Vallecular recess, inferior parathyroid glands thymus gland
IV	Thyroid cartilage, cricothyroid m. superior laryngeal nerve.	Superior parathyroid glands
VI	Cricoid and arytenoid cartilages intrinsic muscles of the larynx recurrent laryngeal nerve	Laryngeal ventricle

325. The answer is c. (*Moore and Dalley, pp 945–947, 954–955.*) One of the risks of the surgical resection is that she may develop right-sided facial muscle paralysis. About 80% of salivary gland tumors originate from within the parotid salivary gland. The facial nerve sends out motor neurons from the stylomastoid foramen. This nerve then branches into 5 to 7 major branches that innervate the muscles of facial expression (derived from the second branchial arch). The branches divide while passing through the substance of the parotid salivary gland. The branches are named for their anatomic regions that they serve: temporal; zygomatic; buccal; mandibular; cervical; and posterior auricular branches. While it is unlikely all of these branches would be cut while removing the parotid tumor, they all are potentially at risk. The tumor is described as superficial within the parotid salivary gland and since the facial nerve normally passes through the middle of the gland, the facial nerve might be spared. She is very unlikely to lose the ability to taste **(answer a)**. That information is carried in the lingual and chorda tympani nerves, which are much deeper and unlikely to be at risk. The mandibular division of the mandible innervates the muscles of mastication and exits the skull at the foramen ovale well deep to the parotid and protected by the lateral pterygoid muscles, so losing the ability to chew on the right side is unlikely **(answer b)**. The hypoglossal nerve innervates tongue muscle **(answer d)** from below the tongue, so is *not* in jeopardy of being cut. The tensor tympani receives innervation from the mandibular division of the trigeminal nerve as it exits the foramen ovale which is well deep to the surgical area, thus in not in danger **(answer e)**.

326. The answer is c. *(Moore and Dalley, pp 1036, 1146.)* Acoustic neuroma. An acoustic neuroma is a benign tumor of the Schwann cells that myelinate the vestibular portion of the VIII cranial nerve. Even though the tumor arises on the vestibular portion of the VIII cranial nerve, hearing loss **(answer a)** is usually the first reported symptom. Tinnitus or ringing in the ear and headaches are also frequently reported. Normally, while the vestibular system may be disrupted (this patient reported a couple of days of dizziness) since the vestibular system on the right side is functioning normally and provides enough information once one is use to the loss. In this case the tumor has started to also affect the VII cranial nerve which controls the muscles of facial expression. Her symptoms go beyond conductive hearing loss [she is also young (53) to be suffering from conductive hearing loss]. Meniere's disease **(answer b)** is an excess accumulation of endolymph, which is usually associated with hearing loss, tinnitus and vertigo (all reported in this woman), but would not be associated with any facial paralysis. This is the second best answer. Tic douloureux (or trigeminal neuralgia) **(answer d)** is characterized by sudden pain along the distribution of the trigeminal nerve and is not a presenting problem.

327. The answer is b. *(Moore and Dalley, p 1007.)* You explain to the mother that the problem could likely be corrected by cutting the lingual frenulum. The boy is currently "tongue-tied". The frenulum of the tongue limits its ability to protrude from the mouth. The inferior aspect of the genioglossus and the geniohyoid muscles contract in order to pull the hyoid bone forward allowing one to stick their tongue out of their mouth. All the intrinsic and three quarters of the extrinsic muscles of the tongue are innervated by the hypoglossal nerve (XII CN). It is very unlikely that the XII cranial nerve never developed **(answer a)**, since the child would then have no tongue movement and the tongue would atrophy. Shortening the posterior belly of the digastric (**answer c**) would worsen the problem by pulling the tongue up and back within the mouth. Cutting the pterygomandibular raphe (**answer d**) would serve no function. Speech therapy (**answer e**) would be the second best answer in that it might stretch the frenulum over time.

328. The answers is a. (*Moore and Dalley, pp 968, 975.*) Aqueous humor is produced at the ciliary process (**answer c**), which is in the posterior chamber of the eye, and then flows out the pupil into the anterior chamber of the eye, where it normally drains through the trabecular meshwork that leads to the scleral venous sinus (or canal of Schlemm). This trabecular meshwork can become plugged with red blood cells, especially if some blood clotting occurs. If the trabecular meshwork plugs then intraocular pressure can build up in the eye, which if excessive, can lead to blindness. This is why the intraocular pressure should be monitored daily until the blood clears. Generally when intraocular pressure increases suddenly (hours) it is very painful, and the pressure must be relieved by inserting a small needle or sharp object at the corner of the cornea and applying pressure elsewhere, thus releasing fluid in a procedure called "burping the eye." Usually as the intraocular pressure is normalized the eye pain subsides. Gradual increases (over days or weeks) in intraocular pressure however, may go undetected because they are not always painful (such as in the case of glaucoma). The ciliary muscle which has zonular fibers (suspensory ligament of the lens) attached to it (**answer b**) controls the shape of the lens, but does *not* drain aqueous humor. It also lies in the posterior *not* anterior chamber of the eye. The lens (**answer d**) is *not* the site of drainage of aqueous humor and is located in the posterior chamber of the eye.

Thorax

Questions

DIRECTIONS: Each item below contains a question or incomplete statement followed by suggested responses. Select the **one best** response to each question.

329. Where would you find the specialized cardiac muscle cells that control the rate of the heartbeat?

a. In the muscular wall of the interventricular septum
b. In the arch of the aorta
c. In the wall of the left atrium between openings of the pulmonary veins
d. In the wall of the right atrium near the opening of the superior vena cava
e. On the surface of the heart

330. Which of the following statements is true of cardiac development?

a. During formation of the heart loop, a single-tube heart remains suspended by a complete dorsal mesocardium (mesentery)
b. The atria are represented by cranial portions of the endocardial tubes
c. The heart bends into an S-shape because the caudal regions of the endocardial tubes grow faster than the cranial regions
d. The left and right sides of the heart result directly from the side-by-side apposition of the left and right endocardial tubes
e. The sinus venosus becomes incorporated into the atrium prior to the formation of the heart loop

331. A mammogram of a woman, age 48, reveals macrocalcification within the right breast, indicating the need for biopsy. The surgeon visually and manually examines the breast with negative results. The surgeon closely examines the nipple for indications of ductal carcinoma. At surgery for the biopsy, a locator needle is inserted into the region of macrocalcification and the position confirmed by mammography. The surgeon incises the skin and dissects a block of tissue. The pathology report indicates ductal carcinoma with microinvasion necessitating surgery. Both patient and surgeon agree that a modified radical mastectomy offers the best prognosis in her case. At surgery for mastectomy, the surgeon carries the dissection along the major pathway of lymphatic drainage from the mammary gland. The major lymphatic channels parallel which of the following?

a. Subcutaneous venous networks to the contralateral breast and abdominal wall
b. Tributaries of the axillary vessels to the axillary nodes
c. Tributaries of the intercostal vessels to the parasternal nodes
d. Tributaries of the internal thoracic (mammary) vessels to the parasternal nodes
e. Tributaries of the thoracoacromial vessels to the apical (subscapular) nodes

332. A 48-year-old woman underwent a complete mastectomy, including removing several axillary lymph nodes. The lymph nodes were all negative for evidence of metastasis. However, the patient is found to have winging of the scapula when her flexed arm is pressed against a fixed object. This indicates injury to which of the following nerves?

a. Axillary
b. Long thoracic
c. Lower subscapular
d. Supraclavicular
e. Thoracodorsal

333. A firefighter, age 34, who is a nonsmoker, complains of bouts of dizziness at times of intense exertion. His history reveals having been exposed to intense smoke 6 months ago when his breathing apparatus malfunctioned during a job. He is scheduled for a pulmonary function test. During deep inspiration the "pump handle" movement results in?

a. A decrease in the anterior-posterior diameter of the chest
b. No movement at the costovertebral joints
c. An increase in the superior-inferior diameter of the chest
d. A primary change in the anterior-posterior diameter of the chest
e. A primary change in the transverse diameter of the chest

334. When you ask a patient to exhale forcibly and maximally, the volume of expiration is constant, but the rate of flow is diminished compared to normal, indicating airway constriction likely due to bronchospasm. The smooth muscle of the bronchial airways is innervated by which of the following?

a. Intercostal nerves
b. Phrenic nerves
c. Thoracic splanchnic nerves
d. Vagus nerve

335. When examining an AP chest film of a 57-year-old man with a systolic ejection-type cardiac murmur, you notice that the arch of the aorta forms a typical aortic knob on the left of the mediastinal border, but also appears as a bulge on the right upper mediastinal border, suggesting an enlarged ascending aorta. In addition, the left ventricular heart border appears prominent. There is *no* evidence of pulmonary hypertension in your patient. Your order an echocardiogram because you suspect your patient has which of the following?

a. Tetralogy of Fallot
b. Pulmonary valve stenosis
c. Atherosclerosis
d. Aortic valve stenosis
e. Defective tricuspid valve

336. Pain referred to the right side of the neck and extending laterally from the right clavicle to the tip of the right shoulder is most likely to involve which of the following?

a. Cervical cardiac accelerator nerves
b. Posterior vagal trunk
c. Right intercostal nerves
d. Right phrenic nerve
e. Right recurrent laryngeal nerve

337. An elderly woman visits the hospital emergency room with the recent onset of grotesque swelling of the right arm, neck, and face. Her right jugular vein is visibly engorged and her right brachial pulse is diminished. On the basis of these signs, her chest x-rays might show which of the following?

a. A left cervical rib
b. A mass in the upper lobe of the right lung
c. Aneurysm of the aortic arch
d. Right pneumothorax
e. Thoracic duct blockage in the posterior mediastinum

338. A 3-year-old child suspected of aspirating a small, cloth-covered metal button is seen in the emergency room. Although the child does *not* complain of pain, there is frequent coughing. Diminished breath sounds are most likely to be heard in which of the following?

a. In both lungs
b. In the lingula of the left inferior lobe
c. In the right inferior lobe
d. In the left superior lobe
e. In the right superior lobe

339. A 58-year-old man comes into your emergency room with difficulty breathing. He also reports some left side chest pain and points to the inferior portion of his ribs. You listen to his lung sounds and there seems to be reduced breath sounds in the inferior half of his left plural cavity. Both PA and lateral chest films confirm what is likely fluid in the inferior 1/3 of the left pleural space. There were *no* obvious rib fractures. You wish to determine the nature of the fluid accumulating in the left pleural cavity, since that will dictate the appropriate treatment. What structures will your 19 g needle penetrate as you pass from skin to fluid at the midaxillary line below the sixth rib?

a. Skin, subcutaneous tissue, external intercostal muscle, internal intercostal muscle, innermost intercostal muscle, parietal pleura
b. Skin, subcutaneous tissue, external intercostal muscle, internal intercostal muscle, parietal pleura, innermost intercostal muscle
c. Skin, subcutaneous tissue, parietal pleura, external intercostal muscle, internal intercostal muscle, innermost intercostal muscle
d. Skin, parietal pleura, external intercostal muscle, internal intercostal muscle, innermost intercostal muscle, subcutaneous tissue
e. Skin, subcutaneous tissue, innermost intercostal muscle, internal intercostal muscle, external intercostal muscle, parietal pleura

340. An otherwise healthy married 25-year-old female medical student is referred to your cardiology practice by her primary care physician for consultation and evaluation. She has told her primary care physician that she is thinking of starting a family. She has an atrial septal defect, diagnosed at age 5, but did not undergo repair because her parents "didn't want their healthy daughter to undergo open-heart surgery." Why are you going to recommend that prior to her planned pregnancy that she at least considers getting her atrial septal defect (ASD) repaired?

a. The pregnancy adds significant additional resistance to the peripheral venous system because of the size of the placenta. This will cause a left to right atrial shunt, which will cause hypertrophy of the left ventricle. In addition, there are clamshell devices that may be inserted intravenously to repair the ASD that do *not* require open-heart surgery

b. The pregnancy adds significant additional resistance to the peripheral venous system because of the size of the fetal circulatory system. This will cause a right to left shunt, which will cause hypertrophy of the left atrium. In addition, there are clamshell devices that may be inserted intravenously to repair the ASD that do *not* require open-heart surgery

c. You would *not* recommend any treatment because living with an ASD carries *no* risk if you have lived with it for 20 years

d. Pregnancy increases the chances of venous emboli, which might lead to stroke because emboli might bypass the lung by passing through the ASD. In addition, there are clamshell devices that may be inserted intravenously to repair the ASD that do *not* require open-heart surgery

e. The pregnancy adds significant additional resistance to the peripheral venous system because of the size of the fetal circulatory system. This will cause a left to right shunt, which will cause hypertrophy of the right atrium. In addition, now that she is older the risks of open-heart surgery are significantly reduced compared to surgery as a child because the heart is much larger

341. Cardiothoracic surgeons must be familiar with bronchopulmonary segments since individual segments of the lung can be removed, leaving the rest of the lung intact and functional. Which of the following is a correct characterization of bronchopulmonary segments?

a. They are arranged with their bases directed toward the hilum of the lung
b. They are separated by parietal pleura
c. The arterial supply is located in the periphery of each segment
d. Each segment is supplied by a secondary or lobar bronchus
e. Veins may be used to localize the planes between segments

342. A 28-year-old woman comes into the emergency room exhibiting dyspnea and mild cyanosis, but *no* signs of trauma. Her chest x-ray is shown below. The most obvious abnormal finding in the inspiratory posteroanterior chest x-ray of this patient (viewed in the anatomic position) is a left pneumothorax (collapsed lung) as indicated by the dark appearance of the left lung and the shifting of the heart to the right. Which of the following structures is indicated by the arrow?

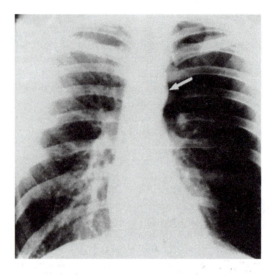

a. Bilateral expansion of the pleural cavities above the first rib
b. Grossly enlarged heart
c. Aortic arch
d. Pulmonary trunk
e. Left ventricle

343. A 23-year-old, semiconscious man is brought to the emergency room following an automobile accident. He is tachypneic and cyanotic. The right lower anterolateral thoracic wall reveals a small laceration and flailing. Air does *not* appear to move into or out of the wound, and it is assumed that the pleura have *not* been penetrated. After the patient is placed on immediate positive pressure endotracheal respiration, his cyanosis clears and the abnormal movement of the chest wall disappears. Radiographic examination confirms fractures of the fourth through eighth ribs in the right anterior axillary line and of the fourth through sixth ribs at the right costochondral junction. There is *no* evidence that bony fragments have penetrated the lungs or of pneumothorax (collapsed lung). The small superficial laceration, once it is ascertained that it has *not* penetrated the pleura, is sutured and the chest bound in bandages; positive pressure endotracheal respiration is maintained. Several hours later, the cyanosis returns. The right side of the thorax is found to be more expanded than the left, yet moves less during respiration. Chest x-rays are shown below.

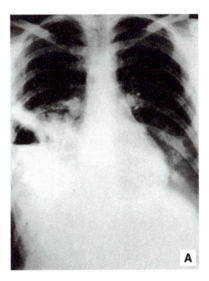
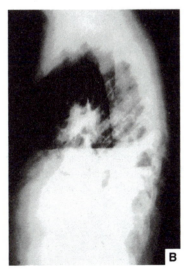

Which of the following is the most obvious abnormal finding in the inspiratory posteroanterior and lateral chest x-ray of this patient (viewed in the anatomic position)?

a. Flail chest
b. Right hemothorax
c. Right pneumothorax
d. Paralysis of the right hemidiaphragm

344. A negative pressure drain (chest tube) must be inserted into the pleural space in order to remove either fluid or air that normally is *not* present. Effective locations for the drain include which of the following?

a. Apex between the clavicle and first rib
b. Costomediastinal recess on the left, adjacent to the xiphoid process
c. Right fourth intercostal space in the midclavicular line (just below the nipple)
d. Right sixth intercostal space in the midaxillary line
e. Right eighth intercostal space in the midclavicular line (about 4 in. below the nipple)

345. The intercostal neurovascular bundle is particularly vulnerable to injury from fractured ribs because it is found in which of the following locations?

a. Above the superior border of the ribs, anteriorly
b. Beneath the inferior border of the ribs
c. Between external and internal intercostal muscle layers
d. Deep to the posterior intercostal membrane
e. Superficial to the ribs, anteriorly

346. The miscarriage rate in humans is estimated to be as high as 15% of all pregnancies. These most often occur very early in pregnancy due to major defects in vital organs. Failure of the sixth aortic arch arteries to form would lead to loss of blood supply to which of the following essential organs?

a. Right side of the heart
b. Face
c. Thyroid gland
d. Lungs
e. Upper digestive tract

347. A 62-year-old man reports to you that at times he has some chest pain and thinks that his heart is *not* beating at an appropriate rate, mainly too slowly, but occasionally too quickly. You send him for a 64 slice helical CT to look at the blood supply to the sinoatrial node. The sinoatrial artery supplies blood to the sinoatrial node. Which of the following is the best description of the blood supply for the sinoatrial nodal artery?

a. Blood always comes from the right coronary artery
b. Blood always comes from the left coronary artery
c. About 60% of the time blood comes from the right coronary artery and about 40% of the time blood comes from the left circumflex artery
d. About 60% of the time blood comes from the right marginal artery and 40% of the time from the left marginal artery
e. Blood usually comes from the posterior interventricular artery regardless of whether that has originated from the right or left coronary artery

348. The major venous return system of the heart, the coronary sinus, empties into which of the following structures?

a. Inferior vena cava
b. Left atrium
c. Right atrium
d. Right ventricle
e. Superior vena cava

349. A 36-year-old male bartender is brought by ambulance to your emergency room because a patron jumped over the bar, grabbed an ice pick, and stabbed him in the chest rather than pay his bar tab at the end of the night. The ice pick entered the chest about 2 cm to the left of the sternum in between the fourth and fifth rib. Upon examining the bartender, you note very little blood is coming from the puncture wound and normal lung sounds from both the right and left lung. However, his heart is beating rapidly at 100 beats per minute, his external jugular veins are bulging, and you have difficulty hearing his heart sounds. You order a PA and lateral chest film because you suspect which of the following?

a. Hemothorax
b. Pneumothorax
c. Cardiac tamponade
d. Aortic valve stenosis
e. Deep venous thrombosis

350. During a bar fight a client was punctured with an ice pick. He is brought to the emergency room because he can *no* longer walk due to weakness, and he is feeling faint. You place him on oxygen as you listen to his heart and lungs. All his heart sounds are distant and muffled and his blood pressure is low despite a very rapid pulse. His lungs sound normal. Using a 3 in. 19 gauge needle you do which of the following?

a. Insert it just under the left tip of the xiphoid process in an effort to remove blood from the pericardial cavity

b. Insert it at the second intercostal space on the left side of the sternum in an effort to inject nitroglycerine in an effort to increase the strength of cardiac contractions.

c. Insert it at the ninth intercostal space at the left midclavicular line in an effort to remove blood from the pleural cavity

d. Insert it at the fourth intercostal space on the right side in an effort to remove blood from the right pulmonary artery

e. Insert it just under the left clavicle in an effort to remove blood from the right cephalic vein

351. Your patient reports he spent two weeks on a desert island as part of a television survival show. It rained and was cool the last 5 days, and he developed a cough. He is now in the ER with a productive cough that produces rusty and bloodstained sputum. He also complains of significant pleural pain. You suspect a pneumococcal lobar pneumonia. From this CT scan at the T4 level, which of the following lung lobes (indicated by the asterisk) is involved with the pneumonia?

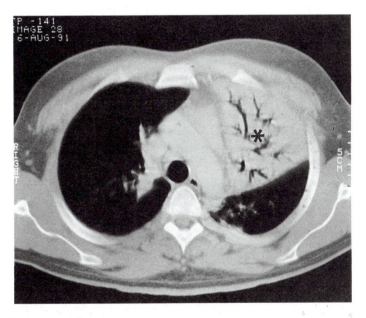

a. Right upper lobe
b. Right middle lobe
c. Right lower lobe
d. Left upper lobe
e. Left lower lobe

352. A 36-year-old male office worker comes to the clinic complaining of general weakness and shortness of breath. He also relates a rapid, throbbing pulse after climbing a flight of stairs. Cardiac auscultation reveals a diastolic rumbling murmur attributable to the mitral valve. The mitral valve is best heard where?

a. Left side adjacent to the sternum in the second intercostal space
b. Left side adjacent to the sternum in the fifth intercostal space
c. Left side in the midclavicular line in the fifth intercostal space
d. Right side adjacent to the sternum in the second intercostal space
e. Right side adjacent to the sternum in the fourth intercostal space

353. A 62-year-old woman comes into your office complaining of a cough and chest cold that she just can't get rid of. While listening to her lungs, which do sound congested, you also listen to her heart. While three of the valves sound normal the valve sound at the second intercostal space just to the right of the sternum sounds stenotic. You order a PA and lateral chest film to evaluate the extent of her pneumonia, you also note that the aortic arch/knob is enlarged, as is the left border of the heart. In addition to mild pneumonia, which one of the following other conditions should be further evaluated for potential treatment?

a. Pneumothorax
b. Ventricular septal defect
c. Aortic valve stenosis
d. Pulmonary valve stenosis
e. Mitral valve prolapse

354. A 6-year-old girl is brought to your pediatric office by her mother. The girl has just joined a recreational soccer team for the first time and she is *not* as fast as most of the girls her age and both of her legs hurt all over during and after soccer practices. The nurse checked her blood pressure upon arrival and was shocked at how high it was, 150/90. Upon physical exam, you reconfirm the hypertension in both arms and feel a weak femoral pulse just below her inguinal ligament. Her leg blood pressure was 85/55. You order a PA chest film to look for which of the following?

a. A patent ductus arteriosus
b. Tetralogy of Fallot
c. Transposition of the great arteries
d. Grooving of the inferior surface of the ribs
e. An enlarged right heart border

355. The heart has nociceptive nerves called c-fibers that sense extracellular ATP that leaks from cells that die due to lack of oxygen. In angina pectoris, the pain that is often referred down the left arm, is mediated by increased activity in the c-fibers in which of the following nerves?

a. Carotid branch of the glossopharyngeal nerves
b. Greater splanchnic nerves
c. Phrenic nerves
d. Cardiac plexus
e. Vagus nerve and recurrent laryngeal nerves

356. You deliver a 6 lb, 6 oz fullterm baby girl. Her breathing rate is slightly elevated, and when she cries her lips turn blue. Her toes are also bluish. You immediately send for a pediatric cardiologist who orders an echocardiogram. The sonographer, who immediately performs the echo study, is convinced that the baby girl has transposition of her great vessels. Which of the following is the most likely additional heart defect that is present in the newborn girl?

a. Overriding aorta
b. Ventricular septal defect
c. Ligamentum arteriosum
d. Coarctation of the aorta
e. Aortic aneurysm

357. To improve the blood flow to the interventricular septum, a coronary bypass procedure is elected. During surgery the anterior interventricular artery is located and prepared to receive a graft. The vessel lying adjacent to the anterior interventricular artery is which of the following?

a. Anterior cardiac vein
b. Coronary sinus
c. Great cardiac vein
d. Middle cardiac vein
e. Small cardiac vein

358. When choosing vessels for bypass surgery for occluded coronary arteries, sections of the internal thoracic artery have been preferred in recent years over lower leg veins, since they seem to last longer. In coronary bypass surgery, the transplanted blood vessel is placed in which of the following positions?

a. The proximal end of the artery is anastomosed to the pulmonary trunk
b. The distal end of the artery is anastomosed to the great cardiac vein
c. The proximal end is attached to the ascending aorta and the distal end is attached distal to the occluded corinary artery
d. The distal end of the artery is anastomosed to the great cardiac vein and the proximal end is attached distal to the occluded corinary artery

359. The first (S_1, or "lub") heart sound and the second (S_2, or "dup") heart sound originate, respectively, from which of the following?

a. Closure of the pulmonary valve followed by closure of the aortic valve
b. Closure of the tricuspid valve followed by closure of the mitral valve
c. Closure of the atrioventricular valves followed by closure of the semilunar valves
d. Closure of the atrioventricular valves followed by opening of the semilunar valves
e. Opening of the atrioventricular valves followed by closure of the atrioventricular valves

360. Structure(s) that normally transit the diaphragm by way of the esophageal hiatus include which of the following?

a. Azygos vein
b. Hemiazygos vein
c. Azygos and hemiazygos veins
d. Anterior and posterior vagal trunk
e. Thoracic duct

361. A 3-month-old girl is seen for the first time by a physician in your free clinic. Her mother reports that she is OK, but she quits physical activity after short bursts of effort, thus likes to be held a lot. The girl recently appears bluish when feeding or trying to crawl sometimes. When you listen to her chest there is an extra sound or murmur, especially during systole. You do a PA chest film and note a general increased density of both lungs and the right inferior heart margin appears enlarged. There is *no* enlargement of the aortic knob, but the left inferior border of the heart margin also appears slightly enlarged. You schedule the girl for an echocardiogram because you suspect which of the following?

a. Tetralogy of Fallot
b. coarctation of the aorta
c. transposition of the great vessels
d. aortic stenosis
e. ventricular septal defect

362. When removing blood from the left pleural space, a chest tube is placed into the pleural space typically below the normal extent of the lung. The chest tubes are most conveniently placed at the midaxillary line through intercostal muscles midway between the ribs to avoid damaging subcostal nerve arteries and veins and their collateral branches. At the midaxillary line, to which rib does the left lung normally extend?

a. Sixth
b. Eighth
c. Tenth
d. Twelfth

363. In the sagittal CT of the thorax below, which of the following is structure 8.

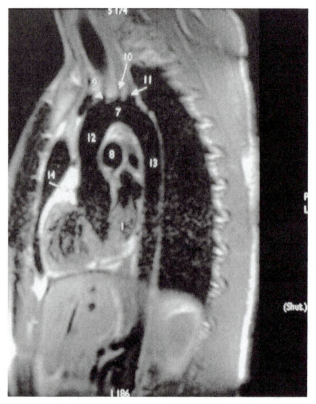

(Image 3304-007 used with permission from the Radiological Anatomy web site, University of Kansas, School of Medicine, http://classes.kumc.edu/som/radanatomy/.)

a. Left subclavian artery
b. Pulmonary trunk (bifurcated)
c. Left atrium
d. Right atrium

364. Circulatory adaptation to the extrauterine, postnatal environment includes which of the following pairs of changes?
a. The interventricular and interatrial foramen close
b. The septum primum closes against the septum secundum and the aorta undergoes coarctation
c. The septum primum closes against the septum secundum and the ductus arteriosus closes
d. The foramen ovale closes and there is transposition of the great vessels
e. The interatrial foramen closes and the interventricular septum closes

365. A 48-year-old man is brought to the emergency room by ambulance due to sudden shortness of breath and left-sided chest and back pain. ECG and blood work suggest normal cardiac function and *no* evidence of a heart attack. He has diminished lung sounds on the left side and extreme tenderness in the mid-back on the left side about 6 cm off the midline. History reveals that he was kneed in the back during a game one week ago while playing goalie. He is 5 ft 10 in. and 165 lb. His urine is normal in color, smell, and volume. An AP chest film suggests fluid in the left pleural space at the costophrenic recess. You order CTs of the thorax and abdomen to look for which of the following?
a. Enlarged right ventricle consistent with pulmonary hypertension
b. A cracked rib
c. Cardiac tamponade
d. Appendicitis
e. Inflamed gallbladder

366. Coronary artery disease is a frequent cause of myocardial infarction in the United States. If an echocardiogram suggests reduced posterior ventricular wall movement, there will be reduced blood flow within which of the following coronary arteries and veins?
a. Circumflex branch of the left artery; great cardiac vein
b. Anterior interventricular artery; great cardiac vein
c. Anterior interventricular artery; middle cardiac vein
d. Right marginal branch of the right artery; small cardiac vein
e. Posterior interventricular artery; middle cardiac vein

367. When examining an axial/horizontal CT of the chest, remember that the origin of the pulmonary trunk just cranial to the right ventricle starts out where?

a. Anterior and to the left of the ascending aorta
b. Posterior and to the left of the ascending aorta
c. Anterior and to the right of the ascending aorta
d. Anterior and to the left of the aorta

368. You are looking at series of axial CTs of one of your patients. Which of the following is the description of structures typically found at the same level as the sternal angle in an axial CT?

a. Junction of the arch of the aorta with right brachiocephalic artery, left common carotid and left subclavian artery
b. Junction of right and left pulmonary arteries with pulmonary trunk
c. Third rib, intervertebral disc T3/4, bifurcation of the trachea, hemiazygos vein draining into superior vena cava
d. Second rib, intervertebral disc T 4/5, bifurcation of trachea, azygos veins joining superior vena cava
e. Second rib, intervertebral disc T 4/5, bifurcation of right and left pulmonary arteries, top of the arch of the aorta

Thorax

Answers

329. The answer is d. (*Moore and Dalley, pp 162–163.*). Specialized cardiac muscle cells, which form the sinoatrial (SA) node, are the pacemakers of the heart. They have the fastest-paced autorhythmicity of all cardiac muscle cells and are located in the wall of the right atrium near the opening of the superior vena cava. Specialized cardiac muscle cells forming the atrioventricular node are also located in the wall of the right atrium, but near the interatrial wall and the opening of the coronary sinus. The left atrium (**answer c**) contains *no* known nodes of pacing cells. Large specialized cardiac muscle cells are the Purkinje cells, which make up the bundle of these that run along the interventricular septum (**answer a**). These cells are found in the subendocardial portion of the interventricular wall and conduct impulses to the ventricular myocytes of both ventricles. The aortic arch (**answer b**) contains baroreceptors that control heart rate through a reflex arc connected to parasympathetic ganglia on the surface of the heart (**answer e**).

330. The answer is c. (*Moore and Dalley, pp 137–138. Sadler, pp 162–165.*) The heart bends into an S-shape because the caudal regions of the endocardial tubes grow faster than the cranial regions. The heart forms during the third week by the apposition of left and right endocardial tubes as the head fold progresses caudally. The endocardial tubes fuse to form a single heart tube. This fusion begins cranially in the region of the bulbus cordis (outflow trunks) and proceeds caudally through the ventricles and the atria to the (**answer e**) sinus venosus, which is incorporated into the atrium (**answer b**) after loop formation. Rapid proliferation of the ventricular region results in the single-tube heart bending into an S-shaped loop. During this process, the dorsal mesocardium (**answer a**) partially breaks down, which leaves the heart suspended only at the cranial and caudal ends; the discontinuity in the mesocardium is the transverse sinus. The left and right sides of the heart (**answer d**) are established by the subsequent division of the single-tube heart, *not* by the apposition of left and right endocardial tubes.

331. The answer is b. (*Moore and Dalley, pp 107–109.*) The lymphatic drainage of the mammary gland, which follows the path of its blood supply, generally parallels the tributaries of the axillary, internal thoracic (mammary), thoracoacromial, and intercostal vessels. Because about 75% of the breast lies lateral to the nipple, the more significant lateral and inferior portions of the breast drain toward the axillary nodes. The smaller medial portion drains to the parasternal lymphatic chain paralleling the internal thoracic vessels (**answers c and d**), whereas the very small superior portion drains toward the nodes associated with the thoracoacromial trunk and the supra-clavicular nodes. Lymph rarely crosses the midline (**answer a**). Lymph generally reaches subscapular (apical axillary) nodes after passing through axillary nodes (**answer e**).

332. The answer is b. (*Moore and Dalley, pp 751–753.*) The serratus anterior muscle (protractor and stabilizer of the scapula) is innervated by the long thoracic nerve (of Bell), which arises from roots C5 to C7 of the brachial plexus. During modified radical mastectomy, this nerve is usually spared to maintain shoulder function. However, its location places it in jeopardy during the lymphatic resection. The suprascapular nerves (**answer d**) are sensory branches of the cervical plexus. The axillary nerve (**answer a**), deep in the brachial portion of the axilla, innervates the deltoid muscle. The thoracodorsal nerve (**answer e**), which arises from the posterior cord of the brachial plexus, innervates the latissimus dorsi. The lower subscapular nerve (**answer c**) innervates the teres major muscle and a portion of the subscapularis muscle.

333. The answer is d. (*Moore and Dalley, pp 89–90.*) Contraction of the intercostal muscles causes rotation of the costovertebral joints (**answer b**) and elevation of the sternal ends of the upper (2 to 6) ribs. Along with slight movement of the sternomanubrial joint, particularly in the young, this "pump-handle movement" increases (**answer a**) the anteroposterior (AP) diameter of the chest. The transverse diameter (**answer e**) of the thoracic cavity increases when contraction of the intercostal muscles also elevates the midportion of the ribs (bucket-handle movement). Contraction of the diaphragm increases the vertical diameter of the thoracic cavity (**answer c**).

334. The answer is d. *(Moore and Dalley, pp 132–133.)* Innervation of the bronchial smooth muscle is mediated by parasympathetic neurons carried by the vagus nerve. Those nerves also stimulate secretion from the bronchial glands. Excessive vagal activity may initiate bronchospasm or the asthmatic syndrome. The intercostal nerves **(answer a)** innervate the intercostal muscles. The phrenic nerve **(answer b)** innervates the diaphragm. Thoracic splanchnic nerves **(answer c)** arise from preganglionic sympathetic nerves that pass through the thorax to go on to innervate the gastrointestinal tract within the abdomen.

335. The answer is d. *(Moore and Dalley, p 155.)* The presence of a systolic ejection-type murmur suggests that blood is becoming turbulent during contraction of the ventricles, consistent with the aortic valve stenosis. Aortic stenosis (often discovered in adults due to a congenital bicuspid aortic valve) produces a jet of blood, which in turn causes the subsequent dilation of the ascending aorta. Secondarily, the left ventricle hypertrophies in size due to the increased resistance of forcing blood through a small valve. Tetralogy of Fallot **(answer a)** would generally be diagnosed in cyanotic newborns. Pulmonary valve stenosis **(answer b)** is unlikely since the pulmonary trunk on this patient is normal. Atherosclerosis **(answer d)** has nothing to do with the findings. A tricuspid valve defect **(answer e)** would *not* probably produce a systolic murmur.

336. The answer is d. *(Moore and Dalley, pp 132–133.)* The phrenic nerve, which arises from cervical nerves C3 through C5, mediates sensation from the diaphragmatic pleura and peritoneum, as well as from the pericardium; in addition, it carries motor fibers to the diaphragm. Therefore, pain from the diaphragmatic pleura or peritoneum, as well as from the parietal pericardium, may be referred to dermatomes between C3 and C5, inclusive. Those dermatomes correspond to the clavicular region and the anterior and lateral neck, as well as to the anterior, lateral, and posterior aspects of the shoulder. Cervical cardiac accelerator nerves **(answer a)** would be sympathetic, generally from T1-5. The vagus **(answer b)** which is a cranial nerve does *not* carry referred pain back to the brain. The right intercostal nerve **(answer c)** may carry referred pain from the parietal pleura to the chest wall. The right recurrent laryngeal nerve **(answer e)** is a branch of the vagus and does *not* carry referred pain to the brain.

337. The answer is b. (*Moore and Dalley, pp 40, 1060. Hansen and Lambert, p 321.*) A Pancoast tumor in the apex of the right lung may compress the right brachiocephalic vein with resultant venous engorgement of the right arm and right side of the face and neck. In addition, there may be compression of the brachial artery, the sympathetic chain, and recurrent laryngeal nerve with attendant deficits. The left cervical rib **(answer a)** is on the wrong side. An aneurysm of the aortic arch **(answer c)** could reduce pulse pressures as the great vessels are occluded, but it could *not* explain the venous congestion. A right pneumothorax **(answer d)** would *not* affect blood flow within the right arm. Thoracic duct blockage in the posterior mediastinum **(answer e)** would be unlikely to affect only the right arm.

338. The answer is c. (*Moore and Dalley, p 126.*) Large aspirated objects tend to lodge at the carina (both lungs affected) **(answer a)**. Smaller objects usually lodge in the right inferior lobar bronchus [not superior **(answer e)**] because the right mainstem (primary) bronchus is generally more vertical in its course than the left **(answers b and d)** and of greater diameter. In addition, the takeoff angle of the right lower lobe bronchus is less acute than that of the right middle lobe, thereby continuing in the general direction of both the right mainstem bronchus and trachea. Blockage of the airway will produce absence of breath sounds within the lobe and eventual atelectasis, collapse.

339. The answer is a. (*Moore and Dalley, pp 118–119.*) The sampling of pleural fluid is called thoracocentesis. The nature of the fluid will determine the appropriate course of treatment. Since the sampling is being performed at the midaxillary line you would pass through all three layers of muscles. Further anteriorly, the external intercostal muscle turns membranous, while near the transverse process of the ribs the innermost intercostal muscle becomes membranous (See *Moore and Dalley p 97*). None of the other answers **(b, c, d, or e)** are correct.

340. The answer is d. (*Moore and Dalley, pp 150–151.*) Pregnancy increases the chances of venous emboli, which might lead to stroke because emboli might bypass the lung by passing through the ASD. In addition, there are clamshell devices that may be inserted intravenously to repair the ASD that do *not* require open-heart surgery. Normally emboli that form in the blood develop within the venous circulatory system, especially with stasis of blood flow. During pregnancy, the weight of the fetus on the inferior vena cavatends to increase the chances of forming emboli. In a normal circulatory system those venous emboli become trapped in the first capillary bed, in the lungs, where they form small pulmonary emboli, which in most young, healthy people are a minor health risk. When an atrial septal defect is present, systemic venous emboli may pass from the right to the left atria, thus by-passing the lung capillary network and move into the brain capillary bed, where even small emboli can cause strokes. There are now "clamshell" devices that can be introduced via catherization that can be inserted to fill the atrial septal defect, thus eliminating the need for open-heart surgery.

341. The answer is e. (*Moore and Dalley, pp 125–130.*) Veins may be used to localize the planes between segments. Although the segmental bronchus and artery tend to be centrally located (**answer c**), the veins do *not* accompany the arteries, but tend to be located subpleurally and between bronchopulmonary segments. Indeed, at surgery the intersegmental veins are useful in defining intersegmental planes. Bronchopulmonary segments, the anatomic and functional units of the lung, are roughly pyramidal in shape, have apices directed toward the hilum of the lung (**answer a**), and are separated from each other by connective tissue septa. Each bronchopulmonary segment is supplied by one tertiary or segmental bronchus (**answer d**), along with a branch of the pulmonary artery. The parietal pleura (**answer b**) only covers the ends of the bronchopulmonary segments.

342. The answer is c. (*Moore and Dalley, pp 185–186.*) The patient has a left pneumothorax. The lucidity of the left pleural cavity with the lack of pulmonary vessels indicates that the left lung has collapsed into a small, dense mass adjacent to the mediastinum. Such a nontraumatic pneumothorax may result from the rupture of a pulmonary bleb, especially in a young person. The right lung is normal. There is *no* pleural fluid level indicative of hemothorax, and the near symmetry of the domes of the two hemidiaphragms on inspiration indicates normal function of the phrenic nerves. The pleural cavities normally extend superior to the first rib into the base of the neck (**answer a**). The heart, measuring less than one-half of the chest diameter, is of normal size **(answer b)**, but is shifted to the right. Both the pulmonary trunk **(answer d)** and the left ventricle **(answer e)** would be inferior to the arrow on the left heart border.

343. The answer is b. *(Moore and Dalley, pp 117–118.)* The fluid level in the right pleural cavity is indicative of hemothorax caused by bleeding into the pleural space. As blood collects, lung tissue is displaced and cannot expand fully, thereby impairing ventilation. However, perfusion continues so that the ventilation-perfusion ratio is altered. There would be *no* fluid line if it were a pneumothorax **(answer c)**. A puncture wound often produces a flailing chest [**(answer a)** moving inward as the rest of the thoracic cage expands during inspiration]. Paralysis of the right hemidiaphragm **(answer d)** would result in the diaphragm becoming stationary near its normal expiration height.

344. The answer is d. *(Moore and Dalley, pp 118–119.)* The usual location of choice for a chest tube drain is in the midaxillary or posterior axillary line, that is, the vertical line commencing at the middle or posterior axillary fold, at the approximate level of the fifth or sixth intercostal space. Since the lung is collapsed toward the hilum the exact level tends *not* to be so important since the lung has pull cranial and medial. The needle is usually inserted just below the level at which percussive dullness occurs (if hemothorax). The apex of the lung **(answer a)** is close to the brachial plexus and subclavian vessels and thus is *not* used. The costomediastinal recess on the left, adjacent to the xiphoid process **(answer b)** is used for pericardiocentesis. The midclavicular line **(answers c and e)** is *not* used because tubes placed this far anteriorly tend to be in the way of the patient.

345. The answer is b. *(Moore and Dalley, pp 97, 102, 118–119.)* The upper two posterior intercostal arteries arise from the costocervical trunk; the remaining arteries arise from the descending thoracic aorta. The posterior intercostal arteries anastomose with the anterior intercostal arteries, which arise from the internal thoracic artery. Laterally, the intercostal neurovascular bundle lies in the costal groove along the internal surface of the inferior border of each rib and between the innermost intercostal and internal intercostal muscles **(answers c and e)**. Indeed, scalloping of the inferior edge of the rib is a radiographic indication of increased collateral circulation through the intercostal arteries that results from a circulatory deficit elsewhere. Just as a subcostal location offers protection to the intercostal neurovascular bundle, fracture of a rib may involve tearing of these structures. The intercostal neurovascular bundle components give off a smaller accessory bundle, which lies adjacent to the upper border of the ribs. Thoracocentesis usually is performed adjacent to the upper border of the ribs (**answer a**) to avoid the main intercostal neurovascular bundle. Deep to the posterior intercostal membrane (**answer d**) is *not* anatomically relevant.

346. The answer is d. *(Sadler, pp 180–183. Moore and Persaud, Developing, pp 361–365.)* Branches of the arteries of the sixth aortic arches form the pulmonary arteries. In addition, the left sixth arch artery forms the ductus arteriosus. The blood supply to the right side of the heart (**answer a**) is primarily derived from the right and left coronary arteries derived from the truncus arteriosus. The face (**answer b**) and thyroid gland (**answer c**) receive blood primarily from the facial and superior thyroid arteries, respectively. These are branches of the common and external carotid arteries which, in turn, are derivatives of the second and third aortic arch arteries. The upper digestive tract (**answer e**) is supplied by the celiac and superior mesenteric arteries, derivatives of the vitelline arteries.

347. The answer is c. *(Moore and Dalley, pp 156–159.)* The sinoatrial artery arises from right coronary artery about 60% of the time and arises from the left circumflex artery about 40% of the time, thus *not* always from either the right (**answer a**) or left (**answer b**) coronary artery. Coronary occlusions involving the right coronary artery are, therefore, often accompanied by rhythm disturbances. The right marginal (**answer d**) is *not* involved in supplying blood to the sinoatrial node. While it is true that the posterior interventricular artery (**answer e**) can receive blood mainly from either the right or left coronary arteries (so called right or left "dominant" patterns) the sinoatrial artery usually does *not* arise from this region.

348. The answer is c. *(Moore and Dalley, pp 159–162.)* With the exception of the anterior surface of the right ventricle, blood returning from the coronary circulation collects in the coronary sinus, which, in turn, empties directly into the right atrium. Both the superior (**answer e**) and inferior (answer a) vena cava bring venous blood to in the right atrium. Oxygenated blood from the lungs is brought to the left atrium (answer b) by the pulmonary veins. The right ventricle (answer d) receives blood from the right atrium.

349. The answer is c. (*Moore and Dalley, pp 140–141.*) The ice pick likely penetrated the left ventricle of the heart, causing blood to leak into the pericardial sac. The rapid filling of the pericardial space does *not* allow the heart to fully expand between contractions leading to increased venous hypertension. The result is filling of the external jugular veins. Since the heart can only pump small quantities of the blood with each beat, it speeds up (tachycardia). The heart sounds and apical heartbeat soften because the blood surrounding the heart absorbs the sounds. A hemothorax (answer a) and pneumothorax (answer b) are unlikely since both right and left lungs sounds are normal and because of the location of the ice pick injury. Aortic valve stenosis (answer d) would *not* result from a puncture wound. Deep venous thrombosis (answer e) generally occurs in the lower extremity and results in leg pain and is *not* caused by a puncture wound.

350. The answer is a. (*Moore and Dalley, pp 140–141.*) Draining blood from the pericardial cavity is performed by inserting a needle just under the left tip of the xiphoid process in an effort to remove blood from the pericardial cavity. This procedure is called pericardiocentesis. Blood within the pericardial sac will cause heart failure as the fluid prevents the heart chambers from expanding properly and filling with blood. Thus, the ability of the heart to pump blood is diminished. Most of the other answers (answers b, c, d, e) are all too cranial and would *not* allow access to the pericardial space.

351. The answer is d. (*Moore and Dalley, pp 120–124.*) The lobe indicated by the asterisk is the left upper (or superior) lobe. The general orientation when viewing CTs is that the observer is looking up from the patient's feet. Therefore, the patient's left is on your right, thus it can't be a part of the right lung (answers a, b, c). In addition, on the left, the inferior (lower) lobe (answer e) begins relatively high in the thoracic cavity and is posterior to the upper lobe.

352. The answer is c. (*Moore and Dalley, pp 167–168.*) The mitral valve is best heard over the apex of the heart, which lies approximately in the fifth intercostal space along the midclavicular line. The tricuspid valve is heard most distinctly in the fifth intercostal space just to the right of the sternum (**answer b**). The aortic (**answer a**) and pulmonary (**answer d**) valves are best auscultated in the right and left second intercostal spaces, respectively, adjacent to the sternum. No valve is heard at the fourth intercostals space on the right of the sternum (**answer e**).

353. The answer is c. (*Moore and Dalley, pp 154–155.*) The other condition that needs be further evaluated is aortic valve stenosis. In individuals over 60, calcifications in the aortic valve can lead to a decrease in its function and restrict blood flow. Aortic valve stenosis often leads to enlargement of the arch of the aorta due to blood turbulence as the blood rushes through the valve and also hypertrophy of the left ventricle as a consequence of increased workload to pump blood to the body. Left ventricle hypertrophy will lead to the enlargement of the left heart border on the PA chest film. There is no evidence for a pneumothorax (**answer a**) or pulmonary valve stenosis (**answer d**). A ventricular septal defect (**answer b**) would produce a systolic murmur and might lead to an increase in the right heart border, not the left. While mitral valve prolapse (**answer e**) would also tend to increase the size of the left border of the heart, there should be no change in the size of the arch of the aorta.

354. The answer is d. (*Moore and Dalley, p 175.*) Coarctation of the aorta often causes grooving of the undersurface of the ribs. Coarctation of the aorta is a constriction of the aorta, often occurring near where the ductus arteriosus had attached. The constriction of the aorta leads to a decrease in the blood pressure within the lower limbs. Often there is a grooving of the inferior surface of the ribs as blood flows into the internal thoracic (mammary) arteries then inferiorly to the anterior portion of the intercostal arteries that subsequently carry blood posteriorly to the thoracic aorta, distal to the coarctation. The increased blood flow from anterior to posterior leads to grooving on the inferior surface of the ribs, which can be seen on a PA chest film. The constriction of the aorta may not be evident on plain films. Echocardiogram or CT of the chest should be used to confirm the diagnosis. Coarctation of the aorta is often seen in conjunction with other heart defects (bicuspid aortic valve, or ventricular septal defect) and is common in Turner's syndrome.

A patent ductus arteriosus (**answer a**) would *not* cause the difference in arm and leg blood pressures. Most people with Tetralogy of Fallot (**answer b**) require surgery prior to age 6. Transposition of the great arteries (**answer c**) requires immediate surgery after birth in most instances. An enlarged right heart border (**answer e**) would *not* occur in this girl.

355. The answer is d. (*Moore and Dalley, pp 63, 166–167.*) Afferent innervation from the heart and coronary arteries travel within the cardiac plexus of nerves along the sympathetic pathways. Once the afferent fibers pass through the cardiac plexus, they run along the cervical and thoracic cardiac nerves to the cervical and upper four thoracic sympathetic ganglia. Having traversed these ganglia, the fibers gain access (via the white rami communicantes) to the upper four thoracic spinal nerves and the corresponding levels of the spinal cord. The visceral afferent fibers associated with the vagus nerve (**answer e**) are associated with reflexes and do *not* carry nociceptive information. The greater (**answer b**), lesser, and least splanchnic nerves convey visceral afferents from the abdominal region. *Neither* the carotid branch of the glossopharyngeal nerve (**answer a**) *nor* the phrenic nerve (**answer c**) carry cardiac pain fibers.

356. The answer is b. (*Moore and Dalley, p 151. Sadler, p 178.*) The additional heart defect the newborn girl also has is a ventricular septal defect. Babies born with transposition of the great vessels normally present with symptoms of cyanosis as the ductus arteriosus closes within the first day of birth. In this defect, the aorta is sitting on top of the right ventricle and the pulmonary trunk is receiving blood from the left ventricle, therefore blood is being pumped mainly to the body by the right side and mainly to the lungs by the left side. The only way oxygenated blood is traveling to the body is if the two sides are connected, often by a patent ductus arteriosus. Babies with this defect are immediately put on oxygen, and prostaglandins are also given to help keep the ductus arteriosus open longer than normal. About 25% of the time that transposition of the great vessels is present, there is also a ventricular septal defect, which aids in the intermixing of blood from the two sides of the heart. This condition must be treated surgically. Defects of the aortic arch are normally *not* present. The presence of a ligamentum arteriosum (**answer c**) would make the problem worse. Coarctation of the aorta (**answer d**) would make the problem worse. An overriding aorta (**answer a**) is the second best answer. An aortic aneurysm (**answer e**) is unlikely to be present in a newborn.

357. The answer is c. (*Moore and Dalley, pp 157–158.*) The great cardiac vein accompanies the anterior interventricular (descending) artery. The anterior cardiac veins (**answer a**) pass across the right coronary sulcus to drain directly into the right atrium. The small cardiac vein (**answer e**) accompanies the right marginal vein and the right coronary artery. The coronary sinus (**answer b**), accompanying the circumflex artery in the left coronary sulcus, receives the great, middle (**answer d**), and small cardiac veins (**answer e**) before draining into the right atrium.

358. The answer is c. (*Moore and Dalley, pp 160–161.*) In a coronary bypass procedure a blood vessel is added to allow blood to flow distal to the occluded coronary artery. This is generally done by removing the internal thoracic artery, which runs along the inner surface of the sternum. Its proximal end is attached to the ascending aorta and its distal end is connected to the occluded coronary artery, just distal to the blockage, thus bypassing the problem. Remember that the internal thoracic artery supplies blood to each subcostal artery, which are branches of the thoracic aorta. All of the other answers (**answers b, d**) involve attaching the blood vessel to a venous structure or in the case of the pulmonary trunk (**answer a**) attaching to relatively unoxygenated blood, which is *not* done.

359. The answer is c. (*Moore and Dalley, pp 167–168.*) Heart sounds originate from the closure of the atrioventricular and semilunar valves as a result of relative pressure reversals during the cardiac cycle. The first heart sound, heard just after the ventricles begin to contract, occurs when ventricular pressures exceed atrial pressures and thereby, closes the atrioventricular valves. Reverberation within the ventricles causes this S_1 sound ("Lub") to have a low frequency and a relatively long duration. The second heart sound is heard at the beginning of ventricular diastole, when the aortic and pulmonary pressures exceed the respective ventricular pressures and snap the aortic and pulmonary semilunar valves shut. This S_2 ("Dup") is relatively sharp when both aortic and semilunar valves close together. However, deep inspiration, which lowers intrathoracic pressure, results in delayed closing of the pulmonary valve and thus produces a split S_2.

Ventricular systole occurs approximately between the S_1 and S_2 heart sounds and diastole between S_2 and S_1. Occasionally, a low, rumbling third heart sound may be heard during diastole and is attributable to ventricular filling. Stenosis or insufficiency of the valves produces turbulence and backflow, respectively, which are heard as murmurs. None of the other combinations (**answers a, b, d, e**) are correct.

360. The answer is d. (*Moore and Dalley, pp 322–323.*) The esophageal hiatus, in addition to allowing passage of the esophagus, also passes the anterior and posterior vagal trunks. The aortic hiatus carries the aorta, the thoracic duct (**answer e**), and occasionally, an azygos (**answer a**) or hemiazygos (**answer b**) vein. Usually, the azygos and hemiazygos veins (**answer c**) either pass lateral to or through a crus of the diaphragm along with the respective left and right sympathetic chains. The phrenic nerves usually penetrate the diaphragm to gain access to the inferior surface; however, the right phrenic may accompany the inferior vena cava through the caval hiatus.

361. The answer is a. (*Sadler, pp 177–178.*) The girl has tetralogy of Fallot. Since the girl is 3 months old it is very unlikely that she would have survived transposition of the great vessels (**answer c**) without surgical intervention. Tetralogy of Fallot consists of three congenital conditions and a fourth acquired condition as a consequence of the first three. Tetralogy of Fallot consists of an overriding aorta that receives blood from both ventricles, pulmonary stenosis that tends to keep blood out of the lungs, and a ventricular septal defect (otherwise the aorta could "override"). As a consequence of the three conditions, the right ventricle tends to hypertrophy since it has to pump blood *not* only into the lungs, but also through the aorta to the rest of the body. Since the girl has normal blood pressure in her upper and lower limbs, coarctation of the aorta (**answer b**) is unlikely. In addition simple aortic stenosis (**answer d**) is unlikely to produce hypertrophy of the right ventricle which appears to be present. A ventricle septal defect (**answer e**) is just part of the problem.

362. The answer is b. (*Moore and Dalley, pp 113, 115.*) Normally the pleural space extends inferiorly about two additional ribs inferior to the lung at each location, thus at the midaxillary line the caudal portion of the lung normally lies at about the eight intercostal space and the pleural space would extend down to about rib 10. The sixth (**answer a**) intercostals space is too cranial and tenth (**answer b**) and twelfth (**answer d**) inter-coastal spaces are too caudal.

363. The answer is b. (*Moore and Dalley, p 189.*) Pulmonary trunk (bifurcated) The pulmonary trunk (8) has just bifurcated and will form the left and right pulmonary artery just inferior to the arch of the aorta. Other labeled structures are: 1, left ventricle; 7 aortic arch; 8 bifurcated pulmonary trunk (most likely left pulmonary artery in this image); 9 brachiocephalic artery; 10, left common carotid artery; 11 left subclavian artery; 12 ascending aorta; 13 descending aorta; and 14 right coronary artery (difficult to see).

364. The answer is c. (*Sadler, p 178.*) The two major changes that occur at birth in the heart or vessels are that the septum primum closes against the septum securdum and the ductus arteriosus closes. At delivery, the blood from the placenta decreases, thus reducing the pressure in the right atrium. As the air fills the lungs there is increased blood flow to the lungs and thus increased blood returning to the left atrium. This increase in left atrial pressure and decrease in right atrial pressure closes the septum primum against the septum secundum, thus closing the foramen ovale, and separating the two atrial chambers. In addition there is smooth muscle constriction within the walls of the ductus arteriosus, also sending more blood to the lungs. (See figures in answer to question 14 in Embryology: Early and General.) None of the other answers (**answers a, b, d, e**) are correct

365. The answer is b. (*Moore and Dalley, pp 79–80.*) One would expect a cracked rib that allows blood from the intercostal vessels to bleed into the pleural cavity, partially collapsing the left lung, causing the shortness of breath. Blood in the pleural cavity is an irritant and causes generalized chest pain. The left-sided, midback pain is from the cracked eleventh rib. Because only one lung appears to have fluid accumulation and he is young and exercises regularly; pulmonary hypertension (**answer a**) is unlikely, especially give his physical findings and history and sudden onset of symptoms. Cardiac tamponade (**answer c**), which is blood within the pericardial sac, is unexpected. Neither gallbladder pain (**answer e**), *nor* an inflamed appendix (**answer d**) would typically cause chest pain. Note: the CT of the abdomen is required to rule out damage to kidneys and spleen.

366. The answer is e. (*Moore and Dalley, pp 156–160.*) A sonogram of the heart (or echocardiogram) that suggests decreased posterior wall movement is most likely due to local infarction or fibrosis of that portion of the heart. Infarcted or fibrotic tissue would reduce blood flow. The major blood supply to the left anterior ventricular wall in most hearts is the posterior interventricular artery (or posterior descending), normally a branch off the right coronary artery. If there is blockage (generally described as a percent of normal) in a coronary artery, then there should be a concomitant decrease in the blood within the vein that serves that region. The middle cardiac vein runs with the posterior interventricular. The circumflex branch of the left coronary artery runs with the great cardiac vein **(answer a)** within the atrial ventricular sulcus for a short distance, but blood flow reduction in those vessels does *not* fit with the echocardiographic results. The right marginal branch of the right coronary artery runs with the small cardiac vein **(answer d)**, but they serve the right ventricle. The anterior interventricular artery runs with the great cardiac vein **(answer b)**, *not* the middle cardiac vein **(answer c)**, but on the anterior aspect of the heart.

367. The answer is c. (*Moore and Dalley, pp 150, 154.*) The origin of the pulmonary trunk is anterior and to the right of the ascending aorta. During embryonic development the outflow tract of the heart (the truncus arteriosus) becomes divided into the ascending aorta and pulmonary trunk by the conotruncal ridges. Remember that semilunar valves form at these outflow tracks. Both the aortic and pulmonary valves have right and left cusps. Remember that the aortic valve has a right and left cusp, but also a posterior cusp, since it is more posterior. In contrast, the pulmonary valve has both right and left cusps and an anterior cusp since it is more anterior (each semilunar valve has the single cusp that the first letter of its name does *not* have); aortic has posterior; pulmonary has anterior. This also reminds you that the aorta is posterior to the pulmonary trunk. Also remember that the right ventricle is the more anterior chamber and thus gives off a more anterior great vessel. The left ventricle is the more posterior chamber as it gives off its outflow tract. As the great vessels proceed cranially, the aorta ends up on the left as it arches over the split of the pulmonary arteries. The other answers **(answers a, b, d)** are *not* correct.

368. The answer is d. (*Moore and Dalley pp 91, 188–189.*) Structures typically found at the same level as the sternal angle in an axial CT include: the second rib; intervertebral disc T 4/5; bifurcation of trachea; and azygos vein joining superior vena cava. Since the tracheal lumen is air filled, it appears black on CT images. The trachea is normally easy to follow inferiorly until it bifurcates into right and left main bronchi. This bifurcation normally occurs at about the sternal angle, where the body of the sternum meets the manubrium and where the second rib attaches, which is also the approximate level of the intervertebral disc T 4/5. The other answers (**answers a, b, c, e**) are *not* correct.

Abdomen

Questions

DIRECTIONS: Each item below contains a question or incomplete statement followed by suggested responses. Select the **one best** response to each question.

369. You deliver a newborn baby girl that has an umbilical hernia with part of another organ attached to its inner surface. What portion of the gastrointestinal tract is most likely to be attached to the inner surface of the umbilical hernia?

a. Anal canal
b. Appendix
c. Cecum
d. Ileum
e. stomach

370. A 46-year-old bakery worker is admitted to a hospital in acute distress. She has experienced severe abdominal pain, nausea, and vomiting for 2 days. The pain, which is sharp and constant, began in the epigastric region and radiated bilaterally around the chest to just below the scapulas. Subsequently, the pain became localized in the right hypochondrium. The patient, who has a history of similar but milder attacks after hearty meals over the past 5 years, is moderately overweight and the mother of four. Palpation reveals marked tenderness in the right hypochondriac region and some rigidity of the abdominal musculature. An x-ray without contrast medium shows numerous calcified stones in the region of the gallbladder. The patient shows no sign of jaundice (icterus). Diffuse pain referred to the epigastric region and radiating circumferentially around the chest is the result of afferent fibers that travel via which of the following nerves?

a. Greater splanchnic
b. Intercostal
c. Phrenic
d. Vagus
e. Pelvic splanchnics

371. Gallbladder pain often presents as epigastric pain that then migrates towards the patient's right side and can even wrap around to the posterior. The referred pain is not the site of the problem. Anatomically where is the gallbladder located?

a. Between the left and caudate lobes of the liver
b. Between the right and quadrate lobes of the liver
c. In the falciform ligament
d. In the lesser omentum
e. In the right anterior leaf of the coronary ligament

372. A woman presents with gallstones and no jaundice. She is prepared for exploratory surgery. The lesser omentum is incised close to its free edge, and the biliary tree is identified and freed by blunt dissection. The liquid contents of the gallbladder are aspirated with a syringe, the fundus incised, and the stones are removed. The entire duct system is carefully probed for stones, one of which is found to be obstructing a duct. In view of her symptoms, where is the most probable location of the obstruction?

a. The bile duct
b. The common hepatic duct
c. The cystic duct
d. Within the duodenal papilla proximal to the juncture with the pancreatic duct
e. Within the duodenal papilla distal to the juncture with the pancreatic duct

373. A full-term 8 lb baby boy was delivered vaginally to a 36-year-old mother. At delivery he had a large scrotum. The delivering OB palpated the enlarged scrotum and determined that both testicles were present. When the OB pressed gently on the newborn's abdomen the scrotum swelled even more. What congenital condition did the OB note in the chart?

a. Abdominal hernia
b. Cryptorchid (maldescended) testes
c. Varicocele
d. Hydrocele
e. Femoral hernia

374. Many cesarean sections are performed by making a horizontal skin incision that is slightly curved (about 15 cm) on the anterior abdominal wall just superior to the pubic hairline (bikini or Pfannerenstiel incision). However, this incision is often only made through the skin down to the perimysium of the rectus abdominis muscle. Which of the following cutaneous nerves are at greatest risk with this type of incision?

a.   Thoracoabdominal (intercostal) nerve (T 10)
b.   Thoracoabdominal (intercostal) nerve (T 11)
c.   Iliohypogastric nerve (L1)
d.   Ilioinguinal nerve (L1)
e.   Lateral (femoral) cutaneous nerve of the thigh (L2–3)

375. A 13-year-old boy was vacationing with his parents in Mexico on spring break. He developed nausea, vomiting 4 days into the trip despite caution about what he ate and drank. He switched to a clear liquid diet. None of the others on the trip were sick. On his flight back to the United States the next day he developed a fever and increased abdominal pain, especially in the paraumbilical region. His parents took him to their pediatrician the next day as he was feeling worse and could barely move. During the physical exam the pediatrician noted tenderness around the umbilicus and rebound tenderness over McBurney's point and was sent for an abdominal CT at a local pediatric hospital. Where is McBurney's point and what is the likely diagnosis?

a.   At the right costal margin at the mid-clavicular line; ruptured gallbladder
b.   On a line drawn between the anterior superior iliac spine and umbilicus on the right; appendicitis
c.   On a line drawn between the anterior superior iliac spine and umbilicus on the left; appendicitis
d.   On a line drawn between the anterior superior iliac spine and the pubic tubercle on the right; kidney stone
e.   On a line drawn between the anterior superior iliac spine and the pubic tubercle on the left; kidney stone

376. A 65-year-old male presents with jaundice for 2–3 weeks, fatigue and increasing epigastric pain. He has no history of peptic ulcers and says the pain does *not* relate to eating in anyway. His epigastric pain is midline and he has had some recent back pain. His urinary bilirubinogen and serum bilirubin are elevated (serum bilirubin 5.8 mg/dl). Helical CT reveals a suspicious mass in the head of the pancreas adjacent to the descending duodenum. The gallbladder is significantly enlarged. Which of the following is the likely cause of the elevated bilirubin?

a. Viral hepatitis
b. Blocked cystic duct
c. Open hepatic duct
d. Blocked duodenal papilla
e. Gilbert syndrome

377. A full-term male infant displays projectile vomiting 1 h after suckling. There is failure to gain weight during the first 48 hours. The vomitus is not bile-stained and no respiratory difficulty is evident. Examination reveals an abdomen *neither* tense *nor* bloated. Which of the following is the most probable explanation?

a. Congenital hypertrophic pyloric stenosis
b. Congenital absence of a kidney
c. Patent ileal diverticulum
d. Imperforate anus
e. Tracheoesophageal fistula

378. In Hirschsprung's disease, there is a loss of peristalsis in the lower colon and often fatal obstruction. Preganglionic neurons, which would innervate the aganglionic segment of bowel, originate in which of the following?

a. The nucleus ambiguus
b. Cervical intermediolateral cell column
c. Sacral levels two to four of the spinal cord
d. The motor nucleus of the vagus nerve (CN X)
e. The ventral horn at spinal levels L1–L2

379. The 65-year-old with pancreatic adenocarcinoma in the head of pancreas was taken to surgery. A PET CT suggested some metastasis to both liver and multiple posterior lymph nodes. It was explained to the patient and his family that the surgery would likely *not* be curative, but rather palliative in that the cancer was already too far advanced for removal. During the surgery ablation of the autonomic innervation that carries pain in this region is also performed to provide pain relief. The surgeon will inject 50% ethanol to kill nerve cells at which of the following locations?

a. At each subcostal nerve under ribs 6–8
b. Around the celiac trunk
c. Around each lateral epigastric fold
d. Around the coronary ligament
e. Around the lateral arcuate ligament

380. An 11-year-old girl is brought into your pediatric office by her mother. She recently learned to do back flips on the balance beam, when her foot slipped off and she landed with her perineum striking the beam. She developed a massive subcutaneous hematoma filling her perineum that posteriorly formed a straight horizontal line just anterior to her anus, and anteriorly extended onto the anterior abdominal wall about half way up to her umbilicus and above the inguinal ligament. No blood entered her thighs. She could still urinate and there was no blood in her urine. The hematoma was contained by what space?

a. Ischioanal fossa
b. Superficial perineal space
c. Deep perineal space
d. Femoral sheath
e. Inguinal canal

381. A slender 53-year-old woman who smokes a pack of cigarettes each day comes to your office complaining of a pulsating sensation in her abdomen with generalized abdominal and back pain. You palpate her abdomen and feel a mid-line pulse with every heart beat. You order an abdominal Doppler ultrasound, which shows a large, high abdominal aortic aneurysm above renal arteries of about 8 cm in diameter. She is admitted to the hospital immediately for repair of her aortic aneurysm because it is life threatening, but you warn her that one of the complications of such surgical repair includes paraplegia. During the procedure the vascular surgeon must completely clamp off the abdominal aorta for about an hour while repairing the aneurysm. Which of the following would explain to the patient why there is a risk of paraplegia?

a. Stopping the blood within the abdominal aorta causes the muscle of the lower limbs to die
b. Stopping the blood within the abdominal aorta causes the peripheral nerves of the lower limb to die
c. Stopping the blood within the abdominal aorta causes loss of blood flow to the major radicular artery (of Adamkiewicz), which causes the motor components in the spinal cord for the lower limb to die
d. Stopping the blood within the abdominal aorta causes microemboli within the lower limb to form during the surgery and those microemboli then pass through the lung and left side of the heart into the brain where they selectively lodge in the motor cortex that controls the lower limbs
e. Stopping the blood within the abdominal aorta causes excessive perfusion of the brain during the surgery, which selectively causes bleeding stroke within the motor cortex that controls the lower limbs

382. The lateral umbilical fold serves as the demarcation for whether an inguinal hernia is direct or indirect. The lateral umbilical fold on each side of the inner surface of the anterior abdominal wall is created by which of the following underlying structures?

a. Falx inguinalis
b. Inferior epigastric artery
c. Lateral border of the rectus sheath
d. Obliterated umbilical artery
e. Urachus

383. A 19-year-old teenager is brought to the emergency room after a single-car accident just 20 minutes earlier in which she lost control of her car on black ice and hit a retaining column of an overpass at about 45 miles per hour. She was wearing a seat belt but looks pale, has tachycardia and positional hypotension, is extremely nauseated, and is lying in the fetal position due to increasingly severe abdominal pain. She has *no* fractures and a cranial nerve test is normal. You order an abdominal CT because you suspect which of the following?

a. Lacerated kidney
b. Ruptured spleen
c. Ruptured gallbladder
d. Diverticulitis
e. Hemorrhoids

384. A posteriorly perforating ulcer in the pyloric antrum of the stomach is most likely to produce an initial localized peritonitis or abscess formation in which of the following?

a. Greater sac
b. Left subhepatic and hepatorenal spaces (pouch of Morison)
c. Omental bursa
d. Right subphrenic space
e. Right subhepatic space

385. A 55-year-old woman arrives at the emergency room the day after St. Patrick's Day coughing up bright red blood. She has frequented your emergency room before. History includes excessive alcohol consumption. Using abdominal percussion you determine that her liver extends 5 cm below the right costal margin at the midclavicular line. You call in a gastroenterologist because you suspect that the bright red blood is most likely the result of which of the following?

a. Hemorrhoids
b. Colon cancer
c. Duodenal ulcer
d. Gastric ulcer
e. Esophageal varices

386. The lesser sac (omental bursa) is directly continuous with which of the following recesses or spaces?

a. Infracolic compartment
b. Left colic gutter
c. Left subphrenic recess
d. Right subphrenic space
e. Hepatorenal recess

387. Mucosal necrosis of the rectum usually will *not* result from occlusion of the inferior mesenteric artery for which of the following reasons?

a. Arterial supply to the rectum is from anastomotic connections from the superior mesenteric artery
b. Arterial supply to the rectum is from the left colic artery with anastomoses to branches of the internal iliac artery
c. The inferior mesenteric artery does not supply the rectum
d. A principal branch of the external iliac artery is a major supplier to the rectum
e. The middle rectal artery, a branch of the internal iliac artery, supplies the rectum

388. Sympathectomy may occasionally relieve intractable pain of visceral origin, in as much as visceral afferent pain fibers run along the sympathetic pathways in the abdomen. The autonomic control of peristalsis in the descending colon should *not* be affected by bilateral lumbar sympathectomy for which of the following reasons?

a. The descending colon is controlled chiefly by parasympathetic innervation from the pelvic splanchnic nerves
b. The descending colon receives its parasympathetic innervation from the vagus nerve
c. The descending colon receives its sympathetic innervation from thoracic splanchnic nerves
d. Lumbar splanchnics from L1, L2, and L3 only innervate the pelvic viscera via the hypogastric nerve
e. Only presynaptic sympathetic fibers have been severed

389. A man, the victim of a superficial knife wound to the lower abdomen during a barroom brawl, subsequently develops a direct inguinal hernia. Damage to which of the following nerves is most likely responsible for the predisposing weakness of the abdominal wall?

a. Genitofemoral nerve
b. Ilioinguinal nerve
c. The subcostal nerve
d. Pelvic splanchnic nerves
e. The nerve of the tenth intercostal space (T10)

390. A multiparous mother brings in her second son, an 18-month-old active toddler, because she has noticed blood (sometimes red, one time "currant jelly") in his stools. Although the toddler is trying new foods, she doesn't think the blood is associated with anything in his diet. Your physical exam, including a digital rectal exam, is normal. You order an upper GI barium swallow with small bowel follow through and radiological report describes a 2-inch-long diverticulum, pointing toward the umbilicus, in the ileum, about 2 ft from the ileocecal valve. You explain to the mother that the blood is most likely from which of the following sources?

a. An appendix that must be removed
b. A Meckel's (ileal) diverticulum
c. Active diverticulitis
d. Internal hemorrhoids
e. A duodenal ulcer

391. Which of the following gives rise to all structures of the kidney?

a. Somitic mesoderm
b. Intermediate mesoderm
c. Splanchnic lateral plate mesoderm
d. Somatic lateral plate mesoderm
e. Neural crest

392. A middle-aged woman describes flushing, severe headaches, and a feeling that her heart is "going to explode" when she gets excited. At the beginning of a physical examination her blood pressure (130/85) is *not* significantly above normal. However, on palpation of her upper left quadrant, the examining physician notices the onset of sympathetic signs. Her blood pressure (200/135) is abnormally high. A subsequent CT scan confirms the suspected tumor of the left adrenal gland. The patient is scheduled for surgery. The symptoms that the patient correlates with the onset of excitement were most likely due to neural stimulation of the adrenal glands. The adrenal medulla receives its innervation from which of the following?

a. Preganglionic sympathetic nerves
b. Postsynaptic sympathetic nerves
c. Preganglionic parasympathetic nerves
d. Postganglionic parasympathetic nerves
e. Somatic nerves

393. A 42-year-oldman presents with an enlarged left adrenal gland on CT scan. He is scheduled for adrenalectomy. The left adrenal gland is located, and the venous drainage is ligated to prevent life-threatening quantities of adrenalin from entering the bloodstream on manipulation of the gland. Normally, the left adrenal venous drainage is into which of the following?

a. Inferior vena cava
b. Left azygos vein
c. Left inferior phrenic vein
d. Left renal vein
e. Superior mesenteric vein

394. Which of the following statements concerning a direct inguinal hernia is correct?

a. It protrudes through the inguinal (Hesselbach's) triangle
b. It is the most common type of abdominal hernia in newborn boys
c. It traverses the entire length of the inguinal canal
d. It contains all three fascial layers of the spermatic cord
e. It exits the inguinal canal via the superficial inguinal ring

395. While moving furniture, an 18-year-old teenager experiences excruciating pain in his right groin. A few hours later he also develops pain in the umbilical region with accompanying nausea. At this point he seeks medical attention. Examination reveals a bulge midway between the midline and the anterior superior iliac spine, but superior to the inguinal ligament. On coughing or straining, the bulge increases and the inguinal pain intensifies. The bulge courses medially and inferiorly into the upper portion of the scrotum and cannot be reduced with the finger pressure of the examiner. It is decided that a medical emergency exists, and the patient is scheduled for immediate surgery. Nausea and diffuse pain referred to the umbilical region in this patient most probably are due to which of the following?

a. Compression of the genitofemoral nerve
b. Compression of the ilioinguinal nerve
c. Dilation of the inguinal canal
d. Ischemic necrosis of a loop of small bowel
e. Ischemic necrosis of the cremaster muscle

396. A 77-year-old woman complains to her doctor about left sided chest pain, difficulty swallowing and the sensation that food is stuck in her esophagus. Antacids don't seem to help much. The symptoms seems to get worse if she lies down shortly after meal and she often has some small reflux of acidic stomach contents. A barium swallow study is performed and one of the late images taken is illustrated below.

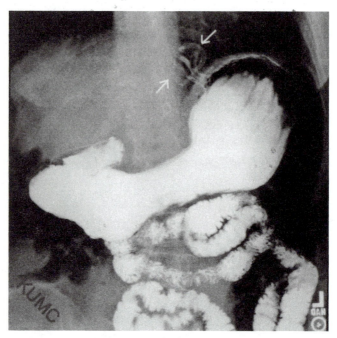

(Image 4910 used with permission from the Radiological Anatomy web site, University of Kansas, School of Medicine, http://classes.kumc.edu/som/radanatomy/.)

   Based on the history and radiological image which of the following is the most likely diagnosis?
a. Sliding hiatal hernia
b. Para esophageal hiatal hernia
c. Congenital Bochdalek hernia
d. Pylorospasm
e. Congenital hypertrophic pyloric stenosis

397. A 24-year old man was a passenger in an automobile broadsided by another vehicle. Although he was wearing a seat belt he felt "terrible," and had left sided abdominal, flank, and shoulder pain. During the ambulance ride into the emergency room his blood pressure kept dropping, he appeared pale, had a rapid heartbeat, with otherwise normal lung and heart sounds. Intravenous saline was started *en route*. Which of the following abdominal organs is most likely damaged?

a. Stomach
b. Duodenum
c. Pancreas
d. Left kidney
e. Spleen

398. Volvulus is most likely to occur within segments of the GI tract that are intraperitoneal, *not* retroperitoneal. Which segments of the GI tract are susceptible to volvulus, and to where does the referred pain of volvulus tend to occur for that segment?

a. Duodenum; epigastric region
b. Jejunum; epigastric region
c. Ascending colon; umbilical region
d. Descending colon; umbilical region
e. Sigmoid colon; suprapubic region

399. You have a patient who has renal failure as a result of Alport's syndrome. While he is currently on dialysis, he is hoping to receive a transplanted kidney. He asks you if they are going to remove one of his bad kidneys and put the new transplanted kidney back in the same place. You tell him which of the following?

a. The right kidney is always removed since it is more inferior and easier to remove and the new kidney will go in its place
b. The left kidney will be removed because it is easier to move the descending colon out of the way and the newly transplanted kidney will go in its place
c. He will keep both of his kidneys, and the newly transplanted kidney will be placed on the left posterior wall just inferior to his left kidney since there is more room because the left kidney is higher
d. The newly transplanted kidney will be placed in the iliac fossa in the greater pelvis, attached to branched iliac vessels and the ureter connected directly to the bladder

400. Allen is a 30-year-old bachelor who frequents "singles" bars. He is cautious and always uses a condom in his sexual encounters. Recently, he has felt "off," experiencing a sore throat, malaise, and a slight fever. When you see him in your office, he has a few swollen lymph nodes and has a large palpable structure in the left upper abdomen indicated by the asterisk in the accompanying radiograph. He had a positive monospot test and an elevated sedimentary rate. The structure you palpated was which of the following?

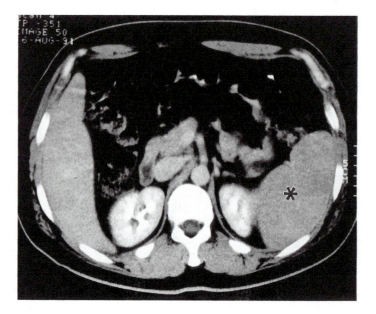

a. Hepatomegaly
b. Splenomegaly
c. The stomach
d. A tumor of the liver
e. Liver cirrhosis

401. A patient complained of severe abdominal pain on several occasions, but *no* cause could be identified. She was recently diagnosed with vasculitis of small and medium muscular blood vessels (polyarteritis nodosa) so you ordered an abdominal arteriogram to determine whether there were abdominal vascular changes that would explain her abdominal pain. On her arteriogram there is a tortuous vessel indicated by the arrow. What is this vessel?

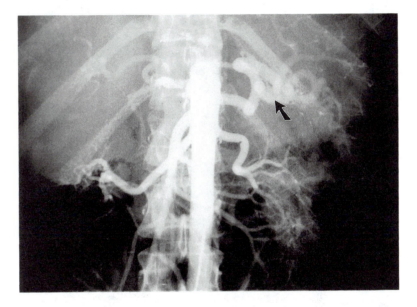

a. Left gastric artery
b. Superior mesenteric artery
c. Splenic artery
d. Right gastric artery
e. Right gastro-omental artery

402. Which of the following is structure 20 in the axial CT of the abdomen with intravenous contrast below?

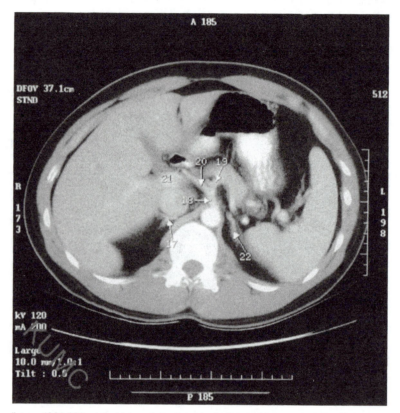

(Image 4201-009 used with permission from the Radiological Anatomy web site, University of Kansas, School of Medicine, http://classes.kumc.edu/som/radanatomy/.)

a. Celiac trunk (artery)
b. Common hepatic artery
c. Left crus of diaphragm
d. Splenic artery
e. Superior mesenteric artery

403. Pathology within some abdominal organs can occasionally cause referred pain in the shoulder and neck regions, C3–C5, because the diaphragm receives its motor and afferent innervation from this level as a result of its cranial embryonic development. Which of the following abdominal organs sometimes causes unilateral shoulder/neck pain?

a. Liver; left side
b. Gallbladder; right side
c. Pancreas; right side
d. Spleen; right side
e. Appendix; left side

404. Sensation of fullness in the rectum involves stretch receptors, which of the following provides innervation for those receptors?

a. Lumbar sympathetic chain
b. Pelvic splanchnic nerves (nervi erigentes)
c. Pudendal nerve
d. Sacral sympathetic chain
e. Vagus nerve

405. A 50-year-old man comes in for a physical so he can attend a boy scout camp with one of his sons. You suggest a colonoscopy after he returns from camp. He agrees, but wants you to describe the procedure and potential risks and complications. You explain that the goal of a colonoscopy is to look at the entire length of the large intestine from the anus to the small intestine (ileocecal junction), observing polyps or diverticuli with a flexible fiber optic colonoscope inserted through the anus. There is a small risk of perforating the bowel especially when the colon takes a sudden turn or twists on itself at regions where it is intraperitoneal rather than attached to the posterior abdominal wall (retroperitoneal). Which of the following regions of the colon generally poses the greatest risk for perforation because the bowel takes either a sudden change in direction or is suspended by a mesentery?

a. Rectum, sigmoid colon and descending colon
b. Sigmoid colon, descending colon and splenic flexure
c. Sigmoid colon, splenic flexure and descending colon
d. Sigmoid colon, splenic flexure and hepatic flexure
e. Descending colon, transverse colon and ascending colon

406. Which of the following is the principal supply to the body and tail of the pancreas?

a. Common hepatic artery
b. Inferior phrenic artery
c. Left gastric artery
d. Splenic artery
e. Superior mesenteric artery

407. A 42-year-old slightly overweight woman comes into your office complaining of recent blood in her stool. She has no fever and feels well otherwise. She generally has 1 or 2 bowel movements daily with no change in frequency or consistency. You ask if she has any painful hemorrhoids and she says she has *none* and *no* pain upon defecation. Prior to examining your patient what should be on your list of potential causes of blood in the stool?

a. Diverticular disease and colorectal cancer
b. Diverticular disease and internal hemorrhoids
c. Diverticular disease, external hemorrhoids, and colorectal cancer
d. External hemorrhoids and fissures, and diverticular disease
e. Diverticular disease, internal hemorrhoids, and colorectal cancer

408. During the physical exam of a 52-year-old man you note internal hemorrhoids. He complains of blood in his stool. Which of the following arteries could be the source of his rectal bleeding?

a. Superior rectal artery off the inferior mesenteric artery
b. Middle rectal artery off the internal iliac artery
c. Inferior rectal artery off the internal pudendal artery
d. Both b and c
e. a, b, and c

409. Several major anatomic structures pass through hiatal openings in the diaphragm. Which of the following lettered openings normally transmits the left vagus nerve?

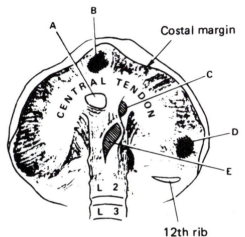

Diaphragm — Inferior Surface

a. A
b. B
c. C
d. D
e. E

410. During the visit of a 73-year-old man to your office for ongoing control of his hypertension (155/90) you note that he has lost about 5 lb since his last visit. He reports that he just doesn't seem to have as much room for food or as much of an appetite. He states that he is getting tired of the food at his nursing home. You palpate his abdomen and note that there is a midline pulse, which you had initially mistaken for a heartbeat, but it is slightly delayed. You grow quite concerned about this pulsating abdominal mass and send him for an abdominal CT with intravenous contrast because you think that he has which of the following?

a. A hiatal hernia
b. Splenomegaly
c. Cirrhosis of the liver
d. An aortic aneurysm
e. A horseshoe kidney

411. Most direct inguinal hernias occur in older men as the conjoint tendon weakens with increased abdominal pressure, often a complication of excessive abdominal weight gain. In contrast, most indirect inguinal hernias occur in which of the following?

a. Teenage females
b. Multiparous women
c. Newborn boys
d. Teenage males
e. Skinny middle aged men

412. As a general surgeon specializing in oncological cases you do a fair number of bowel resections. A 55-year-old man is referred to your office by his gasteroentrogist who recently removed two polyps from his splenic flexure of the colon during an endoscopic exam. The pathology report has confirmed that they are both cancerous and recommends surgical resection of a portion of the bowel from where the polyps were removed. Lymph nodes that receive lymph from this region are removed for sampling to stage the cancer growth. The 55-year-old patient comes to your office to learn what is involved in the surgical procedure. You describe that you are probably going to remove about a foot long section of large intestine, which includes part of the transverse and descending colon and then reattach the cut ends to each other and reconnect a major artery and collect numerous lymph nodes. Which of the following major arteries is going to be reconnected and where are you going to collect lymph nodes from to stage the potential spread of the colon cancer?

a. aorta; splenic and suprarenal lymph nodes
b. splenic artery; splenic and suprarenal lymph nodes
c. marginal artery; splenic and superior mesenteric lymph nodes
d. marginal artery; superior and inferior mesenteric lymph nodes
e. sigmoid artery; left colic and sigmoidal nodes

413. When examining a 48-year-old woman for the first time at a free clinic you note that she is quite slender and tanned. During the physical exam you note that she has prominent veins both on her anterior abdominal wall and also about her nose. During the physical exam you can palpate a fairly large firm organ that extends well below the right costal margin during both inspiration and expiration. There is *no* abdominal tenderness. Which of the following is the most likely explanation for your physical findings?

a. Splenomegaly
b. Hepatomegaly
c. Appendicitis
d. Cholecystitis
e. Abdominal aortic aneurysm

Abdomen

Answers

369. The answer is d. (*Moore and Dalley, pp 270, 271.*) During the first month of development, the midgut communicates over its entirety with the yolk sac. This connection narrows during the second month to form the vitelline duct (yolk stalk, omphalomesenteric duct) as the midgut closes and usually disappears during the ninth week. Because the vitelline duct joins the ileum, this section of the gastrointestinal tract is the last to close. Failure of closure results in a persistent vitelline fistula, whereas partial obliteration results in an ileal diverticulum (of Meckel). The ileal diverticulum and umbilical hernia would most likely be repaired at the same time. Other regions (**answers a, b, c and e**) of the gastrointestinal tract are unlikely to be attached to the anterior abdominal wall.

370. The answer is a. (*Moore and Dalley, pp 257–258, 322–323.*) Visceral afferent pain fibers from the gallbladder travel through the celiac plexus, thence along the greater splanchnic nerves to levels T5–T9 of the spinal cord. Thus, pain originating from the gallbladder will be referred to (appear as if coming from) the dermatomes served by T5–T9, which include a band from the infrascapular region to the epigastrium. If the gallbladder enlarges sufficiently, then pain could be carried by the phrenic nerve (**answer c**), but this would refer pain to the neck. Intercostal nerves (**answer b**) would course above the diaphragm and thus are not involved. The vagus (**answer d**) generally does not transmit pain information. Pelvic splanchinics (**answers e**) receive pain information from pelvic organs and thus are not involved.

371. The answer is b. (*Moore and Dalley, pp 290–291, 295.*) The gallbladder lies on the inferior surface of the liver between the right and quadrate lobes [thus not (**answer a**)]. The caudate lobe lies posteriorly between the right and left lobes. The falciform ligament, a portion of the lesser omentum, attaches to the liver at the incisura between the quadrate and left lobes as well as along the fissure for the round ligament. Toward the superior surface of the liver, the falciform ligament (**answer c**) splits to form the left and right coronary ligaments, which define the bare area of the liver. The coronary ligaments **(answer e)** come together again to form the gastrohepatic ligament of the lesser omentum **(answer d)**.

372. The answer is c. *(Moore and Dalley, p 304.)* Obstruction of any portion of the biliary tree will produce symptoms of gallbladder obstruction. If the common hepatic duct **(answer b)** or bile duct **(answer a)** is occluded by stone or tumor, biliary stasis with accompanying jaundice occurs. In addition, blockage of the duodenal papilla (of Vater), distal to the juncture of the bile duct with the pancreatic duct **(answer e)**, can lead to complicating pancreatitis. If only the cystic duct is obstructed, jaundice will not occur because bile may flow freely from the liver to the duodenum. Bile duct obstruction also may arise as a result of pressure exerted on the duct by an external mass, such as a tumor in the head of the pancreas. **Answser d** is not anatomically correct.

373. The answer is d. *(Moore and Dalley, pp 225–226.)* The newborn boy has a hydrocele. The testicles develop on the posterior abdominal wall and are pulled down and out of the abdominal cavity by the gubernaculum. The final descent through the inguinal canal does not generally occur until the 9th month *in utero.* The testis remains a retroperitoneal organ behind the fluid-filled space which is connected to the abdominal cavity by the process vaginalis (Moore & Dalley, p 218). In this case the testicles successfully migrated into the scrotum on both sides [so he did not have cryptorchid testes **(answer b)**], but rather the processus vaginalis failed to seal itself off from the abdominal cavity. Congenital hydrocele normally resolves itself after 2–3 months without any intervention. An abdominal hernia **(answer a)** is a defect on the anterior abdominal wall and is not present. Varicoceles **(answer c)** are a stasis of venous blood around the testicle and often present as a bluish scrotal mass. Femoral hernias **(answer e)** are defects in both the femoral sheath and fascia lata and present on the anterior thigh below the inguinal ligament.

374. The answer is c. *(Moore and Dalley, pp 207, 209.)* The cutaneous nerves are at risk with this type of incision is the iliohypogastric nerve (L1). The thoracoabdominal (intercostal) nerve T10 **(answer a)** generally supplies the dermatome that includes the umbilicus while the skin over the inguinal ligament is generally served by the L1 spinal level. T11 **(answer b)** is also too cranial to be a risk of injury. Both the subcostal nerve T12 (not listed as choice) and the iliohypogastric nerves are likely cut during the Pfannerenstiel incision. The ilioinguinal nerve **(answer d)** tends to course about an inch superior to the inguinal ligament, thus usually would most likely not be cut. The lateral (femoral) cutaneous nerve of the thigh (from L2 to L3) **(answer e)** runs across the iliacus muscle and under the inguinal ligament well lateral to the femoral sheath to serve the anterolateral aspect of the thigh, thus should not be at risk.

375. The answer is b. (*Moore and Dalley, pp 208–209, 275.*) Rebound tenderness over McBurney's point is the likely diagnosis for an appendicitis. McBurney's point is generally described at 1.5–2 in. superomedial on a line drawn between the patient's right (thus left and **answer c** is wrong) anterior superior iliac spine and the umbilicus. This is the approximate location of the ileocecal junction near where the appendix would lie deep to the anterior abdominal wall. The history of first umbilical pain and nausea and vomiting is consistent with appendicitis, not kidney stones **(answers d and e)**. The inguinal ligament courses between the anterior superior iliac spine and the pubic tubercle, which is the lateral portion of the pubic crest. While kidney stones are very painful they are not always associated with vomiting, nor does the pain locate to either the umbilical region or McBurney's point. Gallbladder pain often presents with rebound tenderness at the right costal margin at the mid-clavicular line **(answer a)**.

376. The answer is d. (*Moore and Dalley, p 288.*) The likely cause of the elevated bilirubin is a blocked pancreatic and bile duct at the duodenal papilla. Pancreatic cancer (usually ductal adenocarcinoma) frequently arises from the head of the pancreas where it blocks the normal flow of bile out of the liver, via the hepatic duct and gallbladder, via the cystic duct which join to form the (common) bile duct that passes through the substance of the head of the pancreas where it joins the main pancreatic duct just before forming the hepatopancreatic ampulla at the second portion of the duodenum (see Moore & Dalley, p 283). As a consequence of the blockage [not open hepatic duct **(answer c)**] of the normal exit of bile from the body bilirubin levels increase and jaundice (yellowing) develops. Blockage of the cystic duct **(answer b)** may just lead to a gallbladder enlargement/inflammation. Viral hepatitis **(answer a)** would normally not be associated with pancreatic cancer. Gilbert syndrome (**answer e**) is due to mild, chronic unconjugated hyperbilirubinemia and is *not* involved.

377. The answer is a. (*Moore and Dalley, p 256.*) Blockage of the foregut in the newborn produces projectile vomiting. Congenital hypertrophic pyloric stenosis, occurring in 0.5–1.0% of males and rarely in females, involves hypertrophy of the circular layer of muscle at the pylorus. This usually does *not* regress and must be treated surgically. During the 5th and 6th weeks of development, the lumen of the duodenum is occluded by muscle proliferation but normally recanalizes during the eighth week. Failure of recanalization results in duodenal atresia. Because this occurs proximal to the hepatopancreatic ampulla, the vomitus will occasionally be stained with bile. Annular pancreas, rare in itself, seldom completely blocks the duodenum. Congenital absence of a kidney (**answer b**) would *not* present with the symptoms described. Imperforate anus (**answer d**) results in intestinal distention with bloating. A newborn with a typical tracheoesophageal fistula (**answer e**) can *not* feed without aspiration. A newborn with a patent ileal diverticulum (**answer c**) would present with stool coming out his umbilicus.

378. The answer is c. (*Moore and Dalley, p 276.*) Preganglionic parasympathetic neurons to the lower colon arise from the spinal cord at sacral levels two to four (thus not **answer b**) and reach the wall of the colon via pelvic splanchnic nerves. The nucleus ambiguus is the source of preganglionic parasympathetic neurons that innervate the heart via the vagus nerve and cardiac plexus (**answer a and d**). Neurons arising in the cervical intermediolateral cell column are sympathetic preganglionics. Preganglionic parasympathetic neurons arising from the motor nucleus of the vagus innervate the upper GI tract. Neurons arising from the ventral horn are primary somatic motor neurons to skeletal muscle (**answer e**).

379. The answer is b. (*Moore and Dalley, pp 284–285, 288.*) The surgeon will inject 50% ethanol to kill nerve cells around the celiac trunk. Palliative pain relief for pancreatic cancer is called chemical splanchnicectomy. The purpose is to kill afferent pain fibers which detect free ATP (from dying cells) and stretch receptors for the foregut area, affected by the cancer. This is best accomplished by injecting ethanol around the celiac trunk at the posterior abdominal wall, thus at the celiac plexus. Injection of each subcostal nerve T 6–8 (**answer a**) would cause a loss of sensation on the upper anterior abdominal wall, but would not cover all the area to which pain is referred. This would be the second best answer. The lateral epigastric folds (**answer c**) are inferior and only house inferior epigastric blood vessels, not nerves. The coronary ligament (**answer d**) holds the liver to the undersurface of the diaphragm. The lateral arcuate ligaments (**answer e**) are connective tissue structures on the posterior abdominal wall that allow the psoas muscles to pass inferiorly. The whipple procedure (performed in this case) removes the head of the pancreas and much of the duodenum and attaches the gallbladder to the descending portion of the duodenum to relieve the back-up of bile.

380. The answer is b. (*Moore and Dalley, pp 440–442.*) The hematoma was contained by superficial perineal space. This is a typical "straddle" injury to the perineum. The blood is collecting in the superficial perineal space, which houses the erectile tissue and is created by the superficial membranous fascia (*see Moore & Dalley, p 440*), which is called Scarpa's on the anterior abdominal wall (where it is attached half way up to the rectus abdominis muscle sheath) and is called Colles' fascia in the perineum. The membranous fascia attaches (deep) to the perineal membrane posteriorly and to the fascia lata of thigh and inguinal ligament. In males the membranous fascia has three names: Scarpa's (anterior abdominal wall); Dartos on penis and scrotum and Colles' on perineum. Following straddle injuries blood does *not* enter the inguinal canal (**answer e**), femoral sheath (**answer d**) and ischioanal fossa (**answer a**). The deep perineal space (**answer c**) is deep to the perineal membrane.

381. The answer is c. (*Moore and Dalley, pp 528–530.*) The lower thoracic and upper lumbar portion of the spinal cord tend to receive a single major radicular artery (of Adamkiewicz), which supplies blood to the anterior longitudinally running spinal artery. The anterior spinal artery mainly supplies the anterior two-thirds of the spinal cord in this region, which includes motor neurons that control the lower limbs. Because the metabolic needs of the spinal cord nerves are so great, the lack of blood during the surgery can lead to nerve cell death and thus paraplegia. Both muscle and peripheral nerves generally can survive the temporary disruption in blood flow. A process of cooling the spinal cord, by perfusing ice cold saline into the extradural space (called epidural cooling), is often performed to reduce the metabolic needs of the spinal nerves, thus often preventing central nervous system cell death during the surgical procedure. Muscles (**answer a**) and nerves (**answer b**) of the lower limb can survive reduced blood flow for an hour. Microemboli would *not* selectively locate in the motor cortex (**answer d**). Bleeding strokes in the motor cortex are unlikely (**answer e**).

382. The answer is b. (*Moore and Dalley, p 231.*) Inferior epigastric artery. The lateral umbilical folds are produced by the underlying inferior epigastric arteries as they course from the external iliac artery in the inguinal region toward the rectus sheath. A direct inguinal hernia starts medial to the lateral ambilical fold and an indirect inguinal hernia starts lateral to the same fold. The medial umbilical folds are peritoneal elevations produced by the obliterated umbilical arteries (**answer d**). In the midline, the median umbilical ligament is formed by the underlying urachus (**answer e**), a remnant of the embryonic allantois. The Falx inguinalis (**answer a**) represents inferomedial attachment of transversus abdominis with some fibers of internal abdominal oblique, also known as: conjoint tendon. The lateral border of the rectus sheath (**answer c**) forms the medial edge of the inguinal triangle.

383. The answer is b. (*Moore and Dalley, pp 191, 284.*) The spleen is a large blood filled organ with a relatively thin capsule that can rupture upon sudden deceleration, causing bleeding into the peritoneal cavity. Appearing pale, the positional hypotension and tachycardia would be consistent with bleeding into the peritoneal cavity, which would lead to generalized abdominal pain, and guarding (**answer c**). A ruptured gallbladder does *not* fit with the blood loss symptoms. Neither diverticulitis (**answer d**) *nor* hemorrhoids (**answer e**) would cause the set of symptoms listed. A lacerated kidney (**answer a**) would *not* bring on the sudden onset of symptoms.

384. The answer is c. (*Moore and Dalley, pp 239–241, 264.*) The omental bursa (lesser sac) is the remnant of the right coelomic cavity, which, owing to rotation of the gut and differential growth of the liver, lies behind the stomach. A posterior gastric perforation or an inflamed pancreas could lead to abscess formation in the lesser sac. The right subhepatic space might become secondarily involved via communication through the omental foramen (of Winslow). The pouch of Morison (**answer b**), which is the combined right subhepatic (**answer d**) and the hepatorenal spaces (**answer e**), may be the seat of abscess formation related to gallbladder disease or perforation of a duodenal ulcer. The right subphrenic space is located between the liver and the diaphragm and communicates with the pouch of Morison. All these spaces are in communication with the greater sac (**answer a**) of the peritoneal cavity.

385. The answer is e. *(Moore and Dalley, pp 305–307.)* Because of an enlarged liver and the history of excessive alcohol consumption, you suspect cirrhosis of the liver, which resulted in portal hypertension. Because the blood is bright red, suggesting that it has *not* been exposed to duodenal or gastric secretions, the most likely source would be esophageal varices, as blood is trying to return from the portal system to the systemic circulatory system. Hemorrhoids (**answer a**) are commonly associated with cirrhosis of the liver, but at the other end of the GI tract. Colon cancer (**answer b**) does *not* present with upper GI bleed, rather lower GI bleeding. *Neither* duodenal (**answer c**) *nor* gastric ulcers (**answer d**) present with bright red blood.

386. The answer is e. *(Moore and Dalley, p 290.)* The omental (epiploic) foramen connects the lesser sac with the hepatorenal (subhepatic) recess of the greater sac (see *Moore and Dalley, p 290* for an excellent picture of this relationship). The hepatorenal recess then communicates with the right subphrenic recess and right paracolic gutter. The subhepatic recess is perhaps the most frequently infected intra-abdominal space as a result of appendicitis, liver abscess, perforated duodenal and gastric ulcers, or perforation of the biliary tree. The infracolic compartment is (**answer a**) part of the greater omentum. The left colic gutter (**answer b**) is further inferior and left. The left subphrenic recess (**answer c**) and right subphrenic space (**answer d**) are further cranial on top of the liver.

387. The answer is e. *(Moore and Dalley, p 430.)* The rectum receives blood from the superior rectal (hemorrhoidal) artery and from the paired middle and inferior rectal arteries. The superior rectal artery is a direct continuation of the inferior mesenteric artery, but the middle and inferior rectal arteries are branches of the internal iliac artery and continue to supply the distal rectum despite occlusion of the inferior mesenteric artery. It should be noted that Sudeck's point, between the last sigmoidal artery and the rectosigmoid artery, is an area of potentially weak arterial anastomoses, but that is further cranial. The superior mesenteric artery **(answer a)** distributes arteries to the small intestine right and middle colic arteries, that supply blood as far distal as the splenic flexure of the transverse colon. The left colic artery **(answer b)** anastomoses with the sigmoidal arteries. The inferior mesenteric artery supplies the superior rectal artery, so **answer c** is *not* correct. The principal branch of the external iliac artery is the femoral artery **(answer e)**.

388. The answer is a. (*Moore and Dalley, p 322.*) The descending colon is controlled chiefly by parasympathetic innervation from the pelvic splanchnic nerves. Control of peristalsis is principally a function of the parasympathetic division of the autonomic nervous system. Although removal of the lumbar sympathetic chain (lumbar sympathectomy) does sever the sympathetic fibers innervating the descending colon as well as the pelvic viscera, [not thoracic splanchnics **(answer c)**] the action of sympathetic fibers to the descending colon is mostly confined to vasoconstriction. Because the parasympathetic innervation to the descending colon is derived from the sacral outflow (S2–S4) through the pelvic splanchnic nerves (nervi erigentes), [not by the vagus **(answer b)**] peristalsis will occur normally after lumbar sympathectomy. Lumbar splanchnics do *not* include L3 **(answer d)**. The **answer e** makes no sense.

389. The answer is b. (*Moore and Dalley, pp 202, 207.*) The ilioinguinal nerve innervates the portion of the internal oblique muscle inserting in the lateral border of the conjoint tendon. Paralysis of these fibers would create weakness in the conjoint tendon, allowing herniation to occur medial to the inferior epigastric vessels. The genitofemoral nerve **(answer a)** supplies sensory innervation to the skin of the femoral triangle and scrotum/labia majora. The subcostal nerve (T12) **(answer c)** supplies lower portions of the external abdominal oblique muscle. The pelvic splanchnic nerves **(answer d)** supply autonomic (parasympathetic) innervation to the pelvic viscera. The tenth thoracic spinal nerve (T10) **(answer e)** supplies abdominal muscles superior to the inguinal region.

390. The answer is b. (*Moore and Dalley, pp 270–271.*) Meckel's (ileal) diverticuli are the most common congenital abnormality of the digestive system. They are a remnant of the herniation and rotation of the midgut and at times the diverticulum remains attached to the umbilicus by a connective tissue stalk, as is mostly likely the case here. The diverticulum generally extends 2 inches from the ileum; about 2 ft from the ileocecal valve and usually manifests itself by bleeding prior to the first 2 years of life. There may be two types of ectopic tissue present in the diverticulum: either acid secreting epithelium (stomach; detected with radioactive technetium injected into the venous blood stream which then accumulates within the diverticulum) or pancreatic epithelium. (The rule of "2" helps remind you of the characteristics of Meckel's diverticulum.) The appendix **(answer a)** is a diverticulum off the cecum, *not* the ileum. Diverticuli **(answer c)** can cause blood in the stool but would be extremely rare in a toddler. Internal hemorrhoids **(answer d)** would generally be detected in a rectal exam, especially in a toddler and is *not* associated with "currant jelly" stools. The blood would more likely be black if a duodenal ulcer **(answer e)** were present, which would also be very rare in a toddler.

391. The answer is b. *(Sadler, pp 229–231.)* The kidney forms in three stages. The pronephric, metanephric, and mesonephric kidneys all form from the urogenital ridge, an extension of intermediate mesoderm into the coelomic cavity. Mesoderm derived from the somites (somatic; **answer a)** gives rise to components of the axial skeleton and associated muscle and connective tissues. Splanchnic lateral plate mesoderm **(answer c)** gives rise to the smooth muscle and connective tissue tunics of the abdominal viscera. Somatic lateral plate mesoderm **(answer d)** contributes substantially to the skeleton, connective tissue, and muscle mass of the appendages. Neural crest **(answer e)** forms the sensory and sympathetic chain ganglia and other structures.

392. The answer is a. *(Moore and Dalley, pp 63–64, 320.)* The adrenal medulla is innervated from thoracic levels of the spinal cord mediated by preganglionic sympathetic nerve fibers traveling in the lesser and least splanchnic nerves, with some contribution from the greater splanchnic and lumbar splanchnic nerves [thus not **(answer b)**]. Because both the adrenal medulla and postganglionic sympathetic neurons are adrenergic and derived from neural crest tissue, the homology of the chromaffin cells and postganglionic sympathetic neurons is apparent. There appears to be *no* parasympathetic innervation **(answers c and d)** to the adrenal medulla or cortex. There is *no* somatic **(answer e)** innervation by the adrenal medulla, by definition a visceral organ.

393. The answer is d. (*Moore and Dalley, pp 316–318.*) The venous drainage from each adrenal gland tends to be through a single vein. The left adrenal gland usually drains into the left renal vein superior [thus not **(answers a and b)**] to the point where the gonadal vein enters the left renal vein. The left adrenal vein usually anastomoses with the hemiazygos vein and may provide an important route of collateral venous return. Left inferior phrenic vein **(answer c)** and superior mesenteric vein **(answer e)** has *no* connections with adrenal veins. The right adrenal gland usually drains directly into the inferior vena cava.

394. The answer is a. (*Moore and Dalley, pp 213, 223–225.*) A direct inguinal hernia protrudes through a space bounded superolaterally by the inferior epigastric vessels, medially by the rectus abdominus muscle, and superior to the inguinal ligament (Hesselbach's triangle). The other statements **(answers b, c, d, e)** are true of an indirect inguinal hernia. A direct hernia traverses only the most medial part of the inguinal canal and is *not* covered by the most internal layers of spermatic cord fascia.

395. The answer is d. (*Moore and Dalley, pp 321–324.*) The diffuse central abdominal pain in the patient presented is probably referred pain from the loop of small bowel incarcerated within the herniated peritoneal sac that then undergoes ischemic necrosis. Compression of the bowel results in compromise of the blood supply and subsequent ischemic necrosis [thus not **(answer e)**]. The visceral afferent fibers from the distal small bowel travel along the blood vessels to reach the superior mesenteric plexus and lesser splanchnic nerves, which they follow to the T10–T11 levels of the spinal cord. The pain, therefore, is referred to (appears as if originating from) the T10–T11 dermatomes, which supply the umbilical region. Because the gut develops as a midline structure, visceral pain tends to be centrally located regardless of the adult location of any particular region of the gut. As a result of dilation **(answer c)** of the inguinal canal by the hernial sac, however, the patient also experiences localized somatic pain mediated by the iliohypogastric, ilioinguinal **(answer b),** and genitofemoral nerves **(answer a),** but this was *not* what the question asked.

396. The answer is a. (*Moore and Dalley, pp 250, 252.*) This patient has a sliding hiatal hernia. Sliding hiatal hernias are more common than paraesophageal hiatal hernias (**answer b**). Sliding hiatal hernias are generally acquired in middle age and lead to chest pain, difficulty swallowing food and acid reflux. A congenital Bochdalek hernia (**answer c**) is unlikely since they usually allow a portion of the small intestine to enter the left pleural cavity and are a medical emergency in newborns. Neither pylorospasm (**answer d**) nor congenital hypertrophic pyloric stenosis (**answer e**) is likely since barium is reaching the small intestine.

397. The answer is e. (*Moore and Dalley, pp 284–285.*) The spleen is one of the most frequently injured organs in the abdomen. This is especially so if the spleen was enlarged as a consequence of infectious mononucleosis making it more susceptible to rupture. Because it has an extensive blood supply, shock and death from bleeding into the peritoneal cavity can occur if a ruptured spleen is left untreated. The symptoms described above are consistent with blood loss most likely associated with a ruptured spleen. None of the other abdominal organs, stomach (**answer a**), duodenum (**answer b**), pancreas (**answer c**), and kidney (**answer d**) are likely to cause the sudden drop in blood pressure.

398. The answer is e. (*Moore and Dalley, pp 277, 257–258.*) Volvulus (twisting of the GI tract on itself) which limits movement of material within the lumen and may compromise blood flow occurs most frequently with the jejunum and ileum and the sigmoid colon. These are intraperitoneal segments of the GI tract. The jejunum and ileum are both midgut derivatives and thus refer pain to the periumbilical region [thus not (**answer b**)]. The sigmoid colon is the most mobile portion of the large bowel and is derived from the hindgut and tends to refer pain to the suprapubic region (especially on the left side) [thus not **answers c and d**]. The duodenum (**answer a**) is retroperitoneal and generally does *not* undergo volvulus.

399. The answer is d. (*Moore and Dalley, pp 311–312.*) The newly transplanted kidney will be placed in the iliac fossa in the greater pelvis, attached to branched iliac vessels and the ureter connected directly to the bladder. Generally unless the kidneys are infected the host kidneys are left in place [thus not (**answers a and b**)]. The newly transplanted kidney is placed in the greater pelvis and connected to the iliac vessels [thus not (**answer c**)]. Often the internal iliac artery is connected to the renal arteries. Normally, anastomotic connections across the midline from the opposite internal iliac artery keep pelvic organs with enough blood to maintain proper function. The transplanted renal vein is often connected to, the external iliac vein, since it is typically larger and thus easier to establish anastomoses.

400. The answer is b. (*Moore and Dalley, p 285.*) The patient in the scenario has infectious mononucleosis, a virus-induced illness, leading to swollen lymph nodes and spleen. The splenomegaly is evidenced by the very rounded contours of the organ. Infectious mononucleosis can exhibit liver involvement; however, the organ indicated is not the liver (not **answers a, d**, and **e**) but the spleen in the upper left hypochondrium. The bright organ between it and the vertebra is the left kidney. The liver is on the opposite side of the abdominal cavity. The stomach (**answer c**) is not seen.

401. The answer is c. (*Moore and Dalley, p 284.*) The splenic artery originates from the celiac trunk and courses tortuously along the posterior aspect of the pancreas. The left gastric artery (**answer a**) is a separate branch of the celiac trunk and courses along the lesser curvature of the stomach where it anastomoses with the right gastric artery (**answer d**), a branch of hepatic artery. The right gastro-omental (gastroepiploic) artery (**answer e**) is a branch of the gastroduodenal artery and courses along the greater curvature of the stomach. The superior mesenteric artery (**answer b**) is more inferior seen running to the right side of the patient.

402. The answer is b. (*Moore and Dalley, p 284.*) Structure 20 is the common hepatic artery. The celiac [18; (**answer a**)] artery (trunk) gives off the splenic [19; (**answer d**)] artery (to the patient's left) and the common hepatic [20; (**answer b**)] artery (to the patient's right). Other labeled structures are as follows: 17, right adrenal gland; 21, portal vein; and 22, left adrenal gland. The crus of diaphragm (**answer c**) is seen covering each side of the abdominal aorta. The superior mesenteric artery (**answer e**) is not seen in this image and would be further inferior with the abdomen.

403. The answer is b. (*Moore and Dalley pp 257–258, 330.*) Enlargement of the gallbladder is a common complication of gallstone development. If the gallbladder enlarges enough and becomes inflamed then it can contact the inferior surface of the diaphragm, leading to right-sided shoulder/neck pain.

The liver, if inflamed, would also produce right-sided shoulder/neck pain [thus not (**answer a**)]. The pancreas (**answer c**) is mainly a midline organ that is retroperitoneal, thus even when infected and inflamed it is unlikely to contact the center of the diaphragm (that portion which carries afferent information back to cervical levels of the spinal cord). An enlarged spleen could cause left sided shoulder/neck pain [thus not (**answer d**)]. Normally the appendix (**answer e**) is too inferior to contact the diaphragm and would cause pain on the left *not* right side.

404. The answer is b. (*Moore and Dalley, p 276.*) Sensation produced by distention of the rectum travels along the pelvic splanchnic nerves to sacral levels S2–S4. Fecal continence is affected by nerves from the S2–S4 segments of the spinal cord. The principal effector, the puborectalis portion of the levator ani muscle, is innervated by somatic twigs from the sacral plexus. The external anal sphincter is controlled by the pudendal nerve (**answer c**), which also carries pain sensation associated with external hemorrhoids. The lumbar (**answer a**) and sacral (**answer d**) sympathetic chain would provide motor innervation to the rectum. The vagus (**answer e**) nerve does *not* innervate the rectum.

405. The answer is d. (*Moore and Dalley, pp 277– 280.*) The colon normally has two regions where it is retroperitoneal: the ascending and descending colon. There are also two normal points of flexure: the hepatic (right) and splenic (left) flexures. Therefore, the sigmoid colon, splenic flexure, and hepatic flexure are the regions where the gastroenterologist has the greatest difficulty passing the fiberoptic scope, and thus have the greatest risk of bowel perforation. This is perhaps most easily visualized by looking at Fig. 2.44 on p 278 of Moore & Dalley. Other answers (**answers a, b, c, and e**) are *not* correct.

406. The answer is d. (*Moore and Dalley, pp 284–287.*) The body and tail of the pancreas receive most of their blood supply from the splenic artery via the great pancreatic, dorsal pancreatic, and caudal pancreatic arteries. The head of the pancreas is supplied by the superior pancreaticoduodenal artery that arises from the gastroduodenal branch of the common hepatic artery. In addition, the pancreatic head is supplied by the inferior pancreaticoduodenal arteries that arise from the superior mesenteric artery. The chief supply to the left side of the gastric (**answer c**) fundus is from the splenic artery via the short gastric branches. The splenic artery also gives rise to the left gastro-omental artery that runs along the greater curvature to anastomose with the right gastro-omental branch that arises indirectly from the common hepatic artery. *None* of the other arteries, common hepatic **(answer a)**, the inferior phrenic **(answer b)**, and superior mesenteric **(answer e)** are close to the pancreas.

407. The answer is e. *(Moore and Dalley, pp 280, 306, 450–451.)* Potential causes of blood in the stool (hematochezia) include diverticular disease, internal hemorrhoids, and colorectal cancer [thus not **(answers a and b)**]. Diverticular disease mainly affects middle age and older adults. It is an outpocketing of the lining of the colon, occurring most frequently in the sigmoid colon. Diverticular disease may be caused by lack of fiber in the diet. If the diverticula get large, they may rupture blood vessels and bleed. Internal hemorrhoids are dilated (varicose) veins that develop above the pectinate line within the internal rectal venous plexus. They can develop as a consequence of hepatic cirrhosis, which could cause portal hypertension as blood resistance within the liver increases. Venous blood within the portal system backflows down the superior rectal veins and into the inferior rectal veins, that are part of the systemic venous system that does *not* have to pass through the liver. Most colorectal cancers initially develop as polyps, which continue to grow and differentiate and in later stages develop increased vascularity and bleed. External hemorrhoids and fissures may result in blood in the stool, but are generally painful [thus not **(answers c and d)**].

408. The answer is e. *(Moore and Dalley, pp 306, 445, 450–451.)* A, b, and c. The rectum receives blood from three different arteries, which come from three different major branches: superior rectal artery off the inferior mesenteric artery; middle rectal artery off the internal iliac artery, and inferior rectal artery off the internal pudendal artery (Moore & Dalley, p 445). Thus *none* of the other answers are complete **(answers a, b, c, and d)**. There are also three sets of veins: superior rectal veins, which drain into the hepatic portal system; middle rectal veins, which drain into the internal iliac veins (part of the systemic venous system); and inferior rectal veins, which drain into internal pudendal veins (also part of the systemic venous system). Because the internal rectal venous plexus is a potential site of portal-systemic anastomoses, internal hemorrhoids may be an indication of liver pathology.

409. The answer is c. (*Moore and Dalley, pp 326–329.*) The diaphragm possesses three principal hiatuses shown in the diagram accompanying the question: the hiatus for the inferior vena cava **(answer a)**, the esophageal hiatus **(answer c)**, and the aortic hiatus **(answer e)**. Potential diaphragmatic developmental defects include the foramen of Morgagni **(answer b)**, just lateral to the xiphoid attachment of the diaphragm, and the pleuroperitoneal canal of Bochdalek **(answer d)**, which is the most common site for congenital hernias. The inferior vena cava and frequently small branches of the right phrenic nerve pass through a hiatus **(A)** slightly to the right of the midline at the T8 level. The left phrenic nerve usually passes through the central tendon of the diaphragm on the left side to innervate the left hemidiaphragm from below. The esophageal hiatus **(C)** just to the left of the midline at the T10 level transmits the esophagus, the left and right vagus nerves, and the esophageal branches of the left gastric artery and vein. An acquired hiatal hernia usually is the consequence of a short esophagus or of a weakened esophageal hiatus.

The two diaphragmatic crura are joined superiorly by the median arcuate ligament to form an opening **(E)** at the T12 level. The aortic hiatus transmits the aorta, thoracic duct, and a continuation of the azygos vein into the abdomen. The splanchnic nerves penetrate the crura on each side of the aortic hiatus to reach the abdomen.

410. The answer is d. (*Moore and Dalley, p 338.*) An aortic aneurysm. This patient may have an abdominal aortic aneurysm. Risk factors for the development of an abdominal aortic aneurysm include hypertension, excessive weight and smoking. Males are about five times more likely to have an aortic aneurysm than females. About 5% of men over 60 years of age have abdominal aortic aneurysms. Ninety percent of the time abdominal aortic aneurysms develop inferior to the renal arteries. About two-third of the time they extend inferiorly to include one of the common iliac arteries. (What blood vessel comes off the aorta inferior to the renal arteries and superior to the bifurcation into common iliac arteries? Answer: gonadal and inferior mesenteric arteries.) Despite the retroperitoneal location of the abdominal aorta, the high-pressure in the vessel typically makes ruptures of abdominal aortic aneurysms fatal. Blood fills the peritoneal cavity and the individual bleeds to death. If discovered prior to rupture they are typically repaired if greater than about 5.5 cm in diameter. Currently they tend to be repaired intravascularly by placing a 6-inch Dacron tube with metal-mesh cylinder into the aorta via the femoral artery. Anecdotally, abdominal aortic aneurysms have been known to rupture with straining, such as during defecation. None of the other conditions, a hiatal hernia (**answer a**), splenomegaly (**answer b**), cirrhosis of the liver (**answer c**), *nor* a horseshoe kidney (**answer d**) would normally pulsate.

411. The answer is c. (*Moore and Dalley, pp 223–225.*) Most indirect inguinal hernias are congenital [present at birth; thus not (**answers d and e**)]. Indirect inguinal hernias recapitulate the passage of the testis through the abdominal wall, and as such, originate lateral to the inferior epigastric vessels and reopen the process vaginalis if it had ever separated from the peritoneal cavity. Large indirect inguinal hernias need to be repaired to prevent intestinal organs from being strangulated within the inguinal canal and the process vaginalis needs to be closed to prevent abdominal peritoneal fluid from accumulating in the scrotum, causing swelling upon increased intra-abdominal pressure. Only about 1 in 20 inguinal hernias occur in females [thus not (**answers a and b**)]; 95% are within males.

412. The answer is d. (*Moore and Dalley, pp 276, 279–281.*) The major artery that is going to be reconnected is the marginal artery and the superior and inferior mesenteric lymph nodes will be collected. About a foot long section of the splenic flexure along with the marginal artery (of Drummond) and vein, paracolic lymph nodes and adjacent mesentery would all be surgically removed. The splenic flexure receives blood from the marginal artery. Blood from the splenic flexure portion of the marginal artery comes from both the middle colic artery, which is a branch off the superior mesenteric artery and from the left colic, which is a branch of the inferior mesenteric artery. Thus, it is essential to collect lymph nodes from the base of both the superior mesenteric and inferior mesenteric arteries. Neither the splenic artery (**answers b and c**) *nor* aorta (**answer a**) would be sectioned. The sigmoid artery (**answer e**) serves the sigmoid colon and would remain intact.

413. The answer is b. (*Moore and Dalley, pp 212, 298, 300.*) The findings are consistent with hepatomegaly. There are two pieces of physical evidence that point towards an enlarged liver as being the likely cause of the physical findings. While the liver lies in the upper right quadrant of the abdomen it is generally fairly well covered by the costal margin. Enlargement of the liver can be caused by chronic alcohol consumption. In addition, the prominent veins on her anterior abdominal wall (called caput medusae) may be a site of portal hypertension as blood backs up within the hepatic portal system and uses alternative routes, rather than through the liver, to return to the systemic circulatory system. In addition to prominent abdominal veins, portal hypertension may also cause esophageal varices and hemorrhoids. Splenomegaly **(answer a)** would be palpated on the left side. While both the gall bladder and appendix are on the right side of the abdomen, both cholecystitis **(answer d)** and appendicitis **(answer c)** should result in abdominal pain, which is absent in this patient. An abdominal aortic aneurysm **(answer e)** would normally appear in the midline and pulsate.

Pelvis

Questions

DIRECTIONS: Each item below contains a question or incomplete statement followed by suggested responses. Select the **one best** response to each question.

414. Which of the following is a characteristic of the female (compared with the male) pelvis?

a. A heart-shaped (as opposed to an oval-shaped) pelvic inlet
b. A relatively deep (as opposed to shallow) false pelvis with ilia that are flared
c. A pelvic outlet of smaller diameter
d. A subpubic angle of about 85°

415. A young couple comes to your urology office because of inability to conceive a wanted child after 1 year of unprotected sex. The wife had already undergone a gynecological workup, including testing for 3 months showing a normal ovulation profile as confirmed by an ovulatory kit. The primary care physician describes the husband's physical exam as normal and had already ordered a semen analysis and had forwarded the results to you. The semen volume was 0.5 mL, pH 6.8, and azospermic without any fructose. The husband has a brother, who has two children, one of whom has confirmed cystic fibrosis. You order a pelvic MRI of the husband to determine whether which of the following exist(s)?

a. Bilateral abdominal testicles
b. Hypospadias
c. Congenital absence of ejaculatory ducts and vas deferens
d. Congenital hydrocele
e. Congenital absence of the prostate gland

416. The gubernaculum is a continuous mesenchymal condensation extending from the caudal pole of each gonad through the inguinal canal to the labioscrotal swelling, inferiorly. In the female the gubernaculum becomes which of the following?

a. Canal of Nuck
b. Ligament of the ovary or proper ligament of the ovary
c. Round ligament of the uterus
d. Round ligament of the uterus and the ligament of the ovary or proper ligament of the ovary
e. Suspensory ligament of the ovary

417. Parts of some human skeletal remains are brought to you as coroner of a rural community. The pelvis is complete, yet the individual bones of the pelvis, the ilium, ischium, and pubis have just started to fuse together. The subpubic angle you estimate at 60° and the pelvic brim has a distinctive heart-shaped appearance. On the basis of this information, you guess the remains are of which of the following?

a. 3-year-old male
b. 4-year-old female
c. 14-year-old male
d. 30-year-old female
e. 80-year-old male

418. Following vaginal childbirth, a woman experienced urinary incontinence, particularly when coughing. This was most likely caused by tearing of which of the following?

a. Puborectalis muscle
b. Obturator internus muscle
c. Pubococcygeus muscle
d. Superficial transverse perineal muscle
e. Piriformis muscle

419. When one touches the upper medial thigh or scrotum of most young males, the testicles are pulled upwards towards the external inguinal ring. This is called the cremasteric reflex. The efferent limb of the cremasteric reflex is provided by which of the following?

a.   Femoral branch of the genitofemoral nerve
b.   Genital branch of the genitofemoral nerve
c.   Ilioinguinal nerve
d.   Pudendal nerve
e.   Temperature differential between core body temperature and scrotal temperature

420. A 36-year-old man complained to his primary care physician of occasional dull, throbbing pain associated with the right testis and scrotum. Examination indicated varicocele of the pampiniform plexus. The physician remarked that in all probability the patient had this condition since adolescence and should *not* be bothered by it. The patient was emphatic that the condition had arisen within the last few months and sought a second opinion from an urologist. The urologist ordered an abdominal and pelvic CT. Factors that the urologist considered include which of the following in regard to varicocele of the pampiniform plexus on the right side?

a.   It is very uncommon
b.   It occurs about as often as that on the left side
c.   It may be the result of testicular torsion
d.   It may be associated with a long, redundant mesorchium

421. A 19-year-old female college student presents to the emergency room at 10:30 PM on a Friday night with severe left side, back, and pelvic pain. While she has never had them before, she states that she thinks she has kidney stones. The pain started in her mid back about a week ago and then subsided and now the pain has decreased somewhat and also extends down into her labia majora. She is on birth control pills, but denies any sexual activity. She is having her period, but denies the pain is menstrual. You have her do a urine pregnancy test while she is waiting to get an abdominal and pelvic computer tomography (CT) to look for ureteric calculi. What specific location(s) will you look for in the CTs for obstructing calculi?

a. At the junction of the renal pelvis with the ureters
b. As the ureters cross the cranial edge of the greater pelvis
c. As the ureters cross the external iliac artery at the pelvic brim
d. As the ureters pass through the wall of the bladder
e. a, b, and c
f. a, c, and d

422. You deliver a full-term baby boy who is healthy and receives an Apgar score of 9 out of 10. You do note that his scrotum is rather large compared to his penis and when he cries and strains, the scrotum gets even bigger. You palpate for testes and epididymides and think both are present and don't feel any abnormal structures. You tell the parents the newborn has which of the following?

a. Cryptorchidism
b. Direct inguinal hernia
c. Varicocele
d. Hydrocele
e. Klinefelter's syndrome

423. A 6-year-old boy badly bruised his perineum on the horizontal bar of his bicycle as he was learning to ride a bike. Blood extended into his scrotum, and onto the anterior abdominal wall from 3 in. below his umbilicus to just anterior to his anus, but did not pass into his thigh. Which anatomical layers most likely explain the distribution of extravasated blood?

a. Superficial membranous fascia and Camper's fascia
b. Superficial membranous fascia and transversalis fascia
c. Dartos fascia and the perineal membrane
d. Superficial membranous fascia and the perineal membrane
e. Deep perineal fascia and inferior fascia of the pelvic diaphragm

424. Fructose, a source of energy for spermatozoa, is found primarily in secretions from which of the following organs?

a. Bulbourethral glands
b. Epididymis
c. Prostate
d. Seminal vesicles
e. Testis

425. In this CT of the pelvis, the muscle indicated by the arrow is which of the following?

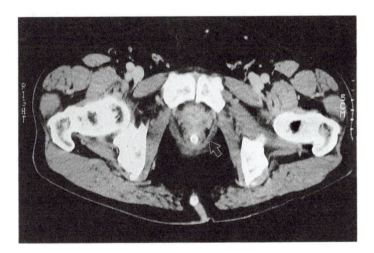

a. Sphincter urethrae/urogenital diaphragm
b. Levator ani/pelvic diaphragm
c. Obturator internus
d. Obturator externus

426. Benign prostatic hypertrophy results in obstruction of the urinary tract. Patients present with weak urine flow, increased difficulty initiating urination, and increase frequency of urination since the bladder often is *not* fully emptied. Benign prostatic hypertrophy is associated with enlargement of which of the following?

a. Entire prostate gland
b. Lateral/posterior lobes
c. Mucosal and submucosal regions
d. Anterior region

427. A rectal cancer that occurs within the anal canal penetrates the mucosa and basement membrane. Which nodes would you most likely harvest at the same time you removed the cancerous growth to send to pathology to determine if there has been metastasis?

a. Superficial inguinal nodes
b. Inguinal nodes and internal iliac nodes
c. Superficial inguinal, internal iliac and preaortic inferior mesenteric nodes
d. Internal iliac and external iliac nodes
e. External iliac, superficial inguinal, and preaortic nodes

428. In the male, the homologue of the vaginal artery is which of the following?

a. Obturator artery
b. Internal pudendal artery
c. Middle rectal artery
d. Umbilical artery
e. Inferior vesical artery

429. A 24-year-old woman seeking assistance for apparent infertility has been unable to conceive despite repeated attempts in 5 years of marriage. She reveals that her husband fathered a child in a prior marriage. Although her menstrual periods are fairly regular, they are accompanied by extreme lower back pain. The lower back pain during menstruation experienced by this woman probably is referred from the pelvic region. The pathways that convey this pain sensation to the central nervous system involve which of the following?

a. Hypogastric nerve to L1–L2
b. Lumbosacral trunk to L4–L5
c. Pelvic splanchnic nerves to S2–S4
d. Pudendal nerve to S2–S4

430. The body of the uterus tends to wander within the pelvic cavity. However the cervix of the uterus tends to remain fairly firmly in place most of the time. Which of the following would be found immediately inferior to the left cardinal (lateral cervical) ligament?

a. Ovarian neurovascular bundle
b. Uterine tube
c. Round ligament of the uterus
d. Ureter
e. Ovarian artery and vein

431. A 50-year-old associate professor is scheduled for a routine physical exam for an increase in the level of coverage for his life insurance. He had never had a digital rectal exam or PSA level determined so you recommend both to him. As you have him hop off the examination table, turn away from you and face the table, then bend at the waist while you gently insert a lubricated gloved finger into his anus you can feel structures through the wall of the rectum. Typically what part of three reproductive organs can you palpate through the anterior wall of the rectum?

a. Main peripheral portion of the prostate gland
b. Ejaculatory ducts
c. Seminal vesicles
d. Epididymal ducts
e. Ampulla of the vas deferens
f. a, b, and c
g. a, b, and d
h. a, c, and e
i. b, c, and d

432. The most important measurement of the pelvic outlet, indicating the SMALLEST dimension, is the transverse midplane diameter. It is measured between which of the following?

a. Ischial spines
b. Ischial tuberosities
c. Lower margin of the pubic symphysis to the sacroiliac joint
d. Sacral promontory to the inferior margin of the pubic symphysis

433. At delivery, caudal analgesia is induced by administration of anesthetic into the epidural space in the sacral region. The needle is introduced via which of the following?

a. Anterior sacral foramina
b. Dural sac
c. Intervertebral foramina
d. Posterior sacral foramina
e. Sacral hiatus

434. Which structure is most susceptible to unintentional damage during a hysterectomy?

a. Uterine artery
b. Ureter
c. Urinary bladder
d. Urethra
e. Kidney

435. The patient is a 45-year-old man with a history of colonic diverticulosis. He complains of fever with pain and swelling in the rectal area. You are concerned that the colonic diverticulum may have become infected (diverticulitis) and ruptured into the space indicated by the asterisk in this CT scan. Which of the following is correct regarding the indicated space?

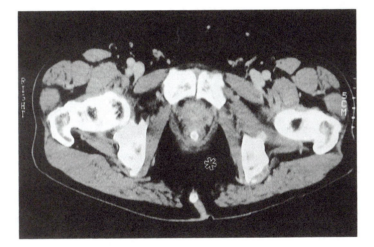

a. It is called the paracolic gutter
b. The space is largely filled with muscle
c. The space is located superior to the pelvic diaphragm
d. Pus from the abscessed diverticuli in that space can extend anteriorly deep to the perineal membrane, but inferior to the urogenital diaphragm
e. Pus from the abscessed diverticuli in that space can extend superiorly, anterior to the sacrum

436. Which of the following arteries may occasionally arise as a branch of the external iliac artery or inferior epigastric artery instead of as a branch of the internal iliac artery?

a. Internal pudendal artery
b. Obturator artery
c. Superior gluteal artery
d. Umbilical artery
e. Uterine artery

437. A couple comes to your office because they have been unable to conceive a child after 1 year of trying. You examine the man and notice a darkish mass and fullness of the left scrotum/spermatic cord compared to the smaller right scrotum/spermatic cord. You suggest he follow up with an urologist because you suspect which of the following?

a. Undiagnosed cryptorchidism of the right testicle
b. Acquired varicocele
c. Acquired left femoral hernia
d. Acquired right direct femoral hernia
e. Congenital absence of the pampiniform plexus on the right side

438. Which of the following is one of the roles of the sympathetic chain in the pelvis?

a. Bladder contraction
b. Cutaneous function (sudomotor, vasomotor, pilomotor)
c. Erection in males
d. Erection in both male and female

439. Both the autonomic and vascular systems need to function properly for successful male sexual function. Which of the following statements concerning erection, emission, and ejaculation in the male is correct?

a. Contraction of the internal urethral sphincter is under control of the parasympathetic nervous system
b. The parasympathetic nerves stimulate closure of helical arteries
c. Sympathetic neurons stimulate the helicine arteries to dilate and increase blood flow to the corpora cavernosum
d. Parasympathetic innervation stimulates emission of seminal fluid
e. Contraction of the bulbospongiosus muscles impedes the drainage of blood from the corpus spongiosum

440. A 45-year-old man was riding a snowmobile and hit a snow-covered rocky outcropping. When standing for the first time after the accident, he slipped and fell on the outcropping and now is experiencing pain in the gluteal region. In this CT scan, the dark linear structure indicated by the arrow is which of the following?

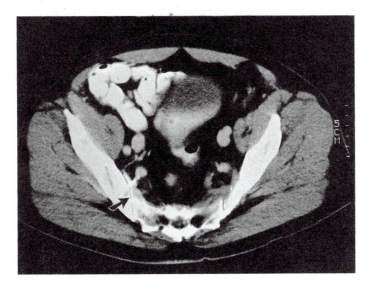

a. A fracture of the sacral body
b. The sacrococcygeal joint
c. A spinal nerve
d. The superior gluteal artery
e. The inferior gluteal artery

441. In the hysterosalpingogram below, the dye at C is within which of the following?

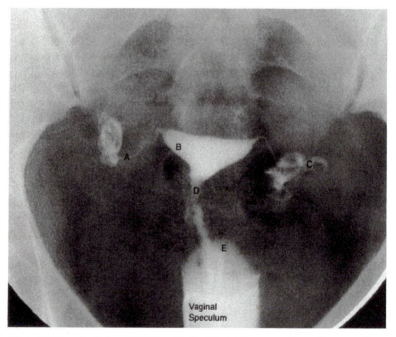

(Image 5001 used with permission from the Radiological Anatomy web site, University of Kansas, School of Medicine, http://classes.kumc.edu/som/radanatomy/.)

a. Ovary
b. Peritoneal cavity
c. Isthmus of the oviduct
d. Uterus
e. Vagina

442. Which of the following locations is optimal for fertilization of an ovulated egg by sperm to occur?

a. Ampulla of the oviduct
b. Uterus
c. Infundibulum of the oviduct
d. Isthmus of the oviduct
e. Cervical canal of the uterus

443. Which of the following contains the ovarian neurovascular bundle?

a. Broad ligament
b. Mesosalpinx
c. Mesovarium
d. Suspensory ligament of the ovary
e. Transverse cervical ligament

444. Following the birth of her third child a 38-year-old woman was undergoing a hysterectomy because of pelvic pain associated with endometriosis. Since she had an android pelvis, cesarean sections had been performed with each delivery of her children. An open (surgical) hysterectomy approach was performed in order to also remove any peritoneal endometrium, in which the ovaries were to be spared. The OB specifically identified and spared a right and left ureter during the clamping and removal of the uterine arteries. After surgery, she developed left sided low back pain. An intravenous pyelogram was ordered and showed normal function of the right kidney and normal function of the upper portion of the left kidney, but there was little kidney function in the inferior pole of the lower portion of the left kidney and two ureters exiting from that kidney. What likely happened during the hysterectomy?

a. Spontaneous kidney failure as a result of the pyelogram
b. Damage to one of the left duplicated ureters
c. Kidney failure as a result of the anesthetic given during surgery
d. Kidney stone development

445. Pap smears are the collection of cells from the uterine cervix to look for cytological evidence of transformation to cancerous forms, most typically due to a viral infection. While most women do not report any discomfort associated with the collection of cervical cells, a few women do. To which of the following somatic areas does the uterine cervix refer pain to?

a. Epigastric region
b. Medial thigh and buttock
c. Inguinal and pubic regions, anterior labia majora, medial thigh
d. Lateral leg and perineum
e. Subcostal and umbilical regions

446. Episiotomies are performed to control tearing that can occur during a vaginal delivery. When performing a mediolateral episiotomy, an OB-GYN will likely cut through several structures of the perineum. What perineal structures must be sutured back together following a typical mediolateral episiotomy?

a. Vaginal wall, pubococcygeus, and piriformis muscles
b. Vaginal wall, pubococcygeus, and iliococcygeus muscles
c. Vaginal wall, bulbospongiosus, and superficial transverse perineal muscles
d. Vaginal wall, prepuce, and rectus abdominis muscle
e. Vaginal wall, sacrospinous and sacrotuberous ligaments

447. A man comes to your office because he thinks he has bilateral hernias and bilateral pain in the inguinal area. Upon physical examination he does *not* have a direct *nor* indirect inguinal hernia, but does have bilateral palpable superficial inguinal lymph nodes, which are tender. You formulate a differential diagnosis of locations from which lymph drains into the superficial inguinal lymph nodes. Which anatomical region or structure does *not* drain into the superficial inguinal lymph nodes and thus should be EXCLUDED from your differential diagnosis list?

a. Penis
b. Scrotum
c. Testicles
d. Anus
e. Epididymides

448. A 35-year-old married woman comes to the emergency room due to sudden onset of nausea, vomiting, positional hypotension, and tachycardia. She also complains of sudden abdominal fullness and generalized pelvic pain. Her period is "late," with the last menses 55 days ago. A pregnancy test is positive. Pelvic sonogram suggests extravasated fluid in the peritoneal cavity and pooling in the rectouterine pouch (of Douglas) and a mass in the left fallopian tube. A culdocentesis yields fresh blood. You correctly suggest that she be admitted for which of the following?

a. D and C (dilation and curettage)
b. Endoscopic exploration to rule out ectopic pregnancy
c. Ovariectomy for ovarian cancer
d. Hysterectomy for fibroids
e. Cystocele repair

449. A 50-year-old multiparous woman comes to your office to rule out cancer. She reports a growing mass or fullness on the anterior wall of her vagina. Upon physical examination you detect a soft, bulging, and a very compressible mass on the anterior surface of the vagina. When you push on the bulging mass she feels the need to urinate. You order a CT because you suspect which of the following?

a. Rectocele
b. Cystocele
c. Cervical cancer
d. Didelphic uterus
e. Indirect inguinal hernia

450. A 30-year-old woman makes her first prenatal visit to your office. She is excited and anxious as this is her first pregnancy. She brings up the topic of pain relief during vaginal delivery. She states that she would like to try "natural birth" but would like to have the option of some pain relief. However, she would prefer *not* to have a caudal epidural block. You suggest a pudendal nerve block. One of the advantages of a pudendal nerve block is that the woman can still feel uterine contractions and thus can actively participate in the birthing process, yet also has some pain relief. What would you tell your patient regarding how to perform a pudendal nerve block and an advantage to performing the injection transvaginally versus injecting through perineal skin?

a. The pudendal nerve serves the skin around the anterior/lateral entrance of the vagina; the nerve wraps around the ischial spine, which is used as landmark; transvaginal administration is less painful since the upper portion of the vagina has fewer pain receptors
b. The pudendal nerve serves the skin around the posterior/lateral entrance of the vagina; the nerve wraps around the ischial spine, which is used as a landmark; transvaginal administration is less painful since the upper portion of the vagina has fewer pain receptors
c. The pudendal nerve serves the skin around the anterior/lateral entrance of the vagina; the nerve wraps around the ischial tuberosity, which is used as landmark; transvaginal administration is less painful since the upper portion of the vagina has fewer pain receptors
d. The pudendal nerve serves the skin around the posterior/lateral entrance of the vagina; the nerve wraps around the ischial tuberosity, which is used as a landmark; transvaginal administration is less painful since the upper portion of the vagina has fewer pain receptors

Pelvis

Answers

414. The answer is d. *(Moore and Dalley, p 361.)* The subpubic angle between inferior pubic rami is significantly greater (about 85°) in the female than in the male (about 60°) and this is perhaps the best identifying feature of the female pelvis. The female pelvis is generally lighter than the male pelvis. The male pelvis generally has more definitive muscle markings, which reflect the larger male musculature and generally heavier male build. In the female the false or greater pelvis tends to be shallower **(answer b)** with flared ilia. The female pelvic inlet tends to be more oval **(answer a)**, rather than the heart-shaped inlet of most male pelves. The female pelvic outlet is generally larger (more suitable for child bearing) than the male pelvis **(answer c)**.

415. The answer is c. *(Casals, pp 1476–1483.)* If the brother has a child with cystic fibrosis, then he must be a carrier of the cystic fibrosis gene, meaning there is a 50% chance that the husband is a CF carrier. Congenital absence of the ejaculatory ducts is increased in carriers of CF. If the ejaculatory ducts are absent, then there should be *no* sperm from the vas deferens (normally 0.5 mL of the semen volume) and *no* products of the seminal vesicles (normally 2.0 mL of the semen volume). The seminal vesicle is responsible for fructose normally present in the ejaculate. Prostatic secretions are normally slightly acidic. The normal physical of the husband rules out hypospadias **(answer b)**, bilateral cryptorchidism **(answer a)**, and hydrocele **(answer d)**. The congenital absence of the prostate gland is extremely rare **(answer e)**.

416. The answer is d. *(Moore and Dalley, pp 218–219.)* In the female, the gubernaculum becomes the round ligament of the uterus and the proper ligament of the ovary. The gubernaculum, which runs from the gonadal anlage to the sexually undifferentiated labioscrotal fold, guides the descent of the testes into the scrotum in the male and the descent of the ovary into the true pelvis in the female. In the female, the developing uterus grows into the gubernacular tract and divides it into the proper ligament of the ovary and the round ligament of the uterus. Thus, the proper ligament of the ovary runs within the broad ligament from the medial pole of each ovary to the uterus. It then continues within the broad ligament as the round ligament of the uterus into the deep inguinal ring. It thereby gains access to the canal of Nuck (the female homologue of the inguinal canal; **(answer a)** to insert into the major labial folds. The suspensory ligament of the ovary **(answer e)** contains the ovarian arteries and veins. **Answers c and d** are thus incomplete.

417. The answer is c. *(Moore and Dalley, pp 358–359, 361.)* The pelvis is most likely that of a 14-year-old male. Because the subpubic angle is about 60° and the pelvic brim is heart shaped, you are looking at a male *not* a female **(answers b and d).** The bones of the pelvis arise from three different centers of ossification and generally fuse together between puberty and the twenty-third year. Therefore, you know you are looking at a 14-year-old male, *not* a 3-year-old **(answer a;** would have 3 separate pelvic bones) *nor* an 80-year-old **(answer e;** pelvic bones would be fused).

418. The answer is c. *(Moore and Dalley, pp 373, 375, 467.)* The pubococcygeus muscle is the most frequently torn muscle that results in female incontinence. The puborectalis, pubococcygeus, and iliococcygeus comprise the levator ani, the main muscular component of the pelvic floor. The pubococcygeus is the part of the levator ani most frequently damaged during parturition. Because the pubococcygeus surrounds and supports the neck of the bladder and the proximal urethra, urinary leakage is a common result, particularly during increased abdominopelvic pressure, as occurs, during coughing. Damage to the puborectalis **(answer a)** results in fecal incontinence under similar situations. Both the obturator internus muscle **(answer b)** and the piriformis **(answer e)** are parts of the lateral wall of the pelvis and assist in lateral rotation of the thigh. Generally damage to the superficial transverse perineal muscle **(answer d)** would be of little significance.

419. The answer is b. *(Moore and Dalley, pp 220–221, 225.)* The efferent portion of the cremasteric reflex is mediated by the genital branch of the genitofemoral nerve, which innervates the cremasteric muscle (skeletal). The femoral branch **(answer a)** supplies the afferent limb, and the genital branch supplies the efferent limb. The ilioinguinal nerve **(answer c)** provides sensory innervation to the medial aspects of the thigh and the anterior aspects of the mons or the base of the penis and can also provide afferent innervation to stimulate the cremasteric response, pulling the testicles upward. The pudendal nerve (**answer d**) provides sensation to most of the skin of the perineum as well as the motor supply to the perineal muscles. The involuntary scrotal reflex can also be based on temperature (**answer e**): warmth causes relaxation of the cremasteric (skeletal) and dartos (smooth) muscle, whereas cold causes contraction of both the cremasteric and dartos muscles.

420. The answer is a. (*Moore and Dalley, pp 228–229.*) It is very uncommon. Varicocele usually occurs on the left side (~95%) and is rare on the right (**answer b**). Left varicocele results from local venous congestion caused by compression of the testicular vein as it passes beneath the usually full sigmoid colon. Testicular torsion (**answer c**), wherein a long mesorchium (**answer d**) is a contributing factor, strangulates the testicular artery, and produces testicular ischemia, not varicocele. Testicular torsion is a medical emergency which normally presents in adolescents as sudden testicular pain (*Moore and Dalley, p 226*).

421. The answer f. (*Moore and Dalley, pp 319–320, 393.*) A, c, and d. Renal and ureteric calculi (laymen's kidney stones) generally are formed in the kidneys and then lodge at one of three locations: 1) at the junction of the renal pelvis with the ureter; 2) as the ureters cross the external iliac vessels at the pelvic brim; and 3) as the ureters pass through the wall of the bladder (*see Fig. 3.14 A, p 393 Moore & Dalley*). Stones generally do not lodge at the edge of the greater pelvis [**answer b**; all other answers (**a, c, d, and e**) are incomplete]. The referred pain from ureteric calculi is usually described as from "loin to groin" in that it often starts in back and side over the kidney and then extends in a band down towards the labia majora or scrotum (from T 11 to L2). Normally the pain is intermittent and comes and goes in waves and may change in location, generally moving inferiorly with time. Since the ureters undergo peristaltic movement, the calculi often move with time. Depending on the chemical composition and shape of the calculi they may either block urine flow or if spiky, stick into the wall of the ureter. Kidney stone pain is often described as being worse than labor pains. Treatments include pain relief and drinking lots of fluids, and either lithotripsy (use of ultrasound waves to break up the stone) or physical removal (surgical) of the stone in severe cases.

422. The answer is d. *(Moore and Dalley, pp 225–226.)* The newborn boy has congenital hydrocele. As the testicles migrate from the posterior abdominal wall to the anterior abdominal wall through the inguinal canal, they bring a process of the peritoneal lining, the processes vaginalis, which is filled with fluid and is connected to the peritoneal cavity. Normally, this process vaginalis disconnects from the abdominal cavity and forms the tunica vaginalis. Sometimes due to the late migration of the testis, the process vaginalis does *not* lose its connection with the peritoneal cavity, so that during straining and coughing or crying the scrotum swells. Normally this condition spontaneously corrects itself a few months after birth. Cryptorchidism **(answer a)** is the failure of the testis to migrate down into the scrotum, but the physical exam indicated the testes were in the scrotum. A direct inguinal hernia **(answer b)** is very rare in newborns. Congenital varicocele **(answer c)** would generally appear bluish and would feel like a bag of worms. Klinefelter's newborn **(answer e)** would have normal-sized testicles and is *not* related to a hydrocele.

423. The answer is d. *(Moore and Dalley, pp 441–442.)* The blood from straddle injuries is generally limited to the superficial perineal space which is bound by the superficial membranous fascia (superficially; including Scarpa's fascia on the anterior abdominal wall, dartos fascia on penis and scrotum, and Colles' fascia on the urogenital triangle) and the deep perineal membrane (deep). The superficial membranous fascia is attached to deep structures at the following locations: superiorly the superficial membranous fascia attaches to the deep fascia of the anterior abdominal muscles about half way between the pubic symphysis and the umbilicus; attaches to the inguinal ligament, and the fascia lata, laterally; and attaches to the posterior edge of the perineal membrane just anterior to the anus. Camper's fascia **(answer a)** is the fatty layer on the anterior abdominal wall, which extends beyond the umbilicus. Transversalis fascia **(answer b)** is the fascia just deep to the peritoneal lining in the abdomen. Dartos fascia **(answer c)** only covers the scrotum and penis. The inferior fascia of the pelvic diaphragm **(answer e)** is deep to the perineal membrane.

424. The answer is d. *(Kierszenbaum, pp 557–558.)* The thick secretion from the seminal vesicles contributes substantially to the ejaculate volume that conveys the spermatozoa. The high fructose content of secretions of the seminal vesicles provides the primary metabolic energy source for sperm motility. The flavins that are contributed to the ejaculate by the seminal vesicles fluoresce strongly in ultraviolet light, a phenomenon that supplies a useful forensic test for the presence of semen. Bulbourethral glands (**answer a**) produce mucus that lubricates the urethra upon erotic stimulus. The epididymis (**answer b**) stores sperm. The prostate gland (**answer c**) produces proteins responsible for semen liquefaction. The testis (**answer e**) produces sperm.

·425. The answer is b. (*Moore and Dalley, pp 396–371, 436–438.*) The muscle indicated is attached to the pubic bone and extends around the rectum. It is the puborectalis portion of the levator ani (pelvic diaphragm). The puborectalis is responsible for fecal continence. The urogenital diaphragm (**answer a**) is positioned inferior to the pelvic diaphragm and includes the deep transverse perineal muscle. The obturator internus (**answer c**) covers the lateral wall of the lesser pelvis. The obturator externus (**answer d**) is found in the deep thigh.

426. The answer is c. (*Moore and Dalley, p 409. Kierszenbaum, p 559.*) Benign prostatic hypertrophy is the result of enlargement of the mucosal and submucosal (median) region, which may compress the prostatic urethra leading to urinary retention [thus not (**answer a**)]. This hypertrophic tissue may also protrude into the urinary bladder to prevent complete emptying. The lateral/posterior lobes (**answer b**) are commonly associated with malignant transformation. The anterior region (**answer d**) tends to be asymptomatic due to its mainly fibrous nature.

427. The answer is c. (*Moore and Dalley, p 431.*) Lymph from the anal region is drained to three different regions because its blood supply comes from three different regions [thus (**answers a and b**) are incomplete]. Superior to the pectinate line the lymph drains into the internal iliac nodes and preaortic nodes (along the path of the superior rectal artery, a branch off the inferior mesenteric artery). Inferior to the pectinate line the lymph drains into the superficial inguinal nodes. Thus the external iliac nodes have nothing to do with the rectum [thus not (**answers d and e**)].

428. The answer is e. (*Moore and Dalley, pp 384–386.*) All of the listed choices are branches of the internal iliac artery. The inferior vesical artery in the male supplies the seminal vesicle, prostate, fundus of the bladder, distal ureter, and the vas deferens. In the female, the vaginal artery supplies the vagina, urinary bladder, and pelvic portion of the urethra. The obturator artery **(answer a)** gives off muscular and nutrient branches within the pelvis and then leaves the pelvis via the obturator canal to supply the thigh. The internal pudendal artery **(answer b)** crosses the piriformis muscle, exits the pelvic cavity via the greater sciatic foramen, and enters the ischiorectal fossa via the lesser sciatic foramen. It supplies the external genitalia (penis and clitoris). The middle rectal artery **(answer c)** supplies the inferior rectum and forms important anastomoses with other rectal arteries. The umbilical artery **(answer d)** gives off the superior vesical artery in both sexes. Its distal portion degenerates to form the medial umbilical ligament.

429. The answer is a. *(Moore and Dalley, pp 423, 425.)* The visceral afferent fibers that mediate sensation from the fundus and body of the uterus, as well as from the oviducts, tend to travel along the sympathetic nerve pathways (via the hypogastric nerve and lumbar splanchnics) to reach the upper lumbar levels (L1–L2) of the spinal cord. Thus, uterine pain will be referred to (appear as if originating from) the upper lumbar dermatomes and produce backache. The visceral afferent fibers that mediate sensation from the cervical neck of the uterus travel along the parasympathetic pathways [via the pelvic splanchnic nerves *(nervi erigentes);* **(answer c)**] to the midsacral levels (S2–S4) of the spinal cord. In this instance, pain originating from the cervix will be referred to the midsacral dermatomes and produce pain that appears to arise from the perineum, gluteal region, and legs. Neither the lumbosacral trunk to L4–L5 **(answer b)** *nor* the pudendal nerve **(answer d)** should be involved.

430. The answer is d. *(Moore and Dalley, pp 387, 414.)* The ureter, lying just medial to the internal iliac artery in the deep pelvis, passes from posterior to anterior immediately inferior to the lateral cervical ligament. This ligament sits at the base of the broad ligament and contains the uterine artery and vein to which the ureters pass inferior approximately midway along their course between internal iliac artery and uterus. The ureter continues inferior to the anterior portion of the lateral cervical ligament (where it can sometimes be palpated through the walls of the vagina at the lateral fornices) to gain access to the base of the urinary bladder. The close association between uterine vessels and ureter is of major importance during surgical procedures in the female pelvis. At the top of the broad ligament would be the ovarian artery and vein (**answers a and e**), which continue on to supply blood to the fundus. The uterine tube (**answer b**) also runs along the top of the broad ligament. The round ligament of the uterus (**answer c**) runs anterior to the broad ligament.

431. The answer is h. (*Moore and Dalley, pp 404, 409, 433.*) In most males, during a digital rectal exam, you can palpate the main peripheral portion of the prostate gland (**answer a**), then just a little more cranially, both the seminal vesicles (**answer c**) and ampulla of the vas (ductus) deferens (**answer e**). The main goal of the digital rectal exam is to palpate the backside of the prostate gland which is the main peripheral portion of the gland; the site of development of most growth of prostate cancer. An additional screening tool is the prostate specific antigen (PSA) level within blood. Generally the PSA level should be below 2.5 ng/mL. Elevated levels of PSA, however, can also indicate inflammation of the prostate in addition to cancerous growth. You can *not* palpate the ejaculatory ducts (**answer b**) as they are embedded within the substance of the prostate gland. You can *not* palpate the epididymis (**answer d**) during a digital rectal exam as it is within the scrotum next to the testicles. All other answers (**f, g, and i**) are wrong or incomplete.

432. The answer is a. (*Moore and Dalley, pp 362–363.*) The transverse midplane diameter is measured between the ischial spines. It can be approximated by the somewhat greater transverse diameter measured between the ischial tuberosities (**answer b**). The distance from the lower margin of the pubic symphysis to the sacroiliac joint (**answer c**) defines the sagittal diameter, which is usually the greatest dimension and, therefore, unimportant. The measurement from the sacral promontory to the inferior margin of the pubic symphysis (**answer d**) is the diagonal conjugate, an estimate of the pelvic inlet.

433. The answer is e. (*Moore and Dalley, pp 422–424, 493.*) Caudal analgesia can be induced by an injection of anesthetic through the sacral hiatus into the sacral epidural space of the vertebral canal well caudal to the termination of the dural sac (**answer b**). The sacral hiatus represents the absence of a complete neural arch of the fifth sacral vertebra. The four anterior (**answer a**) and posterior (**answer d**) sacral foramina on either side of the midline join the intervertebral foramen (**answer c**) and provide egress for the anterior and posterior primary rami of the sacral spinal nerves. The level to which the anesthesia blocks the spinal nerves is a function of the amount of anesthetic delivered.

434. The answer is b. (*Moore and Dalley, pp 387–388.*) The uterine artery (**answer a**) crosses anterior and superior to the ureter near the lateral fornix of the vagina and is deliberately clamped and removed during a hysterectomy. Some clinicians and anatomists once referred to the uterine artery as "the bridge over troubled waters." Because of its close proximity to the artery, the ureter may be accidentally ligated or severed while tying off of the artery. Of course, the bladder (**answer c**) and the kidney (**answer e**) are large structures and should *not* be mistakenly clamped. The urethra (**answer d**) should be far out of the operating field.

435. The answer is d. (*Moore and Dalley, pp 449–451.*) Pus from the abscessed diverticuli in that space can extend anteriorly deep to the perineal membrane, but inferior to the urogenital diaphragm. The ischioanal fossa (asterisk on CT accompanying the question) is a fat-filled space [thus not muscle (**answer b**)] that extends from below the levator ani muscle (puborectalis, pubococcygeus, and iliococcygeus muscles). It also extends anteriorly in the area between the pelvic diaphragm (superiorly) and the perineal membrane (inferiorly). It cannot extend superiorly above the pelvic diaphragm [thus not (**answer c**)] and, therefore, cannot extend superiorly anterior to the sacrum (**answer d**). The paracolic gutter (**answer a**) in *not* on the image.

436. The answer is b. (*Moore and Dalley, p 387.*) The obturator usually arises from the anterior trunk of the internal iliac artery. However, in 25% of the population, it arises from the inferior epigastric or the external iliac artery. There is considerable variation as to the origins of the branches of the posterior and anterior trunks of the internal iliac artery. The internal pudendal artery (**answer a**), umbilical artery (**answer d**), and uterine artery (**answer e**) almost always arise from the anterior trunk. The superior gluteal artery (**answer c**) usually arises from the posterior trunk.

437. The answer is b. (*Moore and Dalley, pp 228–229.*) A dark mass within the scrotum would most likely be one of two things: varicocele or indirect inguinal hernia. Varicoceles are a stasis of blood within the pampiniform plexus and occur most frequently on the left side because the testicular vein on the left drains into the higher pressure left renal vein, whereas the right testicular vein drains into the inferior vena cava. The presence of a varicocele is associated with reduced fertility. A femoral hernia **(answers c and d)** would *not* end up in the scrotum, rather within the thigh. Cryptorchidism **(answer a)**, that is an undescended testicle, on the right side does *not* fit the physical examination findings. The right side is normal [thus *not* **(answer e)**].

438. The answer is b. (*Moore and Dalley, pp 399, 425, 432.*) Postsynaptic sympathetic neurons destined for the skin lie in the ganglia of the sympathetic chain. Although the preganglionic fibers arise between T1 and L2, each of the sacral ganglia has a gray ramus that brings postganglionic fibers to the associated spinal nerve. These sympathetic neurons mediate sweating (sudomotor), vasoconstriction (vasomotor), and piloerection (pilomotor) in dermatomes S1–S5. Male ejaculation is practically mediated by skeletal muscle (contraction of the bulbospongiosus muscle innervated by superficial perineal nerves, branches of the pudendal nerve.) Ejaculation also requires sympathetic discharge to keep the internal urethral sphincter closed, preventing so called retroejaculation into the bladder. Emission (rapid contraction of the vas deferens) is mainly mediated by sympathetic, but mainly by lumbar splanchnic nerves, thereby bypassing the sympathetic chain ganglia. Erection in both male and female **(answers c and d)** is mainly mediated by parasympathetic nerves. Bladder contraction **(answer a)** is also mainly controlled by parasympathetic nerves.

439. The answer is e. (*Moore and Dalley, p 449.*) The bulbospongiosus muscle is innervated by the pudendal nerve (S2–S4) and its contraction helps to keep blood within the shaft of the penis. Contraction of the internal urethral sphincter is under control of the sympathetic nervous system [thus not **(answer a)**]. Concomitant with dilation of the helicine arteries under parasympathetic innervation [thus not **(answers b and c)**], which allows increased blood to flow into the cavernous spaces, contraction of the bulbospongiosus and ischiocavernosus muscles at the base of the cavernous bodies reduce blood from leaving, resulting in engorgement and penile or clitoral erection. Emission of seminal fluid, prostatic secretions, and sperm from the vas deferens is due to contraction of smooth muscle under sympathetic control [thus not (**answer d**)].

440. The answer is b. (*Moore and Dalley, pp 359–360.*) The sacrococcygeal joint. The indicated line represents the sacroiliac joint. These structures are seen bilaterally between the alae of the sacrum and the ilia. The body of the sacrum (**answer a**) is in the midline and normal. The sacroiliac ligaments might have been sprained by the trauma of the fall. The pathway for spinal nerves (**answer c**) is through foramina of the sacrum, *not* through long bony canals. Similarly, the pathway for the gluteal arteries (**answers d and e**) is through the greater sciatic foramen between the ilium and the sacrum.

441. The answer is b. (*Moore and Dalley, pp 424, 469.*) Peritoneal cavity. The purpose of performing a hysterosalpingogram is to determine if the fallopian tubes are open and thus potentially capable of transporting sperm and eggs for conception. The dye is generally introduced via a catheter placed through the cervix and injected into the uterus. In this case it seems as if dye is spilling into the peritoneal cavity at ends of each fallopian tube. The dye would pass the isthmus of the oviduct next to the body of the uterus. Within the image (**E**) is the vagina, (**D**) is the isthmus of the cervix, (**B**) is the body of the uterus, and A is the ampulla of the oviduct just proximal to the infundibulum out of which dye is flowing as curling wisps.

442. The answer is a. (*Moore and Dalley, p 424.*) Ampulla of the oviduct. Fertilization normally occurs in the ampulla of the oviduct within 24 hours of the egg's release from the ovary. The wall of the uterine cavity (**answer b**) is the normal site of implantation about 4 days later. Fertilization normally does *not* occur either in the infundibulum (**answer c**) *nor* isthmus of the oviduct (**answer d**). Sperm must pass through cervical (**answer e**) mucous to reach the uterus.

443. The answer is d. (*Moore and Dalley, pp 428–429.*) The mesosalpinx (**answer b**), mesovarium (**answer c**), and suspensory ligament are all continuous with the broad ligament (**answer a**), which is a reflection of peritoneum over the female reproductive organs. The mesovarium attaches the ovary to the broad ligament. The suspensory ligament of the ovary runs from the pelvic brim to the lateral pole of the ovary. It contains the ovarian artery, ovarian vein, ovarian lymphatics, and ovarian nerves (ovarian neurovascular bundle). Volvulus of the ovary (usually associated with an ovarian tumor) may constrict the neurovascular bundle with ovarian infarct and pain referred to the inguinal and hypogastric regions. The base of the broad ligament has the transverse cervical ligament **(answer e)**.

444. The answer is b. (*Moore and Dalley, p 387. Sadler, p 235.*) Partial or complete duplication of the ureters is a fairly common (1 in 125 births) occurrence. While the OB carefully identified both a right and left ureter and spared them during the clamping and removal of the uterine arteries the duplicated ureter on the left side most likely was *not* noticed and thus damaged. The pain is most likely due to a collection of urine or an "urinoma." Duplicated ureters are at greater risk since they are often smaller than normal ureters. If the site of damage could be identified, then the duplicated left ureters could be connected above the damage to the undamaged ureter and may preserve full kidney function. While a pyelogram **(answer a)** does require injection of an iodine based dye that can cause some kidney damage, this should *not* cause damage specifically to the inferior half of the left kidney. Renal failure following anesthesia **(answer c)** is relatively rare. The development of the kidney stone **(answer d)** within one of the left duplicated ureters would be unlikely, but if present then the stone should be evident on the pyelogram images. Thus, "answer d" is a good second choice answer.

445. The answer is d. *(Moore and Dalley, p 425.)* See table below:

PELVIC VISCERAL AFFERENT INNERVATION			
Organ	**Afferent Pathway**	**Level**	**Referral areas**
Kidneys Renal pelvis Upper ureters	Aorticorenal plexus, least splanchnic nerve, white ramus of T12, subcostal nerve	T12	Subcostal and pubic regions
Descending colon Sigmoid colon Midureters Urinary bladder Oviducts Uterine body	Aortic plexus, lumbar splanchnic nerves, white rami of L1–L2, spinal nerves L1–L2	L1–L2	Lumbar and inguinal regions, anterior mons and labia, anterior scrotum, anterior thigh
None	No white rami between L3–S1	L3–S1	No visceral pain refers to dermatomes L3–S1
Cervix Pelvic ureters Epididymis Vas deferens Seminal vesicles Prostate gland Rectum Proximal anal canal	Pelvic plexus, pelvic splanchnic nerves, spinal nerves S2–S4	S2–S4	Perineum, thigh, lateral leg and foot

446. The answer is c. *(Moore and Dalley, pp 436, 438.)* Vaginal wall, bulbospongiosus, and superficial transverse perineal muscles. Both the pubococcygeus and iliococcygeus muscle **(answers a and b)** are part of the pelvic diaphragm and are much deeper muscles and thus would *not* be cut. The prepuce and rectus abdominis muscle **(answer d)** are superior and lateral to the vagina and an episiotomy is performed in a posterior mediolateral direction, *not* anterior mediolateral direction. Both the sacrospinous and sacrotuberous ligaments **(answer e)** are much deeper structures, which stabilize the pelvis and never cut during an episiotomy.

447. The answer is c. *(Moore and Dalley, pp 392–393, 431, 452.)* Lymph drains from the testicles to preaortic nodes, because remember that the blood supply for the testicles comes directly off the abdominal aorta, where the testicles first develop, prior to their inferior migration into the scrotum. All the other pelvic structures: penis (**answer a**), scrotum (**answer b**), anus (**answer d**), and epididymides (**answer e**) can drain lymphatics to the superficial inguinal nodes. The anus and rectum have drainage to three sites: superficial inguinal nodes, internal iliac nodes, and inferior mesenteric preaortic nodes.

448. The answer is b. (*Moore and Dalley, pp 413, 426–427.*) Endoscopic exploration to rule out ectopic pregnancy. The positive pregnancy test, the blood in the cul-de-sac of Douglas and the mass in the uterine tube all suggest ectopic pregnancy. All the other possible answers (**answers a, c, d, and e**) do *not* fit with a positive pregnancy test and are much lower frequency events.

449. The answer is b. (*Moore and Dalley, p 400.*) Cystocele. Bulges in the anterior wall of the vagina are most likely due to the bladder falling posteriorly into the anterior vaginal wall. A bulge on the posterior wall of the vagina would most likely be a rectocele (**answer b**). Cervical cancer (**answer c**) generally would *not* present as described. A didelphic uterus (**answer d**) is a duplication of the uterus as result of failure of the right and left paramesonephric ducts to fuse in the midline. An indirect inguinal hernia (**answer e**) would generally present as a mass within the labia major.

450. The answer is b. (*Moore and Dalley, pp 422–423, 465–466.*) The pudendal nerve serves the skin around the posterior/ lateral entrance of the vagina; the nerve wraps around the ischial spine, which is used as a landmark; transvaginal administration is less painful since the upper portion of the vagina has fewer pain receptors. The pudendal nerve serves the skin around the posterior/lateral entrance of the vagina; the nerve wraps around the ischial spine, which is used as a landmark; transvaginal administration is less painful since the upper portion of the vagina has fewer pain receptors [thus none of the other (**answers a, c, and d**) are correct].

Extremities and Spine

Questions

DIRECTIONS: Each item below contains a question or incomplete statement followed by suggested responses. Select the **one best** response to each question.

451. The scapula has *no* direct attachment to the axial skeleton. During development, the scapula is formed by which of the following?

a. Splanchnic lateral plate mesoderm
b. Neural crest cells
c. Axial mesoderm
d. Somatic lateral plate mesoderm
e. Somitic mesoderm

452. Innervation to the rotator cuff muscle that medially rotates the arm is provided by which of the following?

a. Axillary nerve
b. Suprascapular nerve
c. Thoracodorsal nerve
d. Upper and lower subscapular nerves

453. A 47-year-old radiology professor suddenly notices that he can no longer hit his normal three-point shot in basketball on his driveway. He reports to your office where you obtain from his history that he has been suffering some mild neck pain of 6 weeks' duration with right arm pain down the back of his right arm and extending to the dorsal surface of his hand, including his middle finger. He has diminished ability to do pushups and you note diminished triceps tendon reflex on the right side only. You order which of the following because you are concerned he has herniated which intervertebral disk?

a. Lateral x-ray; C6–C7
b. Cervical MRI, C6–C7
c. Cervical MRI, C8–T1
d. CT; C5–C6
e. CT; C8–T1

454. The accompanying x-ray shows the shoulder of an 11-year-old girl who fell off the monkey bars, extending her arm in an attempt to break her fall. The small arrows indicate the fracture area. The large arrows indicate which of the following?

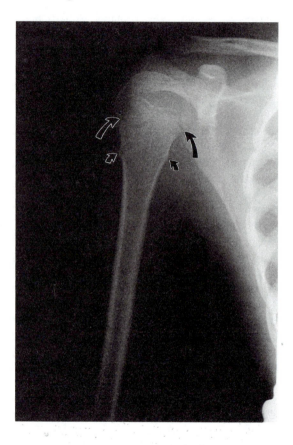

a. A fracture at the anatomic neck of the humerus
b. The glenohumeral joint
c. The joint space between the proximal humerus and the acromion of the scapula
d. The proximal humeral epiphyseal plate
e. What is commonly called a shoulder separation

455. A patient presents in her fifth pregnancy with a history of numbness and tingling in her right thumb and index finger during each of her previous four pregnancies. Currently, the same symptoms are constant, although generally worse in the early morning. Symptoms could be somewhat relieved by vigorous shaking of the wrist. Neurologic examination revealed atrophy and weakness of the abductor pollicis brevis, the opponens pollicis, and the first two lumbrical muscles. Sensation was decreased over the lateral palm and the volar aspect of the first three digits. Numbness and tingling were markedly increased over the first three digits and the lateral palm when the wrist was held in flexion for 30 seconds. The symptoms suggest damage to which of the following?

a. The radial artery
b. The median nerve
c. The ulnar nerve
d. Proper digital nerves
e. The radial nerve

456. A 52-year-old man is brought to the emergency room after being found in the park, where apparently he had lain overnight after a fall. He complains of severe pain in the left arm. Physical examination suggests a broken humerus that is confirmed radiologically. The patient can extend the forearm at the elbow, but supination appears to be somewhat weak; the hand grasp is very weak compared with the uninjured arm. Neurologic examination reveals an inability to extend the wrist (wrist-drop). Because these findings point to apparent nerve damage, the patient is scheduled for a surgical reduction of the fracture. The observation that extension at the elbow appears normal, but supination of the forearm appears weak, warrants localization of the nerve lesion to which of the following?

a. Posterior cord of the brachial plexus in the axilla
b. Posterior divisions of the brachial plexus
c. Radial nerve at the distal third of the humerus
d. Radial nerve in the midforearm
e. Radial nerve in the vicinity of the head of the radius

457. Wrist-drop results in a very weak hand grasp. This is why self-defense classes teach you to flex the wrist of an attacker holding an object to loosen their grip on an object. The strength of the grasp is greatest with the wrist in the extended position for which of the following reasons?

a. Flexor digitorum superficialis and profundus muscles are stretched when the wrist and metacarpophalangeal joints are extended
b. Lever arms of the interossei are longer when the metacarpophalangeal joints are extended
c. Lever arms of the lumbrical muscles are longer when the metacarpophalangeal joints are extended
d. Line of action of the extensor digitorum muscle is most direct in full extension
e. Radial half of the flexor digitorum profundus muscle is paralyzed because it is innervated by the radial nerve

458. When examining muscle function at the metacarpophalangeal (MP), proximal interphalangeal (PIP), and distal interphalangeal (DIP) joints, what findings do you expect in the presence of radial nerve palsy?

a. Inability to abduct the digits at the MP joint
b. Inability to adduct the digits at the MP joint
c. Inability to extend the MP joint only
d. Inability to extend the MP, PIP, and DIP joints
e. Inability to extend the PIP and DIP joints

459. In the upper extremity, each major nerve passes between two heads of a muscle. The median nerve passes between which of the following?

a. Long and medial heads of the triceps brachii muscle
b. Medial and posterior division of the coracobrachialis muscle
c. Ulnar and humeral heads of the flexor carpi ulnaris muscle
d. Ulnar and humeral heads of the pronator teres muscle

460. A spiral fracture of the humerus in the region marked Z on the accompanying radiograph had severely injured a major nerve that passes on the dorsal aspect of the bone. Which of the following is most likely to occur as a result of this injury?

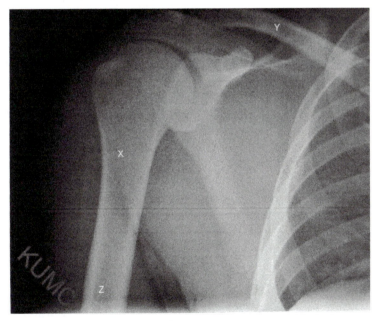

(Image 6101, used with permission from the Radiological Anatomy web site, University of Kansas, School of Medicine, http://classes.kumc.edu/som/radanatomy/.)

a. Wrist-drop palsy
b. Total clawing of the hand
c. Waiter's tip palsy
d. Clawing of digits 4 and 5
e. Dupuytren's contracture

461. Fractures of the humerus in different regions have the potential to damage different nerves. What muscle innervation may be compromised by a fracture of the humerus at the "surgical neck"?

a. Subscapularis
b. Pectoralis major
c. Teres major
d. Deltoid
e. Suprascapularis

462. A 12-year-old boy was riding his bicycle across an intersection when and elderly woman tried to pull out into the busy street just as the boy was riding in front of her, hitting the boy. Fortunately the boy landed on the hood of the car, but the bumper struck the boys legs just below the knee and created a very large cut. The boy presents to the emergency room bleeding and walking with a distinct left foot-drop. The boy has also lost most of his ability to flex his left ankle or evert his left foot and he has lost sensation on the lateral side of his leg distal to the cut. Plain films show that there are *no* broken bones and examination of the knee reveals that is appears intact. You call in a plastic surgeon, to reanastomose which of the following?

a. Sciatic nerve
b. Tibial nerve
c. Common fibular (peroneal) nerve
d. Deep fibular nerve
e. Obturator nerve

463. A 45-year-old plumber presented in the clinic complaining of long-standing pain in the elbow. Subsequent examination revealed normal flexion/extension at both the elbow and the wrist, but weakened abduction of the thumb and extension at the metacarpophalangeal joints of the fingers. Those symptoms were found to be caused by entrapment of the posterior interosseus nerve. Which of the following muscles could itself cause entrapment of the posterior interosseus nerve?

a. Extensor carpi ulnaris
b. Extensor indices
c. Anconeus
d. Extensor digitorum
e. Supinator

464. A 67-year-old woman slipped on a scatter rug and fell with her right arm extended in an attempt to ease the impact of the fall. She experienced immediate severe pain in the region of the right clavicle and in the right distal arm. Painful movement of the right arm was minimized by holding the arm close to the body and by supporting the elbow with the left hand. There is marked tenderness and some swelling in the region of the clavicle about one-third of the distance from the sternum. The examining physician can feel the projecting edges of the clavicular fragments. The radiograph confirms the fracture and shows elevation of the proximal fragment with depression and subluxation (underriding) of the distal fragment. Traction by which of the following muscles causes subluxation (the distal fragment underrides the proximal fragment)?

a. Deltoid muscle
b. Pectoralis major muscle
c. Pectoralis minor muscle
d. Sternomastoid muscle
e. Trapezius muscle

465. Internal bleeding can be a rare complication of a broken clavicle if the broken bone fragment becomes significantly displaced and tears a vessel and punctures the pleura. Normally the subclavius muscle protects the underlying vessels. Which of the following vascular structures is particularly vulnerable in a displaced clavicular fracture?

a. Subscapular artery
b. Cephalic vein
c. Lateral thoracic artery
d. Subclavian vein
e. Thoracocervical trunk

466. A 72-year-old woman trips over the edge of the carpet and falls forward onto the floor. A common reflex reaction to tripping and falling forward is to extend ones hands to ease the impact of striking the floor. She presents to the emergency room holding her left arm with her right hand. There is an obvious posterior displacement of the left distal wrist and hand that looks like a dinner fork. What type of fracture is this called and what bone(s) is/are likely involved?

a. Colles' fracture; always the ulna and sometimes the radius
b. Colles' fracture; always the radius and sometimes the ulna
c. Colles' fracture; always the ulna and sometimes the scaphoid
d. Colles' fracture; always the radius and sometimes the trapezium

467. A 36-year-old man fell while playing soccer 1 week earlier. He fell on his left hand and didn't think he broke anything, but he has a palmar mass and has weakened ability to grasp with that hand and has developed some tingling in his thumb and index finger. He has no pain when you press in the anatomical snuffbox. Which of the following carpal bones is most likely dislocated anteriorly and causing a form of carpal tunnel syndrome?

a. Capitate
b. Hamate
c. Lunate
d. Navicular
e. Scaphoid

468. As a third year medical student on cardiology service you receive a transfer patient from the emergency room. The 52-year-old woman is having chest pain and her cardiac enzymes and ECG suggest that she may have had a Myocardial infarction. The attending cardiologist is about to perform a cardiac catherization to inject dye into her coronary arteries. He tells you to prepare her right inguinal region for insertion of the catheter into her femoral artery. The attending cardiologist asks, "what are the landmarks for finding the femoral artery just under the inguinal ligament and what is on each side of it if you miss?" Which of the following is the best answer?

a. Half way between the anterior superior iliac spine and the pubic tubercle, with the femoral nerve medial and the femoral vein lateral to the femoral artery
b. Half way between the anterior superior iliac spine and the pubic tubercle, with the femoral nerve lateral and the femoral vein medial to the femoral artery
c. Two-thirds of the way between the anterior superior iliac spine and the pubic tubercle, with the femoral nerve lateral and the femoral vein medial to the femoral artery
d. Half way between the anterior inferior iliac spine and the pubic tubercle, with the femoral nerve medial and the femoral vein lateral to the femoral artery
e. Half way between the anterior inferior iliac spine and the pubic tubercle, with the femoral nerve lateral and the femoral vein medial to the femoral artery

469. Which bone on the plain film below is most likely fractured when falling on an outstretched hand?

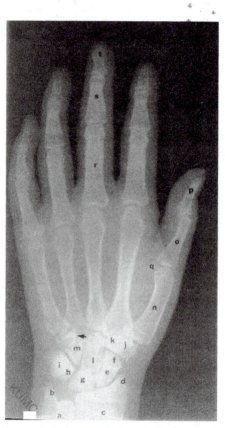

(*Image 6107 used with permission from the Radiological Anatomy web site, University of Kansas, School of Medicine, http://classes.kumc.edu/som/radanatomy/.*)

a. a
b. g
c. ef
d. hi
e. m

470. The carpal tunnel is created by the flexor retinaculum (transverse carpal ligament) and the carpal bones creating a restricted space in which the flexor tendons (9 in all) and the median nerve pass through to get to the hand. The flexor retinaculum (transverse carpal ligament) attaches from the tubercle of the scaphoid and trapezium (laterally) to which of the following bones and hook of the hamate (medially)?

a. Lunate
b. Triquetrum
c. Pisiform
d. Capitate
e. Trapezoid

471. After a night of fraternity parties, a 21-year-old college junior came to the ER the following morning complaining that she could not raise her wrist. There was no history of trauma. On examination, the patient could not extend her fingers or wrist but could flex them. She could also both flex and extend her elbow normally. There were no other motor deficits. The symptoms suggest damage to which of the following?

a. Median nerve
b. Ulnar nerve
c. Radial nerve
d. Axillary nerve
e. Musculocutaneous nerve

472. An 8-year-old boy returns to your pediatric clinic because he has a "pain in his butt" and walks with a limp. He had just been at your office a couple of days ago for a normal summer check up and an update on his vaccinations. When you ask him how this happened the boy said that the pain all started when your nurse gave him his booster shot in his left buttock. You have him demonstrate his walk and you notice that he drops his right hip as he places all the weight on his left leg and swings his right leg forward. You place him prone on the examination table and test the strength of his ability to extend each thigh at the hip and flex his leg at the knee. Both legs flex normally with equal strength, and he can extend his thigh at the hip well, but you notice some falsity of his muscles just under the iliac crest on the left side only. You tell the boy and his mother that the booster shot he got a couple of days ago likely damaged which of the following?

a. Lateral cutaneous nerve of the thigh giving him his pain
b. Superior gluteal nerve partially paralyzing his gluteus medius muscle
c. Superior gluteal nerve partially paralyzing his gluteus maximus muscle
d. Inferior gluteal nerve partially paralyzing his gluteus medius muscle
e. Sciatic nerve partially paralyzing his hamstring muscles

473. A woman falls on an icy sidewalk and complains of her "thumb hurting." You take her x-ray (below) and show her there are *no* fractures. However, she asks you to identify the small light circles (arrow) on the x-ray are. You explain they are sesamoid bones in the tendon of which of the following?

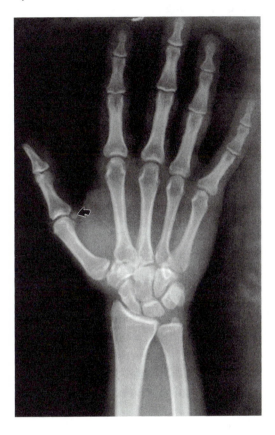

a. Flexor pollicis longus
b. Flexor pollicis brevis
c. Adductor pollicis
d. Abductor pollicis longus
e. Abductor pollicis brevis

474. A workman accidentally lacerated his wrist as shown in the accompanying diagram. On exploration of the wound, a vessel and nerve are found to have been severed, but *no* muscle tendons were damaged. From the indicated location of the laceration and loss of sensation, the involved nerve is which of the following?

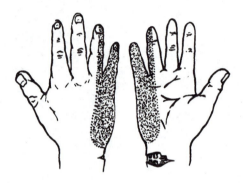

a. Median nerve
b. Recurrent branch of the median nerve
c. Superficial branch of the radial nerve
d. Ulnar nerve

475. A 71-year-old grandmother fell half way down the basement stairs while carrying a laundry basket after dinner. She didn't lose consciousness, but sat at the bottom of the stairs gathering her wits and the scattered laundry. She didn't think she had broken any bones as she could move all her limbs. Her husband, who had heard the noise and came to check on her, helped her stand up. It was then that she felt a slight pain in her left hip when she placed weight on it. She limped about for the rest of the day. The next morning her husband brought her into your family practice office where you could clearly see that she walked with her pelvis tilted as if her left leg was slightly shorter. She still had left hip pain. You order a plain film of the left femur from hip to knee expecting to find which of the following?

a. Femoral neck fracture with compression
b. Femoral neck fracture with complete displacement
c. A spiral fracture of the femoral shaft
d. A transverse supracondylar fracture
e. An intercondylar fracture

476. A 10-year-old boy is brought into your office by his mother. The boy is supporting his left arm at the elbow by using his right hand because he thinks he has "broken his arm." The 10-year-old had been playing tag and tripped over the curb and landed on the grass, catching himself with his hands. Upon physical examination you note a slight drooping of the left shoulder when unsupported, and tenderness over the midclavicular region but *no* palpable fracture or displacement. The jugular notch appears symmetrical. The shoulder has normal movement, but the boy is unwilling to lift his hand above his head because it hurts. Otherwise, hand and arm movements are relatively normal with normal sensation. You order an AP and lateral x-rays of the thorax and upper arm because you suspect which of the following?

a. Colles' fracture
b. Scaphoid fracture
c. Fracture of the surgical head of the humerus
d. Dislocated sternoclavicular joint
e. Greenstick fracture of the clavicle

477. A 16-year-old girl is brought into your orthopedic office because she fell off her bicycle while riding down a steep hill. You examine her left arm and can palpate a displaced midshaft break of her humerus. You note that she can *not* extend her wrist, but you do *not* feel any distal broken bones. She has limited ability to extend and abduct her arm at the shoulder. Her left forearm and hand feel slightly colder than her right arm and you note she seems to have lost some sensation on the posterior lateral portion of her left hand, though she says she can feel with all her fingertips. You are concerned that she has damaged which of the following?

a. Axillary nerve
b. Axillary nerve and posterior humeral circumflex artery
c. Radial nerve
d. Radial nerve and deep artery of the arm
e. Median nerve and brachial artery

478. Hip fractures, especially in the elderly, often do not heal adequately. As a result broken femurs often lead to complete hip replacement with artificial parts. What type of femoral fracture in adults is most likely to result in avascular necrosis of the femoral head?

a. Acetabular
b. Cervical
c. Intertrochanteric (between the trochanters)
d. Subtrochanteric
e. Midfemoral shaft

479. Paresthesia, hyperesthesia, or even painful sensation in the anterolateral region of the thigh may occur in obese persons. It results from an abdominal panniculus adiposus that bulges over the inguinal ligament and compresses which of the following underlying nerves?

a. Femoral branch of the genitfemoral nerve
b. Femoral nerve
c. Iliohypogastric nerve
d. Ilioinguinal nerve
e. Lateral femoral cutaneous nerve

480. Your patient just took up jogging in the evening for exercise and complains that after a mile or so his left leg begins to hurt. You question him on regions of the body or movements that do or do *not* evoke pain and find that it is widespread throughout his left lower limb. Based on the location of the constriction of the artery (indicated by the arrow), what compartment or movement would you think would be LEAST affected by the reduced arterial blood flow?

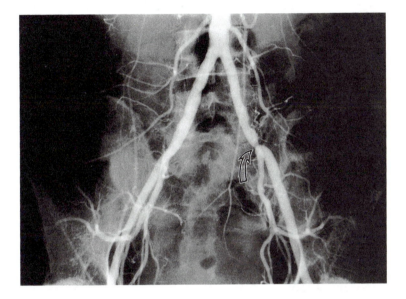

a. Gluteal region
b. Flexion of the thigh
c. Extension of the leg
d. Posterior thigh
e. Plantar flexion of the foot

481. How would you test for the destruction of structure 9 in the Sagittal MRI of the knee shown below?

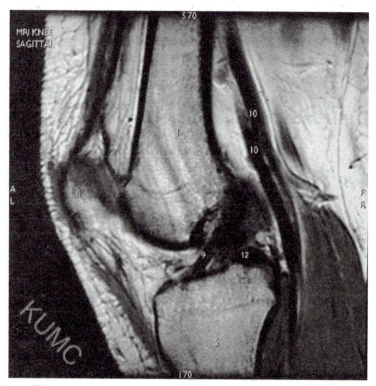

(Image 7304, used with permission from the Radiological Anatomy web site, University of Kansas, School of Medicine, http://classes.kumc.edu/som/radanatomy/.)

a. Excess ability to displace a flexed leg posteriorly
b. Excess ability to displace a flexed leg anteriorly
c. Excess ability to displace the ankle medially
d. Excess ability to displace the ankle laterally

482. A 12-year-old boy is brought to the emergency room by his mother following being pushed out of the neighbor's tree house, about 10 ft off the ground. He can walk but his right heel hurts every time he puts weight on it. When you examine his foot it is tender to pressure on both the medial and lateral aspects of the heel inferior to the tibia. You order plain films of his right lower extremity because you suspect he has fractured which of the following?

a. Calcaneus
b. Fibula
c. Tibia
d. Navicular
e. Cuneiform

483. The process of unlocking the fully extended knee in preparation for flexion requires initial contraction of which of the following?

a. Gastrocnemius, soleus, and plantaris muscles
b. Hamstring muscles
c. Popliteus muscle
d. Quadriceps femoris muscle
e. Sartorius muscle and short head of the biceps femoris muscle

484. A 22-year-old man who belongs to a weekend football league presents in the ER. He was running with the ball when a defender tackled him in the midthigh. The patient reports that when he got up, his thigh hurt, so he sat out the rest of the game. When walking to the car, his posterior thigh was extremely painful and swollen. After his shower, he noticed it was becoming discolored with increased swelling. You are concerned about the presence of a hematoma and a disruption of the arterial blood flow to the hamstring muscles. An arteriogram is performed and the vessels in question (arrows) show good filling by contrast. These blood vessels are which of the following?

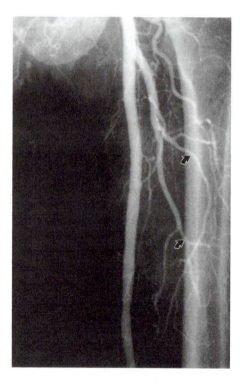

a. Descending branches of the inferior gluteal artery
b. Perforating branches of the deep femoral artery
c. Perforating branches from the obturator artery
d. Perforating branches of the femoral artery

485. A patient experienced a prolonged stay in one position during a recent surgery and postoperative recovery that resulted in compression of the common fibular (peroneal) nerve against the fibular head. Which of the following motor deficits would be most likely to occur?

a. Loss of extension at the knee
b. Loss of plantar flexion
c. Loss of flexion at the knee
d. Loss of eversion
e. Loss of medial rotation of the tibia

486. A 34-year-old woman is brought into the emergency room following her car accident in which she hit a patch of ice and slammed into the back of a trash truck. She can't walk because she has incredible pain in her left knee and hip. She thinks her knee hit the left side of the dashboard as she twisted under the seat belt as she was thrown forward. She reports severe pain as you move her hip. You order a plain film of the leg up to the pelvis and it shows *no* broken bones but posterior displacement of the head of the femur out of the acetabulum. You tell her the good news is that she has *not* broken any bones, but that she has dislocated her hip. She is sedated in order to forcefully relocate her femoral head back into the acetabulum. Despite successful relocation you are concerned that she has damaged which of the following nerves, which may take several months to regain function?

a. Obturator
b. Pudendal
c. Sciatic
d. Femoral
e. Superior gluteal

487. The muscles of the anterior compartment of the leg are innervated primarily by which of the following nerves?

a. Deep fibular
b. Lateral sural cutaneous
c. Saphenous
d. Superficial fibular
e. Sural

488. A 19-year-old teenager was dancing in clogs in an ethnic street festival when she inverted her left foot. She presents to your office the next day with a swollen foot, but mainly complains about tenderness on the lateral aspect of the foot along the plantar surface. You carefully palpate her foot and determine that she has tenderness over the tuberosity of the fifth metatarsal bone. What muscle has avulsed from its insertion on to the tuberosity of the fifth metatarsal?

a. Abductor digiti minimi
b. Fibularis (Peroneus) brevis
c. Fibularis (Peroneus) longus
d. Tibialis anterior
e. Tibialis posterior

489. The bone marked B in the lateral plain film of the right foot is which of the following?

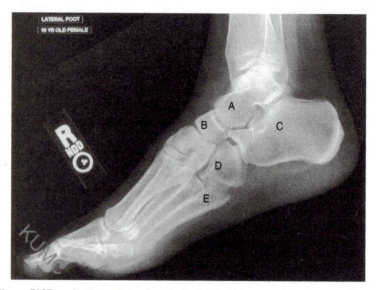

(*Image 7107, used with permission from the Radiological Anatomy web site, University of Kansas, School of Medicine, http://classes.kumc.edu/som/radanatomy/.*)

a. Talus
b. Navicular
c. Calcaneus
d. Cuboid
e. Fifth metatarsal

490. While some people continue to increase in height through their teenage years, most change very little in height for decades. However, many elderly men and women often lose height as a result of which of the following?

a. Lordosis
b. Scoliosis
c. Kyphosis
d. Osteoarthritis
e. Rheumatoid arthritis

491. A 27-year-old man is admitted for neurologic evaluation of a gunshot wound received 5 days previously. A 9-mm bullet had passed through both the medial and lateral heads of the gastrocnemius muscle. The exit wound on the lateral head of the muscle was somewhat deeper than the entrance wound in the medial head. The bullet did not strike bone or significant arteries although significant tissue damage, suppuration, and swelling were found around the exit wound. Neurologic examination reveals losses of dorsiflexion and eversion of the left foot. The patient cannot feel pinprick or touch on the dorsum of the left foot or anterolateral surface of the left leg. Which nerve was most likely involved in the injury?

a. Sciatic nerve
b. Femoral nerve
c. Sural nerve
d. Common fibular (peroneal) nerve
e. Tibial nerve

492. In a presurgical patient, the great saphenous vein was cannulated in the vicinity of the ankle. During the procedure, the patient experienced severe pain that radiated along the medial border of the foot. Which of the following nerves was accidentally included in a ligature during this procedure?

a. Medial femoral cutaneous nerve
b. Saphenous nerve
c. Superficial fibular nerve
d. Sural cutaneous nerve
e. Tibial nerve

493. A pulse in the dorsalis pedis artery may be palpated in which of the following ways?

a. Between the tendons of the extensor digitorum longus and fibularis (peroneus) tertius muscles
b. Between the tendons of the extensor hallucis and extensor digitorum muscles
c. Between the tendons of the tibialis anterior and extensor hallucis longus muscles
d. Immediately anterior to the lateral malleolus
e. Immediately posterior to the medial malleolus

494. Why is the sacral hiatus *not* used as an access point for spinal taps?

a. Because it is covered by a thick anterior sacrococcygeal ligament
b. Because CSF only flows down as inferiorly as S2, and thus is too cranial to be reached
c. Because sacral hiatus is just anterior to anus which contains lots of bacteria, increasing the chances of unintentional contamination
d. Because the filum terminale would likely be damaged
e. Because the caudal posterior sacral foramina would be easier points of access to CSF

495. What pathological condition is illustrated in this plain film of the lumbosacral spine?

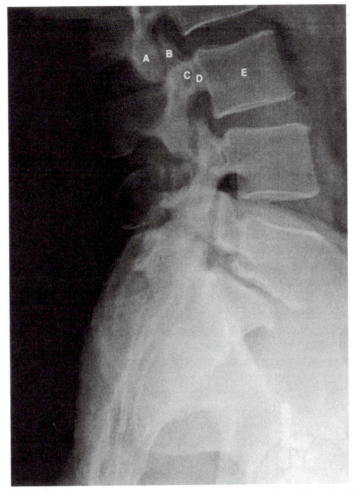

(Image 2115 used with permission from the Radiological Anatomy web site, University of Kansas, School of Medicine, http://classes.kumc.edu/som/radanatomy/.)

a. Kyphosis
b. Scoliosis
c. Lordosis
d. Spondylolisthesis

496. Which part of the vertebra would connect to the three other parts: the body, the lamina and the transverse process?

a. Inferior articular facet (A in the image in question 495)
b. Superior articular facet (B in the image in question 495)
c. Lamina (C in the image in question 495)
d. Pedicle (D in the image in question 495)
e. Body (E in the image in question 495)

497. A 22-year-old man who belongs to a weekend football league was running with the ball when a defender tackled him mid-lower limb from the side. After the tackle, he felt that his knee was hurt and went to the emergency room. From the MRI of the knee shown on the next page, the lateral meniscus is uniformly black; however, the medial meniscus has a tear (lucent area within the meniscus). Which of the following is the reason why the medial meniscus is more susceptible to damage than the lateral meniscus?

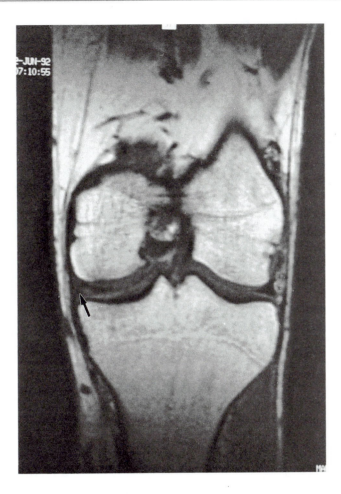

a. The medial meniscus is attached to the popliteus muscle tendon, which can move into a position making it more susceptible

b. The medial meniscus is attached to the medial (tibial) collateral ligament, which holds it relatively immobile, making it more susceptible

c. The medial meniscus is attached to the anterior cruciate ligament, which holds it relatively immobile, making it more susceptible

d. The only reason the medial meniscus is more susceptible to damage is that the knee usually gets hit laterally, causing more torsion on the medial meniscus

498. During a rhizotomy, the denticulate ligament is used as a landmark to distinguish dorsal from ventral roots. The denticulate ligament attaches cranially from the spinal cord to occipital dura and extends caudally to about which vertebral level in most adults?

a. C1
b. T1
c. T8
d. L1
e. S2

499. A physician examines a patient who complains of pain and paresthesia in the left leg. The distribution of the pain, running down the lateral aspect of the leg and the dorsal surface of the foot, is suggestive of a herniated intervertebral disk. The physician links the distribution of symptoms with nerve L5 and concludes that herniation has occurred at which location?

a. L3–L4 intervertebral disk
b. L4–L5 intervertebral disk
c. L5–S1 intervertebral disk
d. S1–S2 intervertebral disk
e. Insufficient data to determine

500. A 25-year-old woman is brought to the emergency room by her roommate because she has a fever of 102°F, stiff neck, and the "worst headache of her life." You check the fundus of her eyes for any evidence of papilledema and there is none. In addition to collecting blood to be sent to the lab for evidence of sepsis, the attending recommends you perform a spinal tap to obtain CSF for evidence of infection. What landmarks and ligaments do you need to remember when performing a spinal tap?

a. The umbilicus, which tells you where dermatome T10 is, and the sacrococcygeal ligament, which you must penetrate
b. The posterior superior iliac crest, which are parallel with spinous process of L4, and supraspinous, intraspinous, ligamentum flavum, which you must penetrate prior to piercing the dura and arachnoid membranes
c. The anterior superior iliac crest, which are parallel with spinous process of L2, and supraspinous, intraspinous, ligamentum flavum, which you must penetrate prior to piercing the dura and arachnoid membranes
d. The sacral cornu, which demarcate the sacral hiatus, and the sacrococcygeal ligament, which you must penetrate to get access to the extradural space
e. The posterior superior iliac crest, which are parallel with spinous process of S2, and supraspinous, interspinous, ligamentum flavum, which you must penetrate prior to piercing the dura and arachnoid membranes

Extremities and Spine

Answers

451. The answer is d. (*Sadler, p 77.*). Somatic lateral plate mesoderm gives rise to the connective tissue, cartilage, and bones of the appendages, including the shoulder and pelvis. The muscles of the appendages, however, originate from somitic mesoderm [(**answer e**) myotome]. Neural crest cells (**answer b**) contribute to the connective tissue of the head but *not* the appendages. Axial mesoderm (**answer c**) forms the notochord, whereas splanchnic lateral plate mesoderm (**answer a**) forms the smooth muscle and connective tissue associated with the viscera.

452. The answer is d. (*Moore and Dalley, pp 755, 761–762, 776.*) The upper and lower subscapular nerves. The upper and lower subscapular nerves innervate the subscapularis muscle, which is the only muscle of the rotator cuff group that medially rotates the arm. The lower subscapular nerve also innervates the teres major muscle, which is *not* part of the rotator cuff group. The suprascapular nerve (**answer b**) innervates the supraspinatus and infraspinatus muscles that abduct and laterally rotate the arm, respectively. The teres minor muscle, innervated by the axillary nerve (**answer a**), also laterally rotates the arm. The thoracodorsal nerve (**answer c**), originating from the posterior cord between the upper and lower subscapular nerves, innervates the latissimus dorsi muscle.

453. The answer is b. (*Moore and Dalley, pp 502–504, 746.*) Herniations of intervertebral disks occur most frequently at L4–L5, L5–S1, and C6–C7. The diminished triceps function in the right arm, as indicated by the inability to shoot three-point shots and do pushups, points to a weakened triceps. The triceps tendon reflex is principally mediated by C7. Spinal nerve C7 comes out between sixth and seventh cervical vertebrae [thus not (**answer c**)] and is most likely compromised by herniation at C6–C7 disk. The dermatomal pattern of pain down the posterior surface of the arm and hand and onto the middle finger is also consistent with C7. MRI [thus not (**answers a, d, and e**)] is the most useful radiological imaging study for viewing soft tissue structures such as herniated disks. CT is much less useful at visualizing soft structures.

454. The answer is d. *(Moore and Dalley, pp 728, 732–733, 876.)* The large arrows indicate the proximal humeral epiphyseal plate. The young girl was only 11 and still growing. The epiphyseal plates show up on x-rays as radiolucent cartilage and should *not* be confused with a fracture. The epiphysis is located at the anatomic neck of the humerus but is *not* discoid-shaped like many epiphyseal plates in long bones. This plate is tent-shaped, which is why it is *not* clearly visible all the way across the proximal humerus. The fracture at the anatomic neck of the humerus is marked by the small arrows **(answer a)**. The glenohumeral joint is more medial **(answer b)**. The joint space between the proximal humerus and the acromion of the scapula **(answer c)** is more superior. The shoulder is *not* dislocated or separated **(answer e)**.

455. The answer is b. *(Moore and Dalley, pp 778, 819–822.)*. The patient has a classic case of carpal tunnel syndrome, in which the median nerve is compressed as it passes through the carpal tunnel formed by the flexor retinaculum in the wrist. Evidence for involvement of the median nerve is weakness and atrophy of the thenar muscles (abductor pollicis brevis, opponens pollicis) and lumbricals 1 to 3. Sensory deficits also follow the distribution of the median nerve. The median nerve enters the hand, along with the tendons of the superficial and deep digital flexors, through a tunnel framed by the carpal bones and the overlying flexor retinaculum. Symptoms are worse in the early morning and in pregnancy because of fluid retention, resulting in swelling that entraps the median nerve. Flexing the wrist for an extended period exaggerates the paresthesia ("Phelan's" sign) by increasing pressure on the median nerve.

Neither the ulnar nerve **(answer c)**, radial nerve **(answer e)**, *nor* radial artery **(answer a)** passes through the carpal tunnel. The ulnar nerve supplies the third and fourth lumbricals and only the short adductor of the thumb. The radial nerve innervates mostly long and short extensors of the digits and the dorsal aspect of the hand. Proper digital nerves **(answer a)** lie distal to the carpal tunnel but are only sensory.

456. The answer is c. *(Moore and Dalley, pp 733–734, 779.)* Radial nerve at the distal third of the humerus. The clinical signs and findings in the patient presented in the question indicate radial nerve damage. The evidence that extension (triceps brachii muscle) at the elbow appeared normal while supination appeared weak can be used to localize the lesion. The innervation to the medial and long heads of the triceps brachii, principal extensor of the arm, arises from the radial nerve (in the axilla) as the medial muscular branches. The innervation to the lateral head, and to a smaller portion of the medial head, arises from the radial nerve as it passes along the musculospiral groove at mid-humerus. The supinator muscle is innervated by muscular twigs from the deep branch of the radial nerve in the forearm, just before the radial nerve reaches the supinator muscle. Thus, paralysis of the supinator muscle, but *not* of the triceps brachii (thus not **answers d** and **e**), localizes the fracture to the distal third of the humeral shaft between the elbow and musculospiral groove. Damage to the posterior cord **(answer a)** or division **(answer b)** of the brachial plexus would also affect the axillary nerve that innervates the deltoid which is *not* affected.

457. The answer is a. (*Moore and Dalley, pp 827–828.*) Muscles are most powerful (disregarding leverage factors) when stretched by extension of the joint(s) over which they pass, because this places the sarcomeres at the optimum tension-producing length in the length-tension relationship. Thus, hand grasp is strongest when the wrist joint and metacarpophalangeal joints are extended, which stretches the digitorum superficialis and profundus flexors to their optimum position [thus not **(answer d)**]. Paralysis of the radial nerve with subsequent wrist-drop will weaken hand grasp because the extrinsic flexor muscles are compelled to operate in a nonoptimum region. The lever arms of the lumbricals **(answer c)** and interossei **(answer b)** are greatest when the metacarpophalangeal joints are flexed, a consideration that does *not* apply to the patient presented in the question. The median nerve innervates the radial side of the flexor digitorum profundus [the **(answer e)** is irrelevant to the question].

458. The answer is c. (*Moore and Dalley, pp 823–824.*) Radial nerve palsy produces an inability to extend the metacarpophalangeal joints, owing to paralysis of the extensor digitorum communis muscle. However, the lumbrical and interossei muscles, which are served by the median and ulnar nerves and insert into the dorsal expansions (extensor hoods) of the proximal phalanges, are able simultaneously to flex the metacarpophalangeal joints and to extend the interphalangeal joints [thus not **(answers d and e)**]. Also, abduction of the digits, a function of the dorsal interossei, and adduction, a function of the palmar interossei, are both mediated by the ulnar nerve and, therefore, unaffected [thus not **(answers a and b)**].

459. The answer is d. (*Moore and Dalley, p 822.*) In the arm, the musculo-cutaneous nerve passes through the coracobrachialis muscle **(answer b)**. The radial nerve, which lies in the musculospiral groove, passes between the long and medial heads of the triceps brachii muscle **(answer a)** in company with the profunda brachii artery. It is here that the nerve and artery are in jeopardy in the event of a mid-humeral fracture. In the forearm, the median nerve courses between the humeral and ulnar heads of the pronator teres. As the ulnar nerve courses behind the medial epicondyle, it passes between the humeral and ulnar heads of the flexor carpi ulnaris **(answer c)** as it enters the forearm. In each instance, the nerve innervates the muscle that it pierces.

460. The answer is a. (*Moore and Dalley, pp 733–734, 795.*) The area marked Z points to the approximate location of the spiral (radial) groove. This shallow depression, on the posterior (dorsal) aspect of the humeral shaft, accommodates the radial nerve and the deep (profunda) brachial vessels. A midline fracture of the humerus may rupture the blood vessels, causing a hematoma that would compress and impair the ability of the radial nerve to conduct information to the extensor muscles of the wrist and digits. A more severe fracture may transect the radial nerve, causing paralysis of the same muscles, resulting in wrist-drop. These muscles include the following: brachioradialis, extensor carpi radialis longus, extensor carpi radialis brevis, extensor digitorum communis, extensor digiti minimi, extensor carpi ulnaris, supinator, abductor pollicis longus, extensor pollicis longus, extensor pollicis brevis, and the extensor indicis. The causes of other palsies listed in this question are injuries due to the nerves within parentheses: total claw hand palsy [median and ulnar nerves; **(answer b)**]; clawing of digits 4 and 5 [ulnar nerve; **(answer d)**]; waiter's tip palsy [C5, C6 roots of the brachial plexus; upper trunk of the brachial plexus; **(answer c)**]; and Erb-Duchenne palsy. Dupuytren's contracture **(answer e)** is caused by a thickening of the palmar aponeurosis and occurs more frequently in diabetrcs.

461. The answer is d. (*Moore and Dalley, pp 760–761.*). The surgical neck of the humerus is the narrow area located just distal to the head and anatomical neck of the humerus (the area marked X in the radiograph for question 460). The posterior (dorsal aspect) of the surgical neck is transversed by the axillary nerve (C5, C6; posterior/dorsal cord of the brachial plexus) and the accompanying posterior circumflex humeral vessels. A fracture of the surgical neck may rupture the posterior circumflex humeral vessels, causing either the compression of the axillary nerve or transection of the same nerve. Injury to this nerve causes weakness (paresis) or paralysis of the deltoid and teres minor muscles. The nerve supply to the other muscles mentioned are shown in parentheses: subscapularis [upper and lower subscapular nerves; (**answer a**)]; pectoralis major [medial and lateral pectoral nerves; (**answer b**)]; teres major [lower subscapular nerve; (**answer c**)]; and supraspinatus [suprascapular nerve; (**answer e**)].

462. The answer is c. (*Moore and Dalley, p 646.*) The common fibular (peroneal) nerve wraps around the fibular shaft just distal to its proximal head. This places it close to the skin, where it is easily damaged. The common fibular nerve then divides into the deep fibular nerve, which innervates the anterior compartment leg muscles and the superficial fibular nerve, which innervates the lateral compartment leg muscles. Both of these nerves also have cutaneous distribution as well. The inability to dorsiflex the ankle and evert the foot is consistent with the boy's clinical presentation. The sciatic (**answer a**) and obturator (**answer e**) nerves are in the thigh. The deep fibular nerve (**answer c**) is also involved, but does *not* explain all the boy's findings. The tibial nerve (**answer b**) runs more medial through the popliteal fossa, thus is *not* involved.

463. The answer is e. (*Moore and Dalley, pp 794–795.*) Each of the muscles listed (**answers a, b, c, and d**) above is innervated by the deep branch of the radial nerve or its terminal portion, the posterior interosseus nerve. The deep radial nerve passes between the deep and superficial layers of the supinator muscle and lies on a bare area of the radius where it may be compressed by action of the supinator or damaged by a fracture of the radius.

464. The answer is b. (*Moore and Dalley, pp 729–730.*) The horizontal direction of the fibers of the clavicular head of the pectoralis major muscle draws the humerus medially and causes the distal fragment of the bone to sublux. The sternal head of this muscle also has the effect of pulling the arm medially, an effect that is normally offset by the strut-like action of the clavicle. The pectoralis minor muscle (**answer c**) is a much smaller muscle and would be the second best answer. The deltoid (**answer a**) muscle would *not* cause inferior subluxation. The subclavian artery (**answer d**) and the thoracoacromial trunk **(answer e)** are blood vessels just below the broken clavicle and are at risk of being injured.

465. The answer is d. *(Moore and Dalley, pp 729–730.)* Subclavian vein. Because large and important neurovascular structures pass between the clavicle and first rib, including the subclavian artery and vein, clavicular fractures may rarely produce life-threatening bleeding into the pleural cavity. The subscapular artery **(answer a)** and lateral thoracic artery **(answer c)** are both branches off the lateral one-third of the axillary artery, so *not* likely injured. The thoracocervical trunk **(answer e)** is medial to the first rib, thus is also *not* likely to be threatened by clavicular fracture. The brachiocephalic artery **(answer a)** is too medial to be damaged. The cephalic vein **(answer b)** is superficial and lateral, thus normally *not* involved in clavicular fractures.

466. The answer is b. *(Moore and Dalley, p 736.)* Colles' fracture is a compression/displacement of the distal end (within 2 to 3 cm) of the radius resulting a classic dinner fork deformity [thus not **(answers a and c)**]. Colles' fracture also may involve the distal portion of the ulna (sometimes just the ulnar styloid process) if osteoporosis is present or if the forces are sufficient. It has been estimated that Colles' fractures represent up to 80% of fractures of the radius bone. While falling on an outstretched hand can result in scaphoid fractures **(answer c)**, they rarely occur at the same time as a distal radial fracture. Fractures of the trapezium bone **(answer d)** are relatively rare.

467. The answer is c. *(Moore and Dalley, pp 870–871.)* Lunate. The lunate bone tends to dislocate anteriorly into the transverse carpal arch, thereby entrapping the tendons of the extrinsic digital flexors and compressing the median nerve, producing symptoms of carpal tunnel syndrome (thenar weakness and paresthesia over the lateral 2.5 fingers). The capitate **(answer a)** is frequently fractured, but does *not* tend to dislocate into the carpal arch. The hamate **(answer b)** provides an anchor for the transverse carpal ligament and is, therefore, located lateral to the carpal tunnel. The scaphoid (navicular) bone **(answers d and e)** has a tendency to fracture but does *not* dislocate into the carpal tunnel. This is a relatively uncommon cause of Carpal tunnel syndrome, but is called "carpal dislocation."

468. The answer is b. (*Moore and Dalley, pp 603–604, 606.*) The way to remember the relationship of the femoral nerve, artery and vein to the inguinal ligament is to remember NAVEL from lateral to medial, for femoral **N**erve, outside the sheath (on top of the iliopsoas muscle), femoral **A**rtery, femoral **V**ein, then an "**E**mpty space" (generally filled with lymph nodes) and then, most medial the **L**acunar ligament as the inguinal ligament attaches to the pubic tubercle at the lateral aspect of the pubic symphysis. Generally, the femoral artery (which is normally easily palpable because of its pulsation) is about half way along the inguinal ligament, which is attached to the pubic tubercle medially and the anterior superior iliac spine laterally. None of the other answers are correct **(answers a, c, d, and e)**.

469. The answer is c. (*Moore and Dalley, p 738.*) (ef; scaphoid) The scaphoid(ef) is the most frequently fractured bone of the hand. Other labeled structures are as follows: **a**, ulna; **g**, lunate; **h**, triquetrum; **i**, pisiform; **m**, hamate; **b**, ulna styloid process; **c**, radius; **d**, radial styloid process; **e**, scaphoid; **f**, tubercle of scaphoid; **j**, trapezium; **k**, trapezoid; **l**, capitate; **m**, ← hook of hamate; **n**, 1st metacarpal; **o**, 1st proximal phalange; **p**, 1st distal phalanges; **q**, sesamoid bones; **r**, third proximal phalange; **s**, third middle phalange; and **t**, third distal phalange.

470. The answer is c. (*Moore and Dalley, p 840.*) The flexor retinaculum (transverse carpal ligament) extends from the tubercle of the scaphoid and trapezium to the pisiform bone (labeled i in the plane film of question 469), which sits anterior to the triquetrum and the hook of the hamate (←) medially. The triquetrum **(answer b)** lies posterior to the pisiform bone. Remember that the transverse carpal ligament traps the flexors of the digits along with the medial nerve and thus creates the carpal tunnel. The lunate **(answer a)**, capitate **(answer d)**, and trapezoid **(answer e)** are boney elements of the carpal tunnel.

471. The answer is c. (*Moore and Dalley, pp 795, 824.*) The radial nerve innervates extensors of the upper extremity. Damage to the radial nerve in the radial groove is frequently caused by supporting the arm in an outstretched position as may be encountered when an inebriated college student passes out on her friend's sofa. This is sometimes referred to as "Saturday night palsy." The median nerve **(answer a)** supplies the pronators (teres and quadratus) and the flexors of the fingers, thumb, and wrist. The ulnar nerve (**answer b**) supplies the flexor carpi ulnaris and a portion of flexor digitorum profundus. The axillary nerve (**answer d**) innervates the deltoid and teres minor and is thus involved in abduction of the arm. The musculocutaneous nerve (**answer e**) innervates flexors of the elbow joint (e.g., biceps brachii).

472. The answer is b. (*Moore and Dalley, pp 621–622.*) The boy has lost partial function of the gluteus medius muscle causing hip drop on the opposite side, which is called a "positive Trendelenburg sign." The gluteus medius (thus not **answer c**) is innervated by the superior gluteal nerve. The nurse who performed the injections likely injected too far medial within the buttock. Normally all injections should be performed in the upper lateral quadrant of the buttock, to stay away from the sciatic nerve and superior and inferior gluteal nerves that exit the pelvis through the greater sciatic notch. The lateral cutaneous nerve of the thigh (**answer a**) would provide general sensation to the anterior region of the thigh. The superior clunial nerves supple the skin over the gluteus maximus and medius muscles. The inferior gluteal nerve (**answer d**) innervates the gluteus maximus muscle. The sciatic nerve (**answer e**) is *not* damaged because the pain does *not* extend down the back of the boy's leg and he has normal function of his hamstring muscles, which flex the leg at the knee.

473. The answer is b. (*Moore and Dalley, pp 21, 831–832, 867, 879.*) The flexor pollicis brevis has two heads and there is a sesamoid bone associated with each of the tendons of these heads. Sesamoid bones are isolated islands of bone that may occur in tendons passing over joints. The patella is the classic example. The adductor pollicis (**answer c**) also has two heads (transverse and oblique), but they are *not* associated with sesamoid bones. [(**Answers a, d, and e**) are not correct.]

474. The answer is d. (*Moore and Dalley, pp 745–747.*) The ulnar nerve descends along the postaxial (ulnar) side of the forearm. It passes lateral to the pisiform bone and under the carpal volar ligament, but superficial to the transverse carpal ligament. In the hand it divides into superficial and deep branches. The median nerve (**answer a**) lies deep to the transverse carpal ligament where it is protected from superficial lacerations. Emerging from the carpal tunnel, it gives off the vulnerable recurrent branch (**answer b**) to the thenar eminence. The superficial branch of the radial nerve (**answer c**) supplies the dorsolateral aspects of the wrist and hand.

475. The answer is a. (*Moore and Dalley, pp 566, 682.*) Fractures of the femoral neck, commonly called "hip fractures" are extremely common in older women as a consequence of osteoporosis. Since the woman was still able to bear some weight on her leg it is very unlikely that she had complete displacement of the femoral neck **(answer b)**, rather a compression fracture with the fall. None of the symptoms are consistent with fracture in either the shaft **(answer c)** or distal portion **(answers d and e)** of the femur.

476. The answer is e. (*Moore and Dalley, pp 21–22, 729–730.*) The clavicle is the most frequently broken bone in body. Greenstick fractures of the clavicle are extremely common in children as a result of falling on outstretched arms. Colles' fracture is also common from falling on outstretched arms, but there are no physical findings to support a Colles' fracture [**(answer a)**; fracture of the distal radius, occasionally including the ulna] in this boy, [nor scaphoid fracture **(answer b)**]. The sternoclavicular joint **(answer d)** is extremely stable and is rarely dislocated. Fracture of the surgical head of the humerus **(answer c)** is *not* indicated by the physical findings.

477. The answer is d. (*Moore and Dalley, pp 733–734.*) Breaks of the midshaft of the humerus are most likely to damage the radial nerve and deep artery of the arm (profunda brachii artery). The radial nerve **(answer c)** runs within the radial groove on the posterior surface of the humerus (midshaft) along with the deep artery of the arm. Because the radial nerve innervates all the extensors of the arm and forearm, the observation that the teenager suffers from wrist drop is expected. Normally the nerve to the posterior compartment of the arm, the extensors of the elbow joint, will be spared in such an injury. Since the left forearm and hand felt slightly cooler than the right this suggests that the deep artery of the arm is also compromised by the displaced fracture. The axillary nerve damage **(answers a and b)** would result in reduced shoulder movement, which is normal. The median nerve and brachial artery **(answer e)**, run along the medial aspect of the arm.

478. The answer is b. (*Moore and Dalley, pp 566, 682.*) Fractures of the femoral neck (cervical) will completely interrupt the blood supply to the femoral head in adults. If the capsular retinaculum also is torn, avascular necrosis of the head will occur because the only remaining blood supply to the head (through the ligamentum teres) is inadequate to sustain it. The nearer the fracture to the femoral head, the more likely the disruption of the retinacular blood supply. None of the other answers are correct.

479. The answer is e. (*Moore and Dalley, pp 585–586.*) The lateral femoral cutaneous nerve passes beneath the inguinal ligament just medial to the anterior superior iliac spine. It innervates the lateral aspect of the thigh. The iliohypogastric nerve (**answer c**) innervates a portion of the gluteal, inguinal, and pubic regions. The ilioinguinal nerve (**answer d**) and the femoral branch of the genitofemoral nerve (**answer a**) supply the upper portions of the anterior thigh. The sensory distribution of the femoral nerve (**answer b**) innervates the anterior thigh and medial leg.

480. The answer is b. (*Moore and Dalley, pp 334, 337–339.*) Flexion of the thigh would be least affected. The lesion involves the common iliac artery just proximal to its division into the internal and external iliac branches. Blood flow would be compromised to the external iliac artery and its downstream branches including the femoral, deep femoral, popliteal, tibial, fibular, and plantar arteries. Blood flow would also be diminished to branches of the internal iliac artery, including gluteal (**answer a**) and visceral arteries. One of the most powerful flexors of the thigh is the psoas muscle, which originates from the lumbar vertebrae and receives most of its blood from the aorta and common iliac artery and thus would be unaffected by the lesion. All functions more distal to the blockage would likely be affected [thus not (**answers c, d, and e**)].

481. The answer is b. (*Moore and Dalley, pp 695–699.*) The excess ability to displace a flexed leg anteriorly is the anterior drawer sign, used to test for disruption of the anterior cruciate ligament (ACL) tear. If the ACL is torn, when the knee is flexed, the cranial part of the leg may be pulled forward excessively. If the posterior cruciate ligament, structure 12 were torn, then (**answer a** would have been correct). Excess ability to displace the ankle medially (**answer c**) or laterally (**answer d**) would arise if the lateral and medial collateral knee ligaments were torn, respectively. The other numbered structures are as follows: 1, femur; 2, tibia; 8, patella; 9, anterior cruciate ligament; 10, popliteal artery and vein; 11, head of the gastrocnemius muscle; and 12, posterior cruciate ligament.

482. The answer is a. *(Moore and Dalley, p 576.)* The calcaneus is the most frequently broken of the tarsal bones. The weight of the body is transmitted down the tibia and onto the talus, which acts as a wedge cracking the calcaneus inferiorly. Unfortunately, this fracture normally involves the cartilaginous articular surface, complicating the healing process, increasing the likelihood of developing an arthritic subtalar joint. These fractures often must be held together with screws or plates for optimal healing. Since the pain was bilateral, and only the calcaneus is bilateral across the heel, none of the other bones **(answers b, c, d, and e)** listed are possible sites of fracture. The distal end of the tibia **(answer c)** would have carried the bulk of the force, but the pain location is inconsistent with a distal tibial fracture.

483. The answer is c. *(Moore and Dalley, pp 653, 694.)* To unscrew a knee from its locked and slightly hyperextended position, the popliteus muscle contracts and causes medial rotation of the tibia or, if the foot is planted, lateral rotation of the femur. This movement frees the medial femoral condyle from its posterior position on the tibial condylar surface. The quadriceps femoris **(answer d)** then relaxes, and knee flexion occurs by contraction of the hamstring muscles **(answer b)**, assisted by the short head of the biceps femoris, sartorius **(answer e)**, gracilis, and gastrocnemius muscles **(answer a)**.

484. The answer is b. *(Moore and Dalley, pp 624–625.)* Perforating branches of the deep femoral artery are the principal blood supply to the posterior thigh. The other arteries supply anterior **(answer d)**, medial **(answer c)**, and gluteal **(answer a)** regions of the thigh.

485. The answer is d. *(Moore and Dalley, pp 643, 646.)* Compression of the common fibular (peroneal) nerve would affect all muscles innervated by this nerve, including tibialis anterior, peroneus longus, and extensor digitorum longus. Loss of dorsiflexion and eversion is usually complete. The extensors of the knee joint [**(answer a)** quadriceps femoris] are supplied by the femoral nerve, whereas the flexors of the knee joint [**(answer c)** the hamstrings and gracilis] are supplied by the tibial nerve and obturator nerve, respectively. The gastrocnemius and soleus muscles are the principal plantar flexors of the foot **(answer b)** and are innervated by the tibial nerve. The popliteus is the prime medial rotator of the tibia **(answer e)** and is also innervated by the tibial nerve.

486. The answer is c. (*Moore and Dalley, p 683.*) About 85% of hip dislocations occur in a posterior direction as the head of the femur slips out of the acetabulum. This stretches the ischiofemoral ligament, which makes up the posterior aspect of the joint capsule. Posterior displacement is also the typical direction of force resulting from the striking of one's knee on the dashboard in a head-on car accident. Anterior hip displacement is unusual since the very strong iliofemoral ligament stabilizes the joint anteriorly and also limits hip extension. The sciatic nerve passes just posterior to the hip joint and may be damaged when the hip is displaced posteriorly, thus compromising innervation to the hamstring and posterior compartment of the leg. The obturator nerve (**answer a**) exits the pelvis through the obturator foramen and into the medial compartment of the thigh, so it is *not* nearby. The pudendal nerve (**answer b**) innervates the external genitalia, so it would also be unaffected. The femoral nerve (**answer d**) exits the pelvis under the inguinal ligament and into the anterior compartment, thus it will be anterior to any damage in this case. The superior gluteal nerve (**answer e**) exits the greater sciatic notch, but is generally cranial to a posteriorly displaced head of the femur and is mobile enough that it is unlikely to be damaged. Therefore this is the second best answer.

487. The answer is a. (*Moore and Dalley, pp 642–643.*) The common fibular (peroneal) nerve bifurcates into superficial and deep branches. The deep fibular nerve innervates all muscles of the anterior compartment of the leg. The lateral sural cutaneous (**answer b**) is a cutaneous branch of the common fibular nerve. The superficial fibular nerve (**answer d**) emerges from the deep fascia and descends in the lateral compartment, where it innervates the fibularis (peroneus) longus and brevis muscles before dividing into median dorsal cutaneous and intermediate dorsal cutaneous nerves, which supply the distal third of the leg, dorsum of the foot, and all the toes. The saphenous nerve [(**answer c**); the terminal branch of the common femoral nerve] distributes cutaneous branches to the anterior and medial aspects of the leg as well as to the dorsomedial aspect of the foot. The sural nerve (**answer e**) follows the course of the lesser saphenous vein and becomes the lateral sural cutaneous nerve to supply the anterolateral aspect of the foot.

488. The answer is b. (*Moore and Dalley, pp 639, 645–646.*) The fibularis (peroneus) brevis, a pronator and everter of the foot, inserts into the tubercle at the base of the fifth metatarsal. Inversion of the foot is a common means of avulsing this tendon from the tuberosity of the fifth metatarsal and is called *Jones fracture* for the doctor that causes his own fracture while dancing around a pole. It is normally treated by placing the patient in a short walking cast. The fibularis (peroneus) longus **(answer c)** passes under the tarsal arch to insert onto the plantar aspect of the first metatarsal. The tibialis posterior **(answer e)** inserts onto the navicular bone, whereas the tibialis anterior **(answer d)** inserts into the first cuneiform and first metatarsal. The abductor digiti minimi **(answer a)** inserts onto the proximal phalanx of the fifth toe.

489. The answer is b. *(Moore and Dalley, pp 572, 711, 719.)* Navicular. The navicular bone **(B)** articulates with both the talus and the three cuneiforms, which are distal. Other labeled structures are as follows: **A,** talus; **C,** calcaneus; **D,** cuboid; and **E,** fifth metatarsal.

490. The answer is c. *(Moore and Dalley, pp 514–515.)* Kyphosis is an excessive anterior curvature of the spine, usually in the upper thoracic and lower cervical regions. Often this abnormal curvature is due to osteoporosis, especially in women, but also may be due to weakening of musculature and decrease height of the intervertebral discs. Lordosis **(answer a)** is an abnormal secondary curvature of the lumbar region of the spine and often occurs with pregnancy. Scoliosis **(answer b)** is abnormal lateral curvature of the spine that often appears during adolescence. Neither rheumatoid arthritis **(answer e)** nor osteoarthritis **(answer d)** is generally associated with height loss in the elderly.

491. The answer is d. *(Moore and Dalley, pp 586–587, 642.)* The common fibular (peroneal) nerve is the lateral terminal branch of the sciatic nerve. After arising near the apex of the popliteal fossa, it descends on the popliteus muscle and winds superficially around the fibular neck. It is extremely vulnerable in this position and is the most often injured nerve in the lower extremity. The common fibular nerve innervates all muscles in the anterior and lateral compartments of the leg. In addition, it provides sensory innervation to the dorsum of the foot and the anterolateral surface of the legs via the superficial and sural **(answer c)**/lateral sural cutaneous nerves, respectively. The tibial nerve innervates plantar flexors of the posterior compartment. The sciatic nerve **(answer a)** generally divides into the tibial **(answer e)** and common peroneal nerves superior to the popliteal fossa. Damage to it might result in deficits in both plantar flexion and dorsiflexion. The femoral nerve **(answer b)** innervates the quadriceps muscles of the anterior thigh. Damage to it would impair flexion of the thigh at the hip.

492. The answer is b. *(Moore and Dalley, pp 672–674.)* The saphenous nerve accompanies the great saphenous vein along the medial aspect of the leg and foot as far as the great toe. The medial femoral cutaneous nerve **(answer a)** innervates the dorsal aspect of the leg. The superficial fibular nerve **(answer c)** innervates the central portion of the dorsum of the foot. The sural cutaneous nerve **(answer d)** innervates the lateral aspect of the foot. The medial and lateral plantar branches of the tibial nerve **(answer e)** supply the sole of the foot.

493. The answer is b. *(Moore and Dalley, pp 639, 670–671.)* The dorsal pedal artery, a continuation of the anterior tibial artery, passes onto the dorsum of the foot between the tendons of the extensor hallucis longus and extensor digitorum longus muscles. The dorsal pedal pulse may be palpated here before the artery passes beneath the extensor hallucis brevis muscle. The posterior tibial artery passes behind the medial malleolus, where the posterior tibial pulse is normally palpable. None of the other answers **(answers a, c, d, and e)** are correct.

494. The answer is b. *(Moore and Dalley, pp 444–445.)* The sacral hiatus is used to gain access to the sacral epidural or extradural space, often to provide caudal epidural anesthesia during childbirth. Because CSF is retained by the arachnoid and dural membranes, which terminate at about S2, the CSF is too cranial to be reached from the sacral hiatus. The needle passed through the posterior *not* anterior **(answer a)** sacrococcygeal ligament. The posterior sacral foramina allow the exit of sacral spinal nerve (dorsal rami), *not* CSF **(answer e)**. The filum terminale externa **(answer d)** is rarely damaged during the procedure. Bacteria **(answer c)** are *not* an issue.

495. The answer is d. *(Moore and Dalley, pp 492–493.)* The fifth lumbar vertebra has shifted anteriorly on top of the sacrum. This condition could also be described as subluxation of the L5 vertebra on the sacrum. Spondylolisthesis is often due to a fracture of the pars interarticularis, that portion of the vertebra arch, which forms the superior and inferior facet joints. This appears to be the case in this image. The inferior facet joint on L5 has broken from the lamina of the L5 and thus allowed the body and L5 to slide anteriorly and inferiorly on top of the sacrum. Kyphosis (**answer a**) is an abnormal anterior curvature, generally in the thoracic region of the elderly. Scoliosis (**answer b**) is an abnormal lateral curvature and rotation of the vertebral column, most frequently initiates during adolescence, and involves both lumbar and thoracic region. Lordosis (**answer c**), an anterior convex curvature of the vertebral column (so-called secondary curvature), most frequently occurs within adults and within the lumbar region. Lordosis generally does *not* involve fracture of the vertebrae, as has occurred here.

496. The answer is d. (*Moore and Dalley, p 437.*) Pedicle (**D** in the image in question 495). The pedicle (**D**) attaches to the vertebral body (**E**) and extends posteriorly and from there both the lamina and the transverse process (**C**) are given off. A is the inferior articular facet of L2. **B** is the superior articular facet of L3.

497. The answer is b. (*Moore and Dalley, pp 695–699.*) The medial meniscus is attached to the medial (tibial) collateral ligament, which holds it relatively immobile, making it more susceptible. It is relatively immovable and, therefore, unable to evade damage such as occurred in this case. The medial meniscus is clearly *not* attached to the popliteus muscle (**answer a**) *nor to* the anterior cruciate ligament (**answer c**). The knee usually gets hit laterally, causing more torsion on the medial meniscus (**answer d**), making this the second best answer.

498. The answer is d. (*Moore and Dalley, pp 524–526.*) L1. The denticulate ligament is generally described as a specialization of the pia layer of the meninges of the spinal cord. It extends laterally from the spinal cord to attach to the dura mater within the spinal canal. It contains connective tissue covered with pia mater. It attaches focally at about 20 spots to the inner surface of the dura mater, thus limiting the mobility of the spinal cord. Since the adult spinal cord ends at about L1–L2 as the medullary cone, the denticulate ligament generally ends by about L1. None of the other answers (**answers a, b, c, and e**) are correct.

499. The answer is b. (*Moore and Dalley, pp 502–504.*) The deep incisure in the inferior border of the pedicle ensures that the spinal nerve associated with that vertebra will exit through the intervertebral foramen well above the intervertebral disk so that it will *not* be affected by a herniation at that level. However, a posterolateral herniation (the usual direction) will impinge on the next lower nerve as it courses toward its associated intervertebral foramen. In this case, pain was distributed along the medial side of the leg and foot as far as the great toe, the distribution of the saphenous branch of the femoral nerve (L5). Herniation of the fourth lumbar intervertebral disk between vertebral bodies L4–L5 would affect nerve L5. None of the other answers (**answers a, c, d, and e**) are correct.

500. The answer is b. (*Moore and Dalley, pp 526–527.*) A horizontal line drawn across the posterior superior iliac crests generally crosses the fourth lumbar spinous process. Lumbar punctures (spinal taps) are generally performed at the L3–L4 or L4–L5 interspinous space since the spinal cord terminates by L2 in greater than 99% of the adult population. The ligaments that need to be penetrated in the midline include the supraspinous ligament, the interspinous ligament and the ligamentum flavum (if slightly off the midline). The needle must pierce both the dura mater and arachnoid mater in order to collect cerebral spinal fluid (CSF), which should be clear. The sacral hiatus, which is marked by the sacral cornu and covered by the sacrococcygeal ligament, is used to gain access to extradural space. None of the other answers (**answers a, c, d, and e**) are correct.

Bibliography

Abbas AK, Lichtman AH: *Basic Immunology: Functions and Disorders of the Immune System,* 2/e. Philadelphia, Saunders/Elsevier, 2006.

Alberts B, Johnson A, Lewis J, Raff M, Roberts K, and Walter P: *Molecular Biology of the Cell,* 4/e. New York, Garland, 2002.

Avery JK (ed): *Oral Development and Histology,* 3/e. New York, Thieme, 2002.

Carpenter MB: *Core Text of Neuroanatomy.* 4/e. Baltimore, Williams & Wilkins, 1991.

Favus MJ (eds): *Disorders of Bone and Mineral Metabolism,* 6/e. Washington, D.C., American Society for Bone and Mineral Research, 2006.

Fawcett DW: *The Cell,* 2/e. Philadelphia, W.B. Saunders, 1981.

Gilbert SF: *Developmental Biology,* 8/e. Sunderland, MA, Sinauer, 2006.

Greenspan FS, Gardner DG: *Basic and Clinical Endocrinology,* 7/e. New York, Lange Medical Books/McGraw-Hill, 2004.

Guyton AC, Hall JE: *Textbook of Medical Physiology,* 10/e. Philadelphia, W.B. Saunders, 2000.

Johnson LR (ed): *Physiology of the Gastrointestinal Tract,* 3/e. New York, Raven, 1994.

Junqueira LC, Carneiro J: *Basic Histology: Text and Atlas,* 11/e. New York, McGraw-Hill, 2005.

Kandel ER, Schwartz JH, Jessell TM: *Principles of Neural Science,* 4/e. New York, McGraw-Hill, 2000.

Kasper DL, Braunwald E, Fauci AS, Hauser SL, Longo DL, Jameson KL (eds): *Harrison's Principles of Internal Medicine,* 16/e. New York, McGraw-Hill, 2005.

Kierszenbaum AL: *Histology and Cell Biology.* St. Louis, Mosby, 2002.

Kindt TJ, Goldsby RA, Osborne BA: *Immunology,* 6/e. New York, W.H. Freeman and Company, 2007.

Kumar V, Abbas AK, Fausto N: *Pathologic Basis of Disease,* 7/e. Philadelphia, Elsevier/Saunders, 2005.

Larsen WJ: *Human Embryology,* 3/e. New York, Churchill Livingstone, 1997.

Lebenthal E: *Human Gastrointestinal Development.* New York, Raven, 1989.

Lobov IB, Brooks PC, Lang RA: Angiopoietin-2 displays VEGF-dependent modulation of capillary structure and endothelial cell survival in vivo, Proc. Natl. Acad. Science (USA) 99:11205–11210, 2002.

Mayne R, Burgeson RE (eds): *Structure and Function of Collagen Types.* New York, Academic, 1987.

Mole SE: The genetic spectrum of human neuronal ceroid-lipofuscinoses. In: Symposium, "The neuronal ceroid-lipofuscinoses (NCL)—a group of lysosomal disease come of age." *Brain Pathol.* 14:70–76, 2004.

Moore KL and Dalley AF: *Clinically Oriented Anatomy,* 5/e Philadelphia, Lippincott Williams & Wilkins, 2006.

Moore KL and Persaud TVN: *Before We Are Born: Essentials of Embryology and Birth Defects,* 6/e. Philadelphia, W.B. Saunders, 2003.

Moore KL and Persaud TVN: *The Developing Human: Clinically Oriented Embryology,* 6/e. Philadelphia, W.B. Saunders, 1998.

Newell FW: *Ophthalmology: Principles and Concepts,* 8/e. St. Louis, Mosby-Year Book, 1996.

Noback CR, Strominger NL, and Demarest RJ: *The Human Nervous System,* 4/e. Philadelphia, Lea & Febiger, 1991.

Reszka AA, Rodan GA: Mechanism of action of bisphosphonates. *Curr. Osteoporosis Rep.* 1:45–52, 2003.

Ross MH, Pawlina W: *Histology: A Text and Atlas,* 5/e. Baltimore, Lippincott Williams & Wilkins, 2006.

Rubin E: *Rubin's Pathology: Clinicopathologic Foundations of Medicine,* 4/e. Baltimore, Williams & Wilkins, 2005.

Sadler TW: *Langman's Medical Embryology,* 10/e. Baltimore, Williams & Wilkins, 2006.

Strauss JF, Mastroianni L, Barbieri R: *Yen and Jaffe's Reproductive Endocrinology,* 5/e. Philadelphia, Saunders/Elsevier, 2004.

Vaughn D, Asbury T, Riordan-Eva P: *General Ophthalmology,* 15/e. East Norwalk, CT, Appleton & Lange, 1999.

Waxman SG: *Correlative Neuroanatomy,* 24/e. New York, McGraw-Hill, 2000.

Young B, Heath JW: *Wheater's Functional Histology,* 4/e. New York, Churchill Livingstone, 2000.

Index